Nurse Writers of the Great War

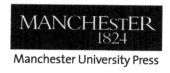

MANCHESTER
1824

Manchester University Press

Nursing History and Humanities

This series provides an outlet for the publication of rigorous academic texts in the two closely related disciplines of Nursing History and Nursing Humanities, drawing upon both the intellectual rigour of the humanities and the practice-based, real-world emphasis of clinical and professional nursing.

At the intersection of Medical History, Women's History, and Social History, Nursing History remains a thriving and dynamic area of study with its own claims to disciplinary distinction. The broader discipline of Medical Humanities is of rapidly growing significance within academia globally, and this series aims to encourage strong scholarship in the burgeoning area of Nursing Humanities more generally.

Such developments are timely, as the nursing profession expands and generates a stronger disciplinary axis. The MUP Nursing History and Humanities series provides a forum within which practitioners and humanists may offer new findings and insights. The international scope of the series is broad, embracing all historical periods and including both detailed empirical studies and wider perspectives on the cultures of nursing.

Previous titles in this series:

NURSE WRITERS OF THE GREAT WAR

CHRISTINE E. HALLETT

Manchester University Press

Published by Manchester University Press
Altrincham Street, Manchester M1 7JA
www.manchesteruniversitypress.co.uk

British Library Cataloguing-in-Publication Data
A catalogue record for this book is available from the British Library

Library of Congress Cataloguing-in-Publication Data applied for

ISBN   978 1 7849 9252 1   hardback

First published 2016

The publisher has no responsibility for the persistence or accuracy of URLs for any
external or third-party internet websites referred to in this book, and does not guarantee
that any content on such websites is, or will remain, accurate or appropriate.

Typeset by Out of House Publishing
Printed in Great Britain by TJ International Ltd, Padstow

To Margaret and David Hallett

Contents

Figures

Preface

During the First World War, tens of thousands of women devoted themselves to the care of the wounded. For many, this involved putting their lives 'on hold' and permitting a military medical machine to control their movements and restrict their freedom. For others, it meant committing themselves – and, for the wealthy, their fortunes – to a 'mission' that was both humanitarian and patriotic: a commitment to saving lives *and* winning the war. A few were pacifists, and others came to embrace pacifism as a result of their wartime experiences. As a group, they made significant contributions to the care of those damaged by war.

Many wrote poignant and moving personal testimonies of their experience – letters, diaries, and narrative accounts. And among them were a few whose writings found their way into print. Some wrote with the deliberate intention of publication. Others found their experience of nursing so powerful that they became determined to publish their memoirs. Still others found themselves under pressure from family and friends to make their personal letters and journals available to a wide audience. This book analyses the published writings of First World War nurses and explores the ways in which authors' backgrounds and motivations influenced the content and style of their writing. In reading their texts and researching their lives and careers, I found that there were significant connections between their social and professional backgrounds and the ways in which they wrote.

One of the most interesting groups consisted of wealthy and well-connected women who funded and directed their own hospital units, most operating under the auspices of the French Red Cross. They adopted two distinct approaches: some wrote in highly traditional styles, emphasising the adventurous and intrepid nature of their 'exploits'. Their writing was infused with a powerful sense of patriotism. Others wrote deliberate exposés of the horrors of war, consciously adopting modernist styles to give a jarring and disturbing feel to their accounts; their projects were almost certainly motivated by pacifist conviction.

Professional nurses were much more likely to write about their patients' sufferings than their own exploits, though their narratives do contain detail about the horrors and dangers of war. Volunteer nurses often wrote reflectively, placing themselves at the centre of their own wartime world and focusing on both their extraordinary encounters with the wounds of war and the transformative nature of their experiences. Their accounts are sometimes filled with awe and wonder; at other times they adopt a pacifist tone, relating encounters with German prisoners of war, or exploring their own feelings of dislocation when reality failed to match the myths that had fed their expectations.

In writing this book, I wanted to capture the patterns of writing within this field – the different genres, styles, and approaches – and also to offer an analysis of the ways in which nurses' and volunteers' backgrounds and pre-war experiences influenced their style. I could have adopted any one of a number of different structures – and did, indeed, experiment with some before deciding on the model here: a structure based on social and professional background. But writers do not fit neatly into categories, and I found myself compromising at times – placing, for example, the important work of professional nurse Ellen La Motte in that section of the book which focuses on the projects of 'independent ladies' who formed their own hospitals. By placing La Motte's work alongside that of Mary Borden, who created and directed the field hospital, L'Hôpital Chirurgical Mobile No. 1; Agnes Warner, who was head nurse of the hospital; and Maud Mortimer, who probably worked there as a volunteer, I hope I have been able to offer a more rounded image of that particular hospital, not only as a centre of healing, but also as a cauldron of literary creativity.

The book contains other compromises, and its content has been influenced by a number of constraints. Only English-language publications have been included, and the focus is on allied nurses, rather than on those who nursed the wounded of the Central Powers. The space constraints of the volume meant that a decision was taken during the editing process to include only British (including one Anglo-Russian) and North American nurse writers; the book thus became a study of transatlantic, rather than global, nursing culture. This is not entirely disadvantageous. The literary outputs of significant Australian and New Zealand authors (notably May Tilton, Edna Pengelly, and Ida Willis) deserve detailed analysis in a completely separate study. The narrower focus of this study permitted a closer analysis of the ways in which British and North American women wove their wartime experiences into their life-writing. It also enabled some comparisons to be made and some distinctions to be drawn among them.

Ultimately, I hope that – for all of its compromises and constraints – this book makes a real contribution to scholarship by bringing together into one volume a detailed exploration of the connections between nurses' social and professional backgrounds and the style and content of their writings. The lengthy biographical overviews of significant nurse writers, such as Kate Luard, Violetta Thurstan, Julia Stimson, and Helen Dore Boylston, have been included to enable readers to understand the complexities and tensions inherent in the lives of female nurses in highly patriarchal and militaristic societies, and in an era well before women's liberation. I hope the combination of collective biography and textual analysis enables readers to understand the extraordinary nature of the ways in which professional and volunteer nurses met the challenges of their times and expressed their sense of the power of war nursing.

Acknowledgements

I should like to thank the Wellcome Trust for awarding the research support grant that enabled some of the research work for this book. The Trust also awarded a further grant to me and Alison Fell (University of Leeds) to conduct a workshop that was attended by some of the best and brightest minds in the research field of First World War nursing. I offer my thanks to all of the attendees at that meeting for helping me better understand nurses' First World War writings: Carol Acton, Margaret Darrow, Alison Fell, Kirsty Harris, Margaret Higonnet, Hazel Hutchison, Jane Potter, Angela Smith, and Janet Watson. Additional thanks to Alison Fell for her friendship and collegiality, Hazel Hutchison for the insight she gave me into the work of Mary Borden, and Jane Potter for introducing me to a number of American nurse writers I would not otherwise have discovered.

The relatives of Kate Evelyn Luard have been extremely generous. Caroline and John Stevens gave me permission to reproduce two family photographs in this book (including the cover image of Kate Luard in the QAIMNS Reserve uniform) and to quote excerpts from Luard's two memoirs: *Diary of a Nursing Sister on the Western Front* and *Unknown Warriors*. Tim Luard forwarded me several transcripts of his great aunt's letters. He and I worked together on an introduction for the new edition of *Unknown Warriors* (edited by John and Caroline Stevens). I am very grateful to him and to his wife, Alison Luard, for their kindness and support. Cathy Fry was also very generous in helping me to trace materials relating to her great aunt.

Melissa Hardie-Budden and her husband, Phil, not only made material relating to Violetta Thurstan available to me, but also offered me generous hospitality in their home while I was in Penzance, studying the archives of the Hypatia Trust. Jonathan Evans, at the Royal London Hospital Archives, was also very helpful in enabling me to access material relating to Violetta Thurstan. Both Sue Light (of 'Scarletfinders' and 'The Fairest Force') and Pete Starling (formerly of the Army Medical Services Museum, UK) were supportive and generous in their assistance with my questions and concerns.

In the USA, Colleen Bowers and Dean Foreman photographed one of the versions of the diary and memoir of Alice Fitzgerald held at the Archives of the Maryland Historical Society. I thank them for this and also for their valuable friendship over many years. The staffs of the Maryland Historical Society (MHS) Archives, Baltimore, and the Alan Mason Chesney (AMC) Archives, Baltimore, were wise and helpful. They assisted me in tracing and researching the five extant versions of Fitzgerald's memoir. I would like to thank, in particular, Patricia Anderson and Damon Talbot (MHS), and Marjorie Kehoe and Phoebe Litocha (AMC). In the USA the support of colleagues at both the Barbara Bates Center (University of Pennsylvania) and the Eleanor Crowder Bjoring Center (University of Virginia) strengthened my understanding of the background to this work.

In Canada, Shawna Quinn and Stephen Claydon enabled me to see the life and work of Agnes Warner in a completely new light. Both were very generous with their time and help.

Image credits are given in the list of illustrations (above, p. ix). Particular thanks for assistance with images go to Caroline Stevens, Richard Willis, Shawna Quinn, Melissa Hardie-Budden, Marjorie Kehoe, Alison Kay, Jane Sparkes, Jonathan Eaker, and Faye Cheung.

I owe thanks to the staffs of libraries and archives around the world, not only for preserving and making available the research materials on which this study is based, but also for assisting my searches. Textual materials, including excerpts from the works of nurse writers, and archive materials were made available by: the John Rylands Library, University of Manchester, UK; the British Library, London, UK; Library and Archives Canada, Ottawa, Canada; The National Archives, Kew, London, UK; the Archive of the Nursing and Midwifery Council, London, UK; the Royal College of Nursing Archives, Edinburgh, UK; the Archives of the Army Medical Services Museum, Aldershot, UK; the Churchill Archives, Churchill College, Cambridge, UK; the Archives of the Royal London Hospital, Aldgate,

Acknowledgements

London, UK; the Archives of the Hypatia Trust, Jamieson Library, Penzance, UK; the Imperial War Museum, London, UK; the Library of the University of Sussex, Brighton, UK; the Liddle Collection, Brotherton Library, University of Leeds, UK; the Red Cross Archive, London, UK; the Maryland Historical Society Archives, Baltimore, Maryland, USA; the Alan Mason Chesney Medical Archives, Johns Hopkins Medical Institutions, Baltimore, Maryland, USA; the Archives of the Barbara Bates Center for the Study of the History of Nursing, Philadelphia, USA; the Archives of the Eleanor Crowder Bjoring Center for Nursing Historical Inquiry, University of Virginia, USA; the Claude Moore Health Sciences Library/ University of Virginia, USA; and the Archives of Saint John, New Brunswick, Canada.

This book contains direct quotations from a number of nurses' memoirs and other personal testimony. I would like to thank the authors and publishers of these texts, for which full references are included in the bibliography. In brief, those quoted are: Anon., *A War Nurse's Diary*; Anon., *The Edith Cavell Nurse from Massachusetts*; Anon., *My Beloved Poilus*; Anon., *Twenty Months a VAD*; Enid Bagnold, *A Diary without Dates*; Enid Bagnold, *Enid Bagnold's Autobiography*; Olive Dent, *A VAD in France*; Vera Brittain, *Testament of Youth*; Florence Farmborough, *Nurse at the Russian Front*; Baroness de T'Serclaes, *Flanders and Other Fields*; Mary Borden, *The Forbidden Zone*; Helen Dore Boylston, 'Sister': *The War Diary of a Nurse*; Mabel St Clair Stobart, *The Flaming Sword in Serbia and Elsewhere*; Mary Britnieva, *One Woman's Story*; Ellen N. La Motte, *The Backwash of War*; Kate Finzi, *Eighteen Months in the War Zone*; Kate Luard, *Unknown Warriors*; Sarah Macnaughtan, *A Woman's Diary of the War*; Sarah Macnaughtan, *My War Experiences in Two Continents*; Shirley Millard, *I Saw Them Die*; Millicent, Duchess of Sutherland, *Six Weeks at the War*; Maud Mortimer, *A Green Tent in Flanders*; Irene Rathbone, *We That Were Young*; Flora Sandes, *An English Woman-Sergeant in the Serbian Army*; Lesley Smith, *Four Years out of Life*; Julia Stimson, *Finding Themselves*; Henrietta Tayler, *A Scottish Nurse at War*; Violetta Thurstan, *Field Hospital and Flying Column*; Violetta Thurstan, *The People who Run*; and Rebecca West, *War Nurse*. Brief excerpts from the following articles are also included: Ellen La Motte, 'Under Shell-Fire at Dunkirk', *The Atlantic Monthly*, 116 (November 1915): 692–700; Ellen N. La Motte, 'A Joy Ride', *The Atlantic Monthly*, 118 (October 1916): 481–90; and Ellen N. La Motte, 'Under a Wine Glass', *The Century Magazine* (December 1918): 150–4. I thank all of these 'nurse writers', and their publishers.

Editorial staff at Manchester University Press have, as always, been unfailingly efficient, patient, and supportive. They ask their authors not to name individuals, so I thank them all.

This book is dedicated to my parents. My dad, David Hallett, died in 2002, but his powerful influence continues to shape my research and writing. My mum, Margaret Hallett, is an unfailing source of wisdom, generosity, and support. Along with them, I thank my husband, Keith Brindle: keen critic, loyal support, and stalwart companion.

Abbreviations

ANC	US Army Nurse Corps
BEF	British Expeditionary Force
BJN	*British Journal of Nursing*
BNA	British Nurses' Association
CCS	casualty clearing station
FFNC	French Flag Nursing Corps
NUTN	National Union of Trained Nurses
NUWSS	National Union of Women's Suffrage Societies
QAIMNS	Queen Alexandra's Imperial Military Nursing Service
VAD	Voluntary Aid Detachment
WSPU	Women's Social and Political Union
WSWCC	Women's Sick and Wounded Convoy Corps

Introduction

The Great War remembered

The First World War was known in its own time as the Great War; its protagonists believed that it would be 'the war to end all wars'.[1] The earliest attempts to recapture it – either as memoir or as history – struggled to put into words a reality that was so complex that it defied expression. Later generations created their own collective cultural understandings but most of these were based on the male, combatant experience. It was not until the 1980s that the perspectives of women gained public attention; even then, the voices of trained nurses remained mostly silent.

This book offers an analysis of the published war memoirs of nurses – both trained and volunteer. It examines the ways in which the cultural and social backgrounds of nurse writers influenced the ways in which they wrote. It is both a collective biography of a small but significant group, and an exploration of a particular type of cultural output. It asks: What were the experiences of nurses who wrote war memoirs? What motivated them to write? What images of themselves and their work did they project? What meanings did they apply to their experiences of the war? And how did these meanings draw upon or challenge existing cultural norms and conventions? It considers both the significance nurses attached to their work and the ways they chose to project their understandings of the war. Many nurses perpetuated the heroic myths of war; others unconsciously challenged these; still others deliberately attacked allied wartime propaganda and began the process of constructing new understandings.

Several nurses' memoirs were published during the First World War; yet, by the end of the 1920s, very few were widely available.[2] The publication of soldiers' memoirs followed a very different pattern. Very few had been produced during the war itself,[3] but the late 1920s and early 1930s saw an outpouring of powerful and moving memoirs, which were produced in large numbers and were widely read. Among them were Edmund Blunden's *Undertones of War*, Siegfried Sassoon's *Memoirs of a Fox-Hunting Man*, Erich Maria Remarque's *All Quiet on the Western Front*, and Robert Graves's *Goodbye to All That*.[4] Soon after the publication of the earliest soldier memoirs, a new group of female writers – among whom Vera Brittain was probably the most successful – began to publish books about their wartime experiences.[5] These early memoirs ended a ten year 'silence' during which very little had been written about the war, and set the tone and content of later generations' understandings of the conflict. But, for the first post-war generation, remembrance was complicated by the looming possibility of another European conflict.

During and immediately after the Second World War, the world's focus was on a very different form of 'total war', and it was not until the 1960s that historians were able to reach back to the early years of the century to re-evaluate the war in which their grandfathers had fought. Authors such as A. J. P. Taylor deliberately placed the common soldier – variously referred to as 'the common man' or 'everyman' – into the historical record.[6] At around the same time, compilations of First World War poetry were published for use in schools, and the darkly satirical *Oh! What a Lovely War* was performed by the Theatre Workshop in London and then developed into a film by Richard Attenborough.[7] It became clear that the writings of those who emerged from the trenches of France and Flanders had changed the culture and expectations of western societies irrevocably, such that, in 1967, Stanley Cooperman could write that 'we are all creatures of the First World War'.[8]

In the 1970s a new genre emerged – a focus on the cultural history of the war. Paul Fussell's *The Great War and Modern Memory* – a remarkable exploration of the cultural significance of First World War literature – still stands as a guidepost for those approaching the subject.[9] Written at a time when the second and third post-war generations were evaluating the meaning of the conflict, Fussell's book surveyed the landscape of the Great War from a vantage point beyond its most far-reaching ramifications, looking back across a historical landscape coloured by the Great Depression, the Second World War and the cultural freedom of the 1960s. Rather than attempting to recapture the mentality of the war generation, Fussell's book produced a creative and imaginative reworking of his own generation's reading of the Great War literary canon. Citing the Second World War memoirist Robert Kee, Fussell observed that 'it is those artists who re-create life rather than try to recapture it who, in one way, prove the good historians in the end'.[10]

In the 1980s the emerging field of women's history – a movement riding the crest of second-wave feminism – addressed women's almost complete absence from the historical record of the First World War. Lyn MacDonald was one of the first to redress the imbalance, through her evocative oral history of First World War nursing, *The Roses of No Man's Land*, published in 1980.[11] A year later, Catherine Reilly's edited anthology of women's war poems gave women a place in the canon of war writings alongside their more famous male counterparts.[12] In 1983, Sandra Gilbert argued emotively that, at the same time as reducing the male combatant to a victim – damaged or destroyed by technology, bureaucracy, and an overbearing military hierarchy – the war had raised women to positions of unprecedented power.[13] Later writers modified Gilbert's thesis, observing, for example, that women's gains – if indeed they were gains – were relinquished after the war, when most returned to their pre-war positions in low-paid work or unpaid domesticity.[14] Margaret and Patrice Higonnet suggested that men's and women's positions in the labour market could be compared to a 'double helix', in which women's roles were always subordinate.[15] The entrenched notion that women were the 'angels of the house' – guardians of the domestic and private life – was too powerful to be overturned by the First World War,[16] however 'topsy-turvy' the world might have become.[17] Joan Scott nevertheless asserted that wars have always been seen as watersheds for women: in wartime women gained new roles and opportunities; won political rights (albeit apparently because of their wartime 'good behaviour'); and became more involved in politics, often through pacifism. In the long term, the effects of war 'revolutionized women's status'.[18]

In 1990, Claire Tylee wrote women irrevocably into the cultural history of the First World War. Drawing upon the work of Fussell, she examined the ways in which the war had altered the consciousness of Western society; but, where Fussell had focused on the writings of men, she highlighted the importance of women as both memoirists and commentators.[19] Her book was part of a growing new focus, adding to an already developing emphasis on women's roles in the First World War.[20] One of her significant themes was the ways in which allied governments – the British in particular – had deliberately used propaganda to promote the war.[21] The propagandist project consciously went well beyond the protection of the public, and Tylee asserted that most women were its 'easy victims'.[22] Even those who served as nurses and deplored the suffering of their patients were still often trapped within the mental straitjacket of their upbringing within a patriarchal and imperialistic society. The Defence of the Realm Act of August 1914 had outlawed the publication of anti-war texts,[23] but for most women such legal restraint was not even required: lack of political and educational opportunity acted as a sufficient brake on their thinking and expression.[24] One of the most constraining images for nurses was that of themselves as a nurturing, Madonna-like figure, reaching, perhaps, its most extreme representation in Alonzo Earl Foringer's poster of a huge Madonna cradling a helpless child-sized wounded soldier, which was published by the American Red Cross at Christmas 1918.[25]

In examining the writings of nurses, I have been influenced by authors such as Jane Schultz, whose work on American Civil War nursing has transformed our perceptions of the influence of female identity on nursing work;[26] Santanu Das, whose incisive analysis of the interplay between nurses' personal trauma and their wartime writings has deepened our understanding of the work of female modernists;[27] and Paul Berry and Mark Bostridge, whose meticulous research on the life of Vera Brittain has made it possible for historians to offer deeper analyses of the significance of her autobiographical writing.[28]

This work also owes a debt to writers such as Margaret Higonnet, Angela Smith, and Janet Watson, who explored nurses' writings among those of other women.[29] It extends their work by deepening the focus on nurses; it offers new insight into well-known nurse authors, and explores the work of previously neglected authors. Most of the published writings of those who nursed the wounded during the First World War were influenced by the cultural tropes and accepted beliefs of their time. But some writers deliberately questioned those tropes and beliefs. This book explores, not only the ways in which nurse writers chose to project themselves as nurses, but also the meanings they gave to their experiences. In caring for those damaged by the First World War, nurses were the most immediate witnesses to the consequences of industrial warfare. Standing between the front lines and the 'home front', and dealing daily with the worst injuries produced by war, they were ideally placed to witness the results of early-twentieth-century modes of combat. This book examines the ways in which some nurse writers were influenced by the myths of their time; it also examines how some demolished those myths, and constructed a new mythology of war, and of war nursing.

Memory and memoir

In 1928, Edmund Blunden wrote of the difficulties associated with remembering the First World War: 'I know that memory has her little ways, and by now she has concealed precisely that look, that word, that coincidence of nature without and nature within which I long to remember.'[30] Thirty-six years later, the Baroness de T'Serclaes sat down to write her own memoir: 'the past comes flooding in', she asserted; 'half-forgotten memories – like the medals in their glass case – seem to demand attention, a good dust, a new look at their significance.'[31] Perhaps the most telling part of her comment is her reference to the 'medals in their glass case'. In writing her memoir, she appears to be engaged in a dual process: of both recreating the past and constructing a narrative – even a myth – of her own life. But not all nurse writers set out deliberately to compose their memoirs. Julia Stimson's *Finding Themselves*, a compilation of the letters she sent home to her family during the war, was clearly written contemporaneously with the events it describes.[32] The letters were composed under difficult conditions in a base hospital in France, where she was sharing a large, partitioned building with her nursing staff. 'I do not know whether I can use this precious type-writer without disturbing all the other nurses on the other side of my room-wall',[33] she commented, and her book was clearly compiled from material written in

5

snatched moments. Nurses – as part of a larger group of middle-class women – appear to have written wherever and whenever they could. Fussell commented that the war coincided with a period in which an education focusing on a canon of 'classical' literature was being extended across social class boundaries.[34] It was also – more slowly – crossing gender ones. British Voluntary Aid Detachment nurse Vera Brittain, more than any other 'nurse writer', epitomises the way in which women embraced the early twentieth century's opportunities for education. But she was not the only nurse writer with such aspiration. Some North American nurse memoirists held bachelor's degrees from prestigious universities such as McGill, Montreal; and Columbia, New York City. In an era in which there was no radio or television, writing and speaking were the most common forms of amusement and entertainment. Nurses kept diaries avidly – even when to do so was in direct contravention of military regulations. They also wrote numerous letters 'home', always in anticipation that those letters would be passed from hand to hand and read by whole families and communities.[35]

Most of the texts considered here were written with publication in mind. Such 'life writings' present a serious challenge to historians. They almost always contain some elements of novel-writing.[36] The reader may even be required to 'suspend disbelief', a process that is alien to historical research. In this book, nurse memoirs are used as windows onto the lived experience of their authors – a lived experience that is taking place at a particular time, the First World War, and that contains embedded, often coded, and sometimes unconscious messages about what it meant to be a nurse during that conflict. Joan Scott emphasises the importance of an acknowledgement of 'experience' as a significant but hitherto neglected element of historical interpretation.[37] In nurse memoirs, the remembered experience of the individual is the lens through which the historical narrative is viewed.

Nevertheless, the problem of veracity remains. Ultimately, as Sidonie Smith and Julia Watson point out: 'autobiographical truth resides in the intersubjective exchange between narrator and reader aimed at producing a shared understanding of the meaning of a life.'[38] In *Nurse Writers of the Great War*, that meaning is multi-layered. The presentation of several lives (or part-lives) chronicled by the writers themselves, interpreted by the historian, and then reinterpreted by the reader, will produce multiple, and only partially shared, understandings.

In their ground-breaking book *Reading Autobiography*, Smith and Watson argue that 'to reduce autobiographical narration to facticity is to strip it of the densities of rhetorical, literary, ethical, political, and cultural dimensions'.[39] In some ways they appear to argue that the value of autobiography – certainly its 'truth value' – goes beyond that of other historical sources. However, they also identify numerous threats to historical accuracy in life writing. Memoirists often present their accounts as histories witnessed from particular perspectives, but their writings go way beyond the mere describing of a remembered past; they also perform 'rhetorical acts'.[40] In their war memoirs, nurses are giving voice to their own perspectives, answering their critics, and projecting desired images of themselves.

Even as they acknowledge the epistemological fragility of life writing, Smith and Watson also challenge the apparent 'truth-value' and factual basis of traditional histories. Historians are assertive in their claims to both accuracy and veracity, stressing, among other claims, that their sources have greater validity than those of other writers. Yet, to focus only on 'traditional' historical sources, such as official documents diaries and letters, is to ignore a large and significant body of evidence. The study of nurses' First World War memoirs has the potential to open a window onto the norms, perspectives, and desires of a hidden occupational and social grouping at a key historical moment. As Susan Friedman has argued, prior to the late twentieth century, autobiography was associated with the white, elite, western male.[41] The perspectives of early-twentieth-century nurses were dissimilar to those of this typical nineteenth- and early-twentieth-century 'individualist'.[42] It was difficult for military nurses, in particular, to find authentic voices. They were a social anomaly: middle-class (for the most part) and female, yet working for a salary. In the pre-war years, their strangeness not only inclined society to ignore them; it also made it more likely that they themselves would hide from view. Yet, at the outbreak of war, they found themselves suddenly acclaimed as a highly respected group: women who took on the roles of carers and nurturers, yet showed a 'toughness' hitherto associated only with men. Some of them chose to place their experiences before wide audiences.

Some nurses' memoirs were both written and published during the war itself. The intention of Violetta Thurstan's *Field Hospital and Flying Column* appears to have been to advertise and promote the work of wartime nurses. Kate Luard's *Unknown Warriors*, by comparison, seems to have been motivated by a need to bear witness to the suffering and heroism of her soldier patients.[43] Ellen La Motte's *The Backwash of War* was a deliberate piece of anti-war propaganda. In 1917 its publication was prohibited in the USA, having already been blocked by the British censor.[44]

A number of books by nurses appeared at about the same time as the most famous soldiers' memoirs, during a five-year period from 1928 to 1933. Historians have commented on the 'great silence' that followed the war: the ten years from 1918 to 1928 when very little was written – as if former combatants were overcoming their shock and assimilating their experiences.[45] Some of the best known nurses' writings – notably Vera Brittain's *Testament of Youth* and Mary Borden's *The Forbidden Zone* – were produced as a direct response to the outpourings of male authors – works such as Robert Graves' *Goodbye to All That*, Richard Aldington's *Death of a Hero*, and Siegfried Sassoon's *Memoirs of a Fox-Hunting Man*.[46] 'Why should these young men have the war to themselves?', asked Vera Brittain.[47] Her *Testament of Youth* gave women a voice in the memorialisation of the war dead, and offered a strong and convincing argument for pacifism. Mary Britnieva's *One Woman's Story* also appears to have been a text with a purpose, reading as a testament to the suffering of the Russian people.[48] Other works appear to have been drawing on the 'girl's own adventure' genre of writing, epitomised by the novels of authors such as Bessie Marchant.[49] Helen Dore Boylston's *'Sister': The War Diary of a Nurse* belongs to this genre; its purpose appears to have been simply to tell a good story.[50]

Two nurses' writings have been viewed as important contributions to the literary modernist movement. Ellen La Motte's *The Backwash of War* and Mary Borden's *The Forbidden Zone* have attracted great interest amongst literary critics. Angela Smith has argued that modernist writings emerged as a means of articulating new modes of thinking and that they were 'self-consciously avant-garde'.[51] And yet she also suggests that nurse writers were 'accidental modernists':[52] that their modernism was part of the struggle to find ways of documenting an experience that had no precedents and was, essentially, disjointed and meaningless. Santanu Das concurs with this view, arguing that the writings of nurse modernists derived from the 'impotence of sympathy'.[53] These arguments have some force; and yet, if one examines the backgrounds of both Borden and La Motte, it becomes clear that both were aspirant authors prior to the war, and that both were acquainted with the influential modernist Gertrude Stein, visiting her salon in the rue de Fleurus in Paris.[54] Although neither Borden nor La Motte can be accused of offering their services to the military medical effort merely to acquire material for publication, both were deeply attached to their writing careers, and Borden, in particular, saw herself primarily as an author, rather than as a nurse. For these women, their experience of nursing fuelled their creativity.

A third period of nurses' writings, in the 1960s and 1970s, was, perhaps, a response to the desire of a new, much later generation to understand the meaning of the war. Memoirs such as the Baroness de T'Serclaes's *Flanders and Other Fields* and Florence Farmborough's *Nurse at the Russian Front* are presented in a very different style from many of the fragmentary diary-based outputs of the earlier periods.[55] Narratives with perspective – permitting us to view their authors' lives before and after the war – these memoirs have clearly been carefully edited to present a particular image of their subjects. In them, the nurse has effectively recreated – or, in the terms of historian Penny Summerfield, 'composed' – herself.[56]

Not all memoirs were published by their authors. In fact, in some cases the author had no knowledge of her work's publication. Agnes Warner's *My Beloved Poilus* was published in her hometown of New Brunswick by her mother and sisters, ostensibly with the purpose of raising funds for the French Field Hospital of which she was head nurse, but possibly also in the interests of family pride.[57] Julia Stimson's letters were brought together after the war and were published at the urging of her father.[58] Ella Mae Bongard's personal writings were published after her death, by her son, Eric Scott, under the title *Nobody Ever Wins a War*.[59] And if some authors were reluctant self-publicists, others remained determinedly anonymous. The author of *A War Nurse's Diary: Sketches from a Belgian Field Hospital* has remained resolutely so, and it is possible only to speculate about her motives for writing a vivid account of her experiences while so effectively concealing her own identity.[60] Maud Mortimer's *A Green Tent in Flanders*, although probably published under her own name, carefully anonymises the details it recounts.[61] Enough information is provided to make it very likely that the hospital she is describing is the field hospital that was offered to the French military medical services by Mary Borden, but her writing is deliberately cryptic, offering an encoded message that is difficult to interpret. Even more mysterious is 'Corinne Andrews', the nurse whose memoir was ghost-written by the successful author Rebecca West.[62]

Nurses' writings of the First World War cannot be viewed as a homogeneous corpus of texts, any more than the nurses of the early twentieth century can be viewed as a homogeneous group of women. And yet, they have numerous characteristics in common. In them, their authors are both recapturing and recreating experience. All contain elements of self-composure: in every case, the nurse projects herself as a strong twentieth-century woman, aware that she is at the vanguard of social change. Most bear deliberate witness to the suffering and courage of their patients; and many offer their own philosophies – some apparently unconsciously, others in highly conscious and deliberate ways – of the nature of industrial warfare. All nurses undoubtedly viewed themselves as healers; most also 'bought into' the cultural tropes of their day, believing their participation in war to be heroic. A few stood back from those cultural tropes and offered their works as counter-arguments to political propaganda, opposing the received wisdom of their day and consciously writing a different 'truth'.

The nurses of the First World War

The First World War began at a time of intense campaigning both for nurses' professional rights and for women's right of political participation. In Britain, the National Union of Women's Suffrage Societies (NUWSS) had been promoting the principle of women's suffrage for decades, while its more militant counterpart, the Women's Social and Political Union (WSPU) – more popularly known as the 'suffragette movement' – had been launching increasingly volatile attacks on male political privilege. In the USA, similar drives for what was referred to as 'woman suffrage' were gaining momentum.[63] And the suffrage campaign was only one part of a wider push for social reform. Women became involved in campaigns for the regulation of capital on both sides of the Atlantic – in America through the 'progressive movement' and in Britain through the campaigns of radicals, such as Sylvia Pankhurst.[64]

The drive for reform went beyond the political and economic spheres. As Sheila Rowbotham has demonstrated, the move towards greater freedom encompassed both the professional and the domestic spheres and included a push for sexual emancipation, which found its greatest expression in the work of American nurse Margaret Sanger and British scientist Marie Stopes. Of those women who were at the vanguard of this movement, 'some were upper middle class and keen to cast off privilege; others were members of the growing in-between strata, educated yet not quite "ladies", uprooted, mobile, and liable to be iconoclastic'.[65] Several professional nurse writers fit into the former category, with Alice Fitzgerald in the USA and Kate Luard in Britain presenting classic examples of women who recognised their privileged status and were anxious to participate in world events even if this meant enduring physical hardship and emotional challenge. Others can be seen as 'educated, yet not quite "ladies"' – indeed, professional nursing, by its very nature as a form of paid employment, cast doubt on the genteel status of those who practised. Large numbers of writers were from Rowbotham's 'in-between strata'. A somewhat impoverished lower-middle-class single mother named Elsie Knocker won fame and recognition during the war for her services on the Belgian Front, later writing a wry memoir under her married name: Baroness de T'Serclaes.[66] Claire Tylee has suggested that the main 'class' difference among women who wrote was not between middle class and working class, but between those who regarded themselves as 'ladies' and those who could be identified as educated 'new women'.[67] Many of the former chose nursing as an acceptable means to earn a 'genteel' living, while the latter moved into public service professions as a way of expressing their growing sense of social responsibility.

The ambiguity and conflict that confronted American women in the years prior to the First World War are captured in Kimberly Jensen's *Mobilizing Minerva*.[68] Her portrait of the 1913 woman suffrage parade reveals the level of hostility faced by those women who fought for citizenship status in the early twentieth century. The parade – held on the day before President Woodrow Wilson's inauguration – was sabotaged by a hostile and violent audience, at best given licence and at worst actively incited by members of the municipal police force. Jensen presents the parade, which took place on the eve of the war's outbreak in Europe, as a powerful symbol of the patriarchal power that had kept American womanhood 'in its place' up to the second decade of the twentieth century.[69] Inspired by British campaigns for women's suffrage, American women had also begun to argue against the assumption that male political dominance was justified by the capacity – assumed to be exclusively male – to defend the State through force of arms.

A powerfully radical strain of feminism infused the nursing profession on both sides of the Atlantic. Emma Goldman, a professional nurse, whose views were coloured by political anarchism, had an important influence on campaigner for sexual emancipation Margaret Sanger.[70] Goldman's views were, in part, developed through her experiences at the Henry Street Settlement, an organisation founded and run by Lillian Wald, which offered a visiting nursing service to the impoverished families of New York's Lower East Side.[71] The same influences and the same strain of radicalism can be found in the writings of influential nurses such as Lavinia Dock, head of the international office of the *American Journal of Nursing*, while the assertive determination of American nurses to make their voices heard can be read through the writings of authors such as Ellen La Motte. British feminist nurses were equally radical, but perhaps less overtly progressive, in their outlook.

In 1914, the nursing profession in Britain was in turmoil – and had been so for twenty-seven years. Prestigious voluntary hospitals in London and other major cities had been turning out highly trained and disciplined 'professional nurses' for over four decades, and senior nurses were organising themselves through the Royal British Nurses' Association and the Matron's Council.[72] Yet, despite these recognised advances, the vast majority of nurses – particularly in Poor Law hospitals – underwent only the most cursory apprenticeship training with almost no theoretical teaching, learning their skills by mirroring the practice of more senior exemplars whilst enduring a harsh disciplinary regime. Paradoxically, the symbolic value of military nursing as a highly regarded – even heroic – feminine pursuit meant that large numbers of wealthy, well-educated ladies took great interest in it, many even going so far as to offer their services at time of war. Indeed, their presence in South Africa during the Second Boer War had caused dismay amongst military medical personnel.[73]

The existence of poorly trained servant-class nurses and of untrained lady volunteers was seen as an affront to their professionalism by elite, fully trained nurses, many of whom were, themselves, well educated and of high social class backgrounds. The campaign for a state register, which would ensure the regulation of the profession and the standardisation of its training, had been simmering since 1887, the year Ethel Gordon Fenwick, a former matron of St Bartholomew's Hospital, had held – in her own drawing room at her house on Wimpole Street – the inaugural meeting of the British Nurses Association (BNA).[74] Although nursing was not a fully recognised profession in the second decade of the twentieth century, it was generally accepted that the term 'trained nurse' referred to a woman with three years' training in a recognised school attached to a general hospital of at least 100 beds.[75] The importance of fully trained nurses' clinical contributions in military contexts was only just beginning to be recognised.[76]

The Queen Alexandra's Imperial Military Nursing Service (QAIMNS) had been officially inaugurated in 1902. At the outbreak of war it had only 297 members.[77] It did, however, have a large 'Reserve' that was available to be 'called up' for active service at short notice. The exact numbers of the Reserve are uncertain, but it seems that approximately 800 nurses were available at the outbreak of war, with a total of 10,404 being recruited during the course of the conflict.[78] Thousands more nurses worked with the Territorial Force Nursing Service, in temporary hospitals,[79] in voluntary hospitals funded by the Red Cross or Order of St John of Jerusalem, and in 'civil hospitals and institutions where military patients were received'.[80]

One of the unique features of the British military nursing landscape in 1914 was the existence of the so-called Voluntary Aid Detachments (VADs), which had been formed in 1909, as part of the Haldane Reforms.[81] A complex and confusing system, the VAD movement ran under the auspices of two longstanding and powerful organisations: the British Red Cross and that section of the Order of St John of Jerusalem known as the 'St John's Ambulance Association'. In the early months of the war, recognising the need to cooperate, the two organisations created a single 'Joint Committee' to oversee the work of the VADs. Large numbers of detachments had already formed, and 8,495 volunteer nurses were available for service.[82] These women, somewhat confusingly, took on the acronym of their detachments, becoming known as 'VADs'. Tens of thousands served during the war, mostly at home, but some overseas, and the works of powerful writers such as Vera Brittain and Irene Rathbone have ensured that their status has been enshrined in the mythology of the British war effort. For trained nurses they were a mixed blessing. Many enjoyed working with them and found them genuinely helpful; others found they had to watch these 'well-meaning girls ... like a cat watches mice, to see that no terrible accidents happen'.[83]

In an indignant article, published in the *BJN* in January 1914, trained nurse Violetta Thurstan observed that many Red Cross VADs paid too much attention to the 'military' side of things, adding that, 'though flagging, signalling, riding, &c., are doubtless very attractive, it certainly has given a large section of the public the idea that the members are rather "playing at soldiers" than training in first aid work'.[84] Power was in the hands of detachment commandants, who took on volunteer nurses from among the ranks of their own social class, hiring trained nurses to teach them a range of skills and enable them to obtain certificates in subjects such as basic hygiene, invalid cookery, wound dressing, and first aid.[85]

One of the ways in which some trained British nurses circumvented both the constraints of military officialdom and the vagaries of the British volunteer services was to offer their services to the French and Belgian Societies of the Red Cross. One of the most intriguing ways in which this was accomplished was through the French Flag Nursing Corps, an organisation created by a British woman, Grace Ellison, and supported by Ethel Gordon Fenwick, which, through the auspices of an 'Anglo-French Committee' of the Red Cross, offered trained nurses to French military hospitals.[86] Although a number of secular schools had been launched over the previous decades, much of the nursing care in France was still offered by religious orders, and most nurses received no formal training.[87] The French Flag Nursing Corps appears to have been a success, although much of what we know of it is reported through the pages of that somewhat partial organ of nursing professionalization, the *BJN*. The Corps was brought under the auspices of the British Committee of the French Red Cross in March 1917.[88]

The development of the nursing professions in self-governing British dominions such as Australia, New Zealand, and Canada had been heavily influenced by that of the British nursing profession itself.[89] The training of nurse probationers and the conditions under which they worked were remarkably similar to those of British nurses. Their Army Nursing Services were modelled on the QAIMNS, and yet, when mobilised for war, did not incorporate large contingents of volunteer nurses. The dominions did not experience the depletion of their male orderlies in the same way as did Britain and France, where most young able-bodied men were eventually moved into active front-line service, and it was possible for Australian, New Zealand, and Canadian units to take on large contingents of military order-lies – rather than female VADs – when they travelled to Europe in 1914 and 1915.[90]

The US Army Nurse Corps (ANC) was established as a permanent corps of the US Army Medical Department on 2 February 1901, and pre-dated by a year the formation of the British QAIMNS.[91] It had, from its inception, very stringent entry criteria. Each applicant was obliged to submit a certificate of health, and a reference from the superinten-dent of her training school, attesting to her success in training and her good moral character. She was also obliged to pass an examina-tion. For promotion to the rank of chief nurse, she faced an even more rigorous written examination on hygiene, medications management, and military protocol.[92] By 1912 there were 125 members of the Corps, with a reserve list of approximately 3,000.[93] By March 1914 there were 403 army nurses, with a reserve of 8,000, and by 11 November 1918 the total number of ANC members had risen to 21,480.[94]

In April 1916, a year before the USA declared war on Germany, George W. Crile, a professor of surgery at Western Reserve University in Cleveland, Ohio had advocated the formation of 'base hospi-tals'. Several discrete units had been created, each staffed by doc-tors and nurses from a single institution.[95] The first six units arrived in France, well before any US combat troops, and began by work-ing with British Expeditionary Force staff in British hospitals.[96] By

15

August 1918, fifty base hospitals were in place, and in that month several more were planned.[97] One of the most difficult issues faced by the Committee on Nursing of the General Medical Board of the Council of National Defense, chaired by Adelaide Nutting, was whether to employ female volunteers as nurses' aides. After much debate, it was agreed that untrained nurses should not be sent to Europe. The relationship between nurses and corpsmen (orderlies drawn from the ranks of serving troops) had not been officially defined prior to the war, but a circular letter from the surgeon general's office, dated 14 April 1918, stated unequivocally that the 'head nurse is in charge'.[98] American nurses thus – at least in principle – found themselves in a clearer position in relation to their assistant nurses than British ones. Nevertheless, they too were subject to the vulnerabilities of a female profession operating in a distinctly male-centred world without officer status.[99]

Surprisingly few nurses' memoirs of the Great War were written by members of the official military nursing services. Most were authored either by female volunteers (often operating under the auspices of the Red Cross), by independent trained nurses who travelled to wherever they perceived their services were most required, or by women working under the auspices of the French Flag Nursing Corps. A number of writings relate to experiences under bombardment in Belgium during the rapid German advance of 1914, and then to subsequent service in the narrow strip of Belgium that remained in allied hands. Others describe the retreat across Albania from the Bulgar advance into Serbia, or work with Russian Red Cross flying columns on the Eastern Front. One remarkable cluster of writings relates to the work of one hospital: L'Hôpital Chirurgical Mobile No. 1 at Rousbrugge in Belgium, one of the most independent hospital units of the First World War. It would appear that those nurses who worked most independently were the ones who were also most likely to write memoirs and war narratives. Although only a minority of nurses were employed in 'freelance' or 'voluntary' units, a disproportionately large number of these chose to publish books about their experiences.

English-speaking nurses from Britain, its dominions, and the USA came from a range of social backgrounds. Some were from a wealthy social elite; others were genteel but impoverished; still others were from socially mobile and highly aspirant sections of society. All were well educated, whether 'at home' by governesses or in private or public schools. Many were extremely well versed in the literary canon of their day. They chose a range of different life-writing styles – some traditional, others quite idiosyncratic – as vehicles to bring their experiences to wide readerships. While some wanted to present portraits of themselves, others were keen to bring the heroism of their patients to the world's attention. Still others simply used autobiographical writings as an outlet, to give vent to their feelings of trauma and anxiety. In this book, their writings are presented as part of a vibrant, feminine, transatlantic culture that, during the First World War, drew on the raw immediacy of experience within the protective discipline of army nursing to convey both the realities of industrial warfare and a range of 'truths' about its impact on human life.

Notes

1 Adrian Gregory, *The Last Great War: British Society and the First World War* (Cambridge: Cambridge University Press, 2008): 5.

2 See, for example: Anon., *Diary of a Nursing Sister on the Western Front 1914–1915* (Edinburgh and London: William Blackwood and Sons, 1915); Violetta Thurstan, *Field Hospital and Flying Column: Being the Journal of an English Nursing Sister in Belgium and Russia* (London: G. P. Putnam's Sons, 1915); Ellen N. La Motte, *The Backwash of War: The Human Wreckage of the Battlefield as Witnessed by an American Hospital Nurse* (New York: G. P. Putnam's Sons and The Knickerbocker Press, 1916).

3 Henri Barbusse's *Le feu* is a notable exception: Henri Barbusse, *Under Fire* (London: Penguin Classics, 2003 [1917]).

4 Edmund Blunden, *Undertones of War* (London: Penguin, 2010 [1928]); Siegfried Sassoon, *Memoirs of a Fox-Hunting Man* (London: Faber and Gwyer, 1928). See also: Siegfried Sassoon, *Memoirs of an Infantry Officer* (London: Faber and Faber, 1930); Siegfried Sassoon, *Sherston's Progress* (London: Faber and Faber, 1936). Erich Maria Remarque, *All Quiet on the Western Front*, trans. Brian Murdoch (London: Random House, 1996 [1929]); Robert Graves, *Goodbye to All That* (London: Jonathan Cape, 1929).

5 Vera Brittain, *Testament of Youth* (Glasgow: Collins and Sons, 1980 [1933]). See also: Irene Rathbone, *We That Were Young: A Novel* (New York: The Feminist Press, 1989 [1932]).

6 A. J. P. Taylor, *The First World War: An Illustrated History* (Harmondsworth: Penguin, 1963). See also: Marc Ferro, *The Great War, 1914–1918* (London: Routledge, 1973 [1969]): 94–107; George Panichas (ed.), *Promise of Greatness: The War of 1914–1918* (London: Cassell, 1968).

7 Claire Tylee, *The Great War and Women's Consciousness: Images of Militarism and Womanhood in Women's Writings, 1914-64* (Houndmills and London: Macmillan, 1990): 1-4.

8 Stanley Cooperman, *World War I and the American Novel* (Baltimore: Johns Hopkins University Press, 1967): viii. Cooperman's words are also cited in Tylee, *The Great War and Women's Consciousness*: 5.

9 Fussell, Paul, *The Great War and Modern Memory* (Oxford: Oxford University Press, 2000 [1975]). On the cultural history of the First World War, see also: Eric Leed, *No Man's Land: Combat and Identity in World War One* (New York: Cambridge University Press, 1979); Modris Eksteins, *Rites of Spring: The Great War and the Birth of the Modern Age* (Boston, MA: Houghton Mifflin, 1989); Jay Winter, *Sites of Memory, Sites of Mourning: The Great War in European Cultural History* (Cambridge: Cambridge University Press, 1995); Jay Winter, 'Shell Shock and the Cultural History of the Great War', *Journal of Contemporary History*, 35.1 (2000): 7-11; Jeffrey Reznick, *Healing the Nation: Soldiers and the Culture of Caregiving in Britain during the Great War* (Manchester: Manchester University Press, 2004); Alan Kramer, *Dynamic of Destruction: Culture and Mass Killing in the First World War* (Oxford: Oxford University Press, 2007); Michael Roper, *The Secret Battle: Emotional Survival in the Great War* (Manchester: Manchester University Press, 2009); Leo van Bergen, *Before My Helpless Sight: Suffering, Dying and Military Medicine on the Western Front, 1914-1918* (Farnham: Ashgate, 2009).

10 Fussell, *The Great War and Modern Memory*, citing Robert Kee, 'Mercury on a Fork', *Listener* (18 February 1971): 208.

11 Lyn MacDonald, *The Roses of No Man's Land* (Harmondsworth: Penguin, 1993 [1980]).

12 Catherine Reilly (ed.), *Scars upon my Heart: Women's Poetry and Verse of the First World War* (London: Virago, 1981).

13 Sandra Gilbert, 'Soldier's Heart: Literary Men, Literary Women and the Great War', *Signs*, 8.3 (1983): 422-50 (425). This paper was later reprinted as: Sandra Gilbert, 'Soldier's Heart: Literary Men, Literary Women and the Great War', in Margaret Randolph Higonnet, Jane Jenson, Sonya Michel, and Margaret Collins Weitz (eds), *Behind the Lines: Gender and the Two World Wars* (New Haven: Yale University Press, 1987): 197-226. Page numbers in further citations are to the reprint.

14 See, for example, the 'Introduction' to Higonnet, Jenson, Michel, and Weitz, *Behind the Lines*.

15 Margaret Higonnet and Patrice Higonnet, 'The Double Helix', in Higonnet, Jenson, Michel, and Weitz, *Behind the Lines*: 31-47.

16 On the power of the Victorian myth of the female as the 'angel of the house', see: M. Jeanne Peterson, 'No Angels in the House: The Victorian Myth and the Paget Women', *The American Historical Review*, 89.3 (1984): 677-708. On

the link between this myth and imperialism, see: Anna Davin, 'Imperialism and Motherhood', *History Workshop*, 5 (1978): 9–65.

17 A verse by Nina Macdonald summed up this feeling: 'All the world is topsy-turvy / Since the War began', quoted by Gilbert, 'Soldier's Heart': 200.

18 Joan Scott, 'Rewriting History', in Higonnet, Jenson, Michel, and Weitz, *Behind the Lines*: 21–30. On the role of women in the war, see also: Miriam Cooke and Angela Woollacott (eds), *Gendering War Talk* (Princeton, NJ: Princeton University Press, 1993); Sharon Ouditt, *Fighting Forces, Writing Women: Identity and Ideology in the First World War* (London: Routledge, 1994).

19 Tylee, *The Great War and Women's Consciousness*: 5.

20 See, for example, Gail Braybon, *Women Workers in the First World War: The British Experience* (London: Croom Helm, 1981); Sandra Gilbert and Susan Gubar, *No Man's Land: The Place of the Woman Writer in the Twentieth Century* (New Haven: Yale University Press, 1988); Jane Marcus, 'Corpus/ Corps/Corpse: Writing the Body in/at War', in Helen M. Cooper, Adrienne Auslander Munich, and Susan Merrill Squier (eds), *Arms and the Woman: War, Gender and Literary Representation* (Chapel Hill: University of North Carolina Press, 1989): 124–67. Several important outputs followed within a few years of Tylee's work. See, for example, Cooke and Woollacott, *Gendering War Talk*; Dorothy Goldman, *Women and World War I: The Written Response* (New York: St Martin's Press, 1993); Agnès Cardinal, Dorothy Goldman, and Judith Hattaway, *Women's Writing on the First World War* (Oxford: Oxford University Press, 1999); Susan Grayzel, *Women's Identities at War: Gender, Motherhood, and Politics in Britain and France during the First World War* (Chapel Hill, NC: University of North Carolina Press, 1999).

21 Tylee, *The Great War and Women's Consciousness*: 252. On the formation of the secret bureau of propaganda in 1914, see Peter Buitenhuis, *The Great War of Words: Literature as Propaganda, 1914–18 and After* (London: B. T. Batsford, 1989 [1987]): 5–20. On propaganda, see also: Trudi Tate, *Modernism, History and the First World War* (Manchester: Manchester University Press, 1998): 41–62.

22 Tylee, *The Great War and Women's Consciousness*: 48.

23 On the Defence of the Realm Act and censorship, see: Tylee, *The Great War and Women's Consciousness*: 53; Angela Smith, *The Second Battlefield: Women, Modernism and the First World War* (Manchester: Manchester University Press, 2000): 36.

24 On the limitations of women's education, see: Sarah Jane Aiston, 'Women, Education and Agency, 1600–2000', in Jean Spence, Sarah Jane Aiston, and Maureen M. Meikle (eds), *Women, Education and Agency, 1600–2000* (London: Routledge, 2010): 1–8.

25 Gilbert, 'Soldier's Heart': 210–11; Tylee, *The Great War and Women's Consciousness*: 67.

26 Jane Schultz (ed.), *Women at the Front: Hospital Workers in Civil War America* (Chapel Hill: University of North Carolina Press, 2004); Harriet Eaton, *This Birth Place of Souls: The Civil War Nursing Diary of Harriet Eaton, ed. Jane E. Schultz* (Oxford: Oxford University Press, 2010).

27 Santanu Das, *Touch and Intimacy in First World War Literature* (Cambridge: Cambridge University Press, 2005).

28 Paul Berry and Mark Bostridge, *Vera Brittain: A Life* (London: Virago Press, 2001).

29 Margaret Higonnet, 'Not So Quiet in No-Woman's Land', in Cooke and Woollacott, *Gendering War Talk*: 205–26; Margaret Higonnet, *Lines of Fire: Women Writers of World War I* (Harmondsworth: Penguin, 1999); Margaret Higonnet, *Nurses at the Front: Writing the Wounds of the Great War* (Boston, MA: Northeastern University Press, 2001); Margaret Higonnet, 'Authenticity and Art in Trauma Narratives of World War I', *Modernism/Modernity*, 9.1 (2002): 91–107; Higonnet, Jenson, Michel, and Weitz, *Behind the Lines*; Smith, *The Second Battlefield*; Angela Smith, *Women's Writings of the First World War: An Anthology* (Manchester: Manchester University Press, 2000); Janet S. K. Watson, *Fighting Different Wars: Experience, Memory and the First World War* (Cambridge: Cambridge University Press, 2004).

30 Blunden, *Undertones of War*: xli.

31 Baroness de T'Serclaes, *Flanders and Other Fields* (London: George G. Harrap, 1964): 15.

32 Julia Stimson, *Finding Themselves: The Letters of an American Army Chief Nurse at a British Hospital in France* (New York: Macmillan, 1927).

33 Stimson, *Finding Themselves*: 35.

34 Fussell, *The Great War and Modern Memory*: 178.

35 Christine Hallett, 'The Personal Writings of First World War Nurses: A Study of the Interplay of Authorial Intention and Scholarly Interpretation', *Nursing Inquiry*, 14.4 (2007): 320–9; Christine Hallett, 'Portrayals of Suffering: Perceptions of Trauma in the Writings of First World War Nurses and Volunteers', *Canadian Bulletin of Medical History*, 27.1 (2010): 65–84.

36 On truth and fact in memoir, see: Victoria Joule, '"Heroines of Their Own Romance": Creative Exchanges between Life-Writing and Fiction, the "Scandalous Memoirists" and Charlotte Lennox', *Journal for Eighteenth-Century Studies*, 37.1 (2014): 37–52; Erin Bartels Buller, 'Vouching for Evidence: The New Life of Old Writing in Lillian Hellman's Memoirs', *Arizona Quarterly*, 70.1 (2014): 109–34.

37 Joan Scott, 'Experience', in Sidonie Smith and Julia Watson (eds), *Women, Autobiography, Theory* (Madison: University of Wisconsin Press, 1998): 57–71. On the importance of experience in the life writing of colonial nurses, see: Jessica Howell, Anne Marie Rafferty, and Anna Snaith, '(Author)

ity Abroad: The Life Writing of Colonial Nurses', *International Journal of Nursing Studies*, 48.9 (2011): 1155–62.

38 Sidonie Smith and Julia Watson, *Reading Autobiography: A Guide for Interpreting Life Narratives* (Minneapolis: University of Minnesota Press, 2010): 16. See also: Sidonie Smith, *Interfaces: Women, Autobiography, Image, Performance* (Ann Arbor: University of Michigan Press, 2002).

39 Smith and Watson, *Reading Autobiography*: 13.

40 Smith and Watson, *Reading Autobiography*: 13.

41 Susan Stanford Friedman, 'Women's Autobiographical Selves: Theory and Practice', in Smith and Watson, *Women, Autobiography, Theory*: 72–82 (72).

42 On the autobiographical 'individualist', see: Sidonie Smith and Julia Watson, 'Introduction: Situating Subjectivity in Women's Autobiographical Practices', in Smith and Watson, *Women, Autobiography, Theory*: 3–52 (27). On life writing more generally, see: Smith, *Interfaces*; Linda Anderson, *Autobiography (The New Critical Idiom)* (London: Routledge, 2010); Max Saunders, *Self Impressions: Life-Writing, Autobiografiction and the Forms of Modern Literature* (Oxford: Oxford University Press, 2013). For an analysis of classic, male autobiographical writing, see: Thomas Chase Hagood, ' "Literature to him was a recreation": A Life of Writing on the Southwestern Frontier', *Alabama Review*, 67.4 (2014): 374.

43 Kate Luard, *Unknown Warriors: Extracts from the Letters of K. E. Luard, R.R.C., Nursing Sister in France* (London: Chatto and Windus, 1930). A new edition of this book was published in 2014: Kate Luard, *Unknown Warriors: The Letters of Kate Luard, R.R.C. and Bar., Nursing Sister in France 1914–1918*, ed. John Stevens and Caroline Stevens (Stroud: History Press, 2014).

44 On the censoring of this text, see: Smith, *The Second Battlefield*: 77–8; Tylee, *The Great War and Women's Consciousness*: 94.

45 Juliet Nicholson, *The Great Silence: 1918–1920. Living in the Shadow of the Great War* (London: John Murray, 2009).

46 Brittain, *Testament of Youth*; Mary Borden, *The Forbidden Zone* (London: William Heinemann, 1929); Richard Aldington, *Death of a Hero* (London: Hogarth, 1984 [1929]); Graves, *Goodbye to All That*; Sassoon, *Memoirs of a Fox-Hunting Man*.

47 Vera Brittain, *Testament of Experience: An Autobiographical Story of the Years 1925–1950* (London: Fontana, 1980 [1957]): 77. See also: Christine E. Hallett, *Veiled Warriors: Allied Nurses of the First World War* (Oxford: Oxford University Press, 2014): 1–4.

48 Mary Britnieva, *One Woman's Story* (London: Arthur Baker, 1934).

49 Michelle Smith, 'Adventurous Girls of the British Empire: The Pre-War Novels of Bessie Marchant', *The Lion and the Unicorn*, 33.1 (2009): 1–25; Michelle Smith, *Empire in British Girls' Literature and Culture: Imperial Girls 1880–1915* (London: Palgrave Macmillan, 2011).

50 Helen Dore Boylston, 'Sister': The War Diary of a Nurse (New York: Ives Washburn, 1927).

51 Smith, The Second Battlefield: 6. Smith identified the most significant modernist characteristics in the writings of both Borden and La Motte: 'aesthetic self-consciousness, fragmentation, paradox and uncertainty, dehumanisation, sense of crisis and an engagement with issues of sexuality': 72.

52 Smith, The Second Battlefield: 8, 70.

53 Das, Touch and Intimacy: 175–203.

54 Gertrude Stein, The Autobiography of Alice B. Toklas (London: Penguin, 2001 [1933]): 172; 184–5.

55 de T'Serclaes, Flanders and Other Fields; Florence Farmborough, Nurse at the Russian Front: A Diary 1914–18 (London: Book Club Associates, 1974). The Farmborough work was originally published in New York, in 1974, by Stein and Day. It was later republished as: Florence Farmborough, With the Armies of the Tsar: A Nurse at the Russian Front in War and Revolution, 1914–1918 (New York: Cooper Square Press, 2000).

56 Penny Summerfield, Reconstructing Women's Wartime Lives (Manchester: Manchester University Press, 1998): 16–23.

57 Anon., My Beloved Poilus (Saint John, NB: Barnes, 1917).

58 Stimson, Finding Themselves.

59 Eric Scott (ed.), Nobody Ever Wins a War: The World War I Diaries of Ella Mae Bongard, R.N. (Ottawa: Janeric Enterprises, 1997).

60 Anon., A War Nurse's Diary: Sketches from a Belgian Field Hospital (New York: Macmillan, 1918).

61 Maud Mortimer, A Green Tent in Flanders (New York: Doubleday, Page, 1918).

62 Rebecca West, War Nurse: The True Story of a Woman who Lived, Loved and Suffered on the Western Front (New York: Cosmopolitan Book Corporation, 1930).

63 On the NUWSS and the WSPU, see: Smith, The Second Battlefield: 7. On the women's movement, see: Alison S. Fell and Ingrid Sharp (eds), The Women's Movement in Wartime: International Perspectives 1914–1918 (Basingstoke: Palgrave, 2007). On the woman suffrage movement in the USA, see Ellen Carol Dubois, Woman Suffrage and Women's Rights (New York: New York University Press, 1998).

64 Sheila Rowbotham, Dreamers of a New Day: Women who Invented the Twentieth Century (London: Verso, 2010): 6–9, 187. On women's involvement in the 'progressive' movement, see: Dorothy Schneider and Carl Schneider, American Women in the Progressive Era: 1900–1920 (New York: Facts on File, 1993).

65 Rowbotham, Dreamers of a New Day: 3–4. On gender and class in nursing, see: Arlene Young, 'Entirely a Woman's Question? Class, Gender and the Victorian Nurse', Journal of Victorian Culture, 13.1 (2008): 18–41; Carol Helmstadter, 'Old Nurses and New: Nursing in the London Teaching Hospitals before and after the Mid-Nineteenth-Century Reforms', Nursing History

Review, 1 (1993): 43–70; Carol Helmstadter, 'From the Private to the Public Sphere: The First Generation of Lady Nurses in England', *Nursing History Review*, 9 (2001): 127–40; Carol Helmstadter, 'Doctors and Nurses in the London Teaching Hospitals: Class, Gender, Religion and Professional Expertise, 1850–1890', *Nursing History Review*, 5 (1997): 61–97; Carol Helmstadter, '"A Real Tone": Professionalizing Nursing in Nineteenth-Century London', *Nursing History Review*, 11 (2003): 3–30; Eva Gamarnikow, 'Nurse or Woman: Gender and Professionalism in Reformed Nursing, 1860–1923', in Pat Holden and Jenny Littlewood (eds), *Anthropology and Nursing* (London: Routledge, 1991): 110–29; Sue Hawkins, 'From Maid to Matron: Nursing as a Route to Social Advancement in Nineteenth-Century England', *Women's History Review*, 19.1 (2010): 125–43; Sue Hawkins, *Nursing and Women's Labour in the Nineteenth Century: The Quest for Independence* (London: Routledge, 2010).

66 T'Serclaes, *Flanders and Other Fields*.

67 Tylee, *The Great War and Women's Consciousness*: 16.

68 Kimberly Jensen, *Mobilizing Minerva: American Women in the First World War* (Urbana and Chicago: University of Illinois Press, 2008).

69 Jensen, *Mobilizing Minerva*: 1–10.

70 Rowbotham, *Dreamers of a New Day*: 91–3. On Emma Goldman, see: Cynthia Connolly, '"I am a trained nurse": The Nursing Identity of Anarchist and Radical Emma Goldman', *Nursing History Review*, 18 (2010): 84–99. Goldman's own autobiography is available online: Emma Goldman, *Living My Life* (New York: Alfred A. Knopf, 1931); available at http://theanarchistlibrary.org/library/Emma_Goldman_Living_My_Life.html (accessed 14 December 2012).

71 Karen Buhler-Wilkerson, *No Place like Home: A History of Nursing and Home Care in the United States* (Baltimore: Johns Hopkins University Press, 2001).

72 Brian Abel-Smith, *A History of the Nursing Profession* (London: Heinemann, 1960); Susan McGann, *The Battle of the Nurses: A Study of Eight Women who Influenced the Development of Professional Nursing, 1880–1930* (London: Scutari Press, 1992); Anne Marie Rafferty, *The Politics of Nursing Knowledge* (London: Routledge, 1996).

73 Anne Summers, *Angels and Citizens: British Women as Military Nurses, 1854–1914* (London: Routledge and Kegan Paul, 1988): 205–36; Richard J. Kahn, 'Women and Men at Sea: Gender Debate aboard the Hospital Ship "Maine" during the Boer War, 1899–1900', *Journal of the History of Medicine and Allied Sciences*, 56 (2001): 111–139.

74 Ethel Bedford Fenwick is variously referred to by historians as 'Mrs Bedford Fenwick' or 'Ethel Gordon Manson'. See: Eve Bendall and Elizabeth Raybould, *A History of the General Nursing Council for England and Wales, 1919–1969* (London: H. K. Lewis, 1969): 3; Winifred Hector, *The Work of Mrs Bedford Fenwick and the Rise of Professional Nursing* (London: Royal College of Nursing, 1973): 3–4. On the battle for registration, see also: D. P. Griffon, '"Crowning

the Edifice": Ethel Fenwick and State Registration', *Nursing History Review*, 3 (1995): 201–12; Susan McGann, 'The Wind of Change Is Blowing', *Nursing History Review*, 10 (2002): 21–32; Christine E. Hallett, '"Intelligent interest in their own affairs": The First World War, *The British Journal of Nursing* and the Pursuit of Nursing Knowledge', in Patricia D'Antonio, Julie A. Fairman, and Jean C. Whelan (eds), *Routledge Handbook on the Global History of Nursing* (London: Routledge, 2013): 95–113. On Fenwick's editorship of the *British Journal of Nursing* (hereafter *BJN*), see: Laurel Brake and Marysa Demoor, *Dictionary of Nineteenth-Century Journalism* (London: Academic Press and the British Library, 2009): 464.

75 Violetta Thurstan, 'The British Red Cross Society', *BJN* (24 January 1914): 65–6 (66).

76 On the ambivalence of nurses' gendered roles, see: Kara Dixon Vuic, 'Wartime Nursing and Power', in D'Antonio, Fairman, and Whelan, *Routledge Handbook on the Global History of Nursing*: 22–34.

77 Sue Light, 'British Military Nurses and the Great War: A Guide to the Services', *The Western Front Association Forum* (7 February 2010): 4; available at www.westernfrontassociation.com (accessed 30 October 2012); Christine E. Hallett and Alison S. Fell, 'Introduction: New Perspectives on First World War Nursing', in Alison S. Fell and Christine E. Hallett, *First World War Nursing: New Perspectives* (New York: Routledge, 2013): 1–14; Hallett, *Veiled Warriors*: 20.

78 Anon. (ed.), *Reminiscent Sketches, 1914 to 1919 by Members of Her Majesty Queen Alexandra's Imperial Military Nursing Service* (London: John Bale, Sons, and Danielsson, 1922): iii. This anonymous text appears to have been edited by A. Beadsmore Smith, Matron-in-Chief of the QAIMNS. Sue Light puts the initial figure lower, at fewer than 200, and the final figure (of total numbers of serving Reserve nurses) higher, at 'more than 12,000': Light, 'British Military Nurses and the Great War': 4.

79 The Territorial Force Nursing Service was founded as part of the Haldane Reforms in 1908. On its establishment, see: Dame Sidney Browne Papers, Queen Alexandra's Royal Army Nursing Corps (QARANC) Collection, Box I, Army Medical Services Museum Archives, Aldershot, UK. On the Haldane Reforms, see also: Jenny Gould, 'Women's Military Services in First World War Britain', in Higonnet, Jenson, Michel, and Weitz (eds), *Behind the Lines*: 114–25. Sue Light places the total number of Territorial Force nurses to serve during the war at 8,140: Light, 'British Military Nurses and the Great War': 4.

80 Anon., *Reminiscent Sketches*: iv.

81 On the foundation of the VADs, see: Summers, *Angels and Citizens*: 237–70. On the work of the VADs, see: Sara Amy Zackheim Adams, 'Creating Amateur Professionals: British Voluntary Aid Detachment Nurses and the First World War' (unpublished Ph.D. thesis, University of Rochester, NY, 1998); Hazel Bruce Basford, 'Kent VAD: The Work of Voluntary Aid Detachments in Kent

during the First World War' (unpublished M.Phil. thesis, University of Kent, 2004). On VADs, see also: Hallett, *Veiled Warriors*: 18–20.

82 Anon., *Reminiscent Sketches*: iv.

83 Anon., Column, *BJN* (18 March 1916): 243. On the tensions between nurses and VADs, and the role of social class in exacerbating these, see: Margaret Vining and Barton C. Hacker, 'From Camp Follower to Lady in Uniform: Women, Social Class and Military Institutions before 1920', *Contemporary European History*, 10.3 (2001): 353–73; Janet S. K. Watson, 'Wars in the Wards: The Social Construction of Medical Work in First World War Britain', *Journal of British Studies*, 41 (2002): 484–510. See also Watson, *Fighting Different Wars*; Christine E. Hallett, '"Emotional Nursing": Involvement, Engagement, and Detachment in the Writings of First World War Nurses and VADs', in Fell and Hallett, *First World War Nursing*: 87–102.

84 Thurstan, 'The British Red Cross Society': 66. On women's involvement in paramilitary organisations, see: Lucy Noakes, 'Eve in Khaki: Women Working with the British Military, 1915–1918', in Krista Cowman and Louise A. Jackson (eds), *Women and Work Culture* (Aldershot: Ashgate, 2004); Lucy Noakes, *Women in the British Army: War and the Gentle Sex, 1907–1948* (New York: Routledge, 2006).

85 Summers, *Angels and Citizens*: 261.

86 Laurence Binyon, *For Dauntless France: An Account of Britain's Aid to the French Wounded and Victims of the War. Compiled for the British Red Cross Societies and the British Committee of the French Red Cross* (London: Hodder and Stoughton, 1918): 32–7. On the French Flag Nursing Corps, see: Hallett, *Veiled Warriors*: 32, 71, 101, 163, 164–70, 256.

87 Katrin Schultheiss, *Bodies and Souls: Politics and Professionalization of Nursing in France, 1880–1922* (Cambridge, MA: Harvard University Press, 2001). On French nursing during the First World War, see also: Margaret Darrow, 'French Volunteer Nursing and the Myth of War Experience in World War I', *American Historical Review*, 101.1 (1996): 80–106; Margaret Darrow, *French Women and the First World War: War Stories from the Home Front* (New York: Berg, 2000). See also: Hallett, *Veiled Warriors*: 24–5.

88 Binyon, *For Dauntless France*: 327.

89 On nursing in Canada, see: Kathryn McPherson, *Bedside Matters: The Transformation of Canadian Nursing, 1900–1990* (Toronto: University of Toronto Press, 2003 [1996]). For insight into the work of Canadian nurses during the First World War, see 85 and 94. See also: Susan Mann, *Margaret Macdonald: Imperial Daughter* (Montreal and Kingston: McGill-Queens University Press, 2005). On the Australian Army Nursing Services, see: Jan Bassett, *Guns and Brooches: Australian Army Nursing from the Boer War to the Gulf War* (Melbourne and Oxford: Oxford University Press, 1992); Ruth Rae, *Scarlet Poppies: The Army Experience of Australian Nurses during World War One* (Burwood, NSW: College of Nursing, Australia, 2004); Ruth Rae, *Veiled*

Lives: Threading Australian Nursing History into the Fabric of the First World War (Burwood, NSW: College of Nursing, 2009); Kirsty Harris, *More than Bombs and Bandages: Australian Army Nurses at Work in World War I* (Newport, NSW: Big Sky Publishing, 2011). On the New Zealand Army Nursing Service, see: Jan Rodgers, 'Potential for Professional Profit: The Making of the New Zealand Army Nursing Service 1914–1915', *Nursing Praxis in New Zealand*, 11.2 (1996): 4–12; Anna Rogers, *While You're Away: New Zealand Nurses at War 1899–1948* (Auckland: Auckland University Press, 2003).

90 Although, it is noteworthy that Canada did send a number of VADs. See: Linda Quiney, 'Assistant Angels: Canadian Voluntary Aid Detachment Nurses in the Great War', *Canadian Bulletin of Medical History*, 15 (1998): 189–206; Cynthia Toman, '"Help Us, Serve England": First World War Military Nursing and National Identities', *Canadian Bulletin of Medical History*, 30.1 (2013): 156–7.

91 Mary T. Sarnecky, *A History of the US Army Nurse Corps* (Philadelphia: University of Pennsylvania Press, 1999): 1, 51–2.

92 Sarnecky, *A History of the US Army Nurse Corps*: 51–4.

93 Sarnecky, *A History of the US Army Nurse Corps*: 73.

94 Sarnecky, *A History of the US Army Nurse Corps*: 91–2. Kimberly Jensen observes that: 'Over the course of the war 10,660 ANC nurses served with the American Expeditionary Force in Europe': Kimberly Jensen, 'A Base Hospital Is Not a Coney Island Dance Hall: American Women Nurses, Hostile Work Environment, and Military Rank in the First World War', *Frontiers*, 26.2 (2005): 206–35 (208–9). A very small number of volunteer nurses were incorporated into the US Army Medical Services.

95 Kimberly Jensen, 'A Base Hospital Is Not a Coney Island Dance Hall': 211.

96 Sarnecky, *A History of the US Army Nurse Corps*: 80–1.

97 Sarnecky, *A History of the US Army Nurse Corps*: 83. Brief histories of a number of base hospitals were written shortly after the war. See, for example: Anon., *History of the Pennsylvania Hospital Unit (Base Hospital No. 10, USA) in the Great War* (New York: Paul B. Hoeber, 1921); Anon., *The University of Virginia Base Hospital Forty-One* (unpublished account, 1925); box-folder 001-001, Historical Collection, Claude Moore Health Sciences Library, University of Virginia, Charlottesville, USA.

98 Sarnecky, *A History of the US Army Nurse Corps*: 57 (quote 92–3). See also: Hallett, *Veiled Warriors*: 216.

99 United States military nurses were granted 'relative rank' in the 1920s: Jensen, 'A Base Hospital Is Not a Coney Island Dance Hall': 207, 212–16. British military nurses acquired officer status in 1943. See: Penny Starns, *The March of the Matrons: Military Influence on the British Civilian Nursing Profession, 1939–1969* (Peterborough, DSM: 2000): 25–52.

Part I

Independent ladies

Britain's entry into the First World War was accompanied by a remarkable outpouring of enthusiasm for volunteer nursing, one of the most significant features of which was the emergence of entire hospital units supplied and funded by wealthy, upper-class women. Such 'freelance' units, were partly supported by the Red Cross or Order of St John of Jerusalem and were offered to the army medical services of several allied nations. Ironically, it was often the best organised and potentially most effective of these that were rejected out-of-hand. Elsie Inglis, a doctor and the founder of the Scottish Women's Hospitals, is famously reported to have offered fully equipped and staffed hospitals to the British Army in 1914, but to have been told to 'go home and keep quiet'.[1] She went on to supply highly effective units to the military medical services of several countries, including France and Serbia. Several 'freelance' operations found their way to both Western and Serbian fronts during the early months of the war. But these were organised and funded by wealthy – often aristocratic – ladies and operated under the auspices of the Red Cross.

One of the most unusual hospital units of the war was l'Hôpital Chirurgical Mobile No. 1 at Rousbrugge in Belgium. Offered to the French Service de Santé des Armées by American millionaire Mary Borden Turner, it was not only one of the most successful French field hospitals of the war (in terms of survival and recovery rates) but also an extraordinarily fertile field for the development of female writing talent. Three of its nurses wrote highly acclaimed memoirs of the war, while a fourth published a remarkably vivid, but carefully anonymised account of what appears to be the same hospital.

Note

1 Claire Tylee, *The Great War and Women's Consciousness: Images of Militarism and Womanhood in Women's Writings, 1914–64* (Houndmills and London: Macmillan, 1990): 7.

1

Heroines in Belgium and Serbia

Introduction: plucky nurses

At the outbreak of the First World War British women volunteered for war service in such numbers that organisations such as the Red Cross and the Order of St John of Jerusalem found themselves, initially, overwhelmed. Many of those who offered to nurse the wounded held no nursing qualifications of any kind, and had to wait until they had passed VAD examinations, or acquired full nurse-training in recognised training hospitals, before they could gain acceptance for military service. American women, too, were eager for participation in war – even though their country was to remain neutral until 1917. American writer Margaret Deland observed that 'of all the amazing things that have come bubbling and seething to the surface of life during these last three and a half years, there has been nothing more amazing to me than this exodus of American girls', adding that she believed that such things could only have happened in the USA, 'where fathers and mothers have so very little to say as to the behavior of their daughters'.[1] But British women, too, anxious to prove their 'pluck' and worth, offered themselves for military nursing service in their tens of thousands. Some were so wealthy and powerful that, far from finding themselves barred by parental – or any other – authority, they were able, in the early months of war, to take entire hospital units overseas to France and Belgium. It was only in early 1915, after the official military medical and nursing services had established a structured network of hospitals and transport services on the Western

Front, that such volunteer units began to come under more formal military control.

In the summer of 1914, the sympathies of the British people were as much with Serbia as with Belgium.[2] Many of the volunteer units that had travelled to Belgium during the earliest months of the war, only to be forced out again by the advancing German army, transferred their services to Serbia in 1915. Both nations had a significant hold upon the popular imagination. Whilst Belgium was the victim – the country from which refugees poured in their thousands – Serbia was seen as the small and defenceless, but noble and patriotic, nation that had defied tyranny. The plight of the Serbian people moved several women's volunteer groups to offer their services. The prospect of travelling thousands of miles from home to support a people who were seen as fierce defenders of a noble cause seemed to some a romantic adventure. Yet, the leaders of such expeditions – women such as Elsie Inglis, and Leila, Lady Paget – were very serious in their approaches to what they saw as, at heart, a patriotic endeavour.[3] Their efforts, unsurprisingly, ended in disaster. Some were imprisoned by their German and Bulgarian adversaries; others found themselves on a desperate and life-threatening trek across the Albanian Alps.

The duchess-directrice: Millicent Sutherland and her ambulance

Some wealthy and aristocratic women found that war nursing could be a welcome dramatic episode in an otherwise safe and privileged life. For Millicent, Duchess of Sutherland, war-torn Belgium and northern France were so far removed from anything she had previously known that her involvement seemed a great adventure – an epic journey through an unknown terrain. It is not clear whether her book *Six Weeks at the War* was written with deliberately propagandist intent.[4] It may be that her account unreflectively reproduces the perceptions of her own class. If so, it illustrates how submerged those perceptions were in nationalism. Her beliefs in the right of the British cause and the brutality of the German nation run through her short account of the time she spent in Belgium in the first weeks of war. She bemoans the power that is wielded by 'Prussia's rulers' over the German people.[5]

It is not the millions of soldiers who should be blamed for the catastrophe of war: they are under the control of their military masters. Yet, British men and women drawn into the same war remain pure – and this is particularly true of the nurses she has enlisted into her ambulance, whose courage and selflessness are a recurring theme of her narrative. For her, only the annihilation of the German army can bring the war to an end, and that goal is a just one.[6]

Lady Millicent St Clair-Erskine was born in 1867, and married into the British aristocracy, to become Duchess of Sutherland, in 1884. Although she began her wartime nursing service by enrolling with the French Red Cross in Paris on 9 August 1914, she soon decided that she could best serve the allied war effort by forming her own hospital unit.[7] The 'Millicent Sutherland Ambulance' was established under the auspices of the Belgian 'Service de Santé des Armées' and was formed with the support of the Belgian Red Cross. Dr Antoine Depage, an influential Brussels surgeon, who at that time was working closely with Edith Cavell, gave strong support to the initiative, and was declared by Millicent to be 'a man to brush away all red tape and ineptitude'.[8] Millicent sent to Britain for Guy's Hospital surgeon Oswald Morgan, eight nurses, and a stretcher-bearer.

Memoirist Elsie Knocker (Baroness T'Serclaes) was to comment years later that many of the First World War's earliest field hospitals were 'splendidly freelance' in a way that would never again be possible.[9] The British class system was, in Paul Fussell's words, 'intact and purring smoothly',[10] and significant numbers of upper-class British women appear to have taken it for granted that they should be at the heart of the war effort, whether they possessed the required skills or not. In this sense, they were mirroring the behaviours of their French counterparts, many of whom entered hospitals to work as 'lady-nurses' with no qualifications of any kind.[11] The wealth, social influence, and confidence of even the most aristocratic volunteers were not sufficient to persuade their own compatriots in the British Royal Army Medical Corps to incorporate them into its ranks at the outbreak of war (except as VADs). But a severe shortage of fully trained nurses on the European Continent meant that the beleaguered Belgian and French Services de Santé were only too anxious to accept offers, which ranged from individual service in existing military hospitals to the establishment of whole field hospitals and ambulance units. The impression is given by some accounts that, in the early weeks of the war, Belgium was teeming with groups of wealthy eccentrics, working as hospital directors, nurses, doctors, and ambulance drivers.[12] Amongst the most colourful were the First Aid Nursing Yeomanry, a unit of wealthy, upper-middle-class and aristocratic female ambulance drivers who were said to have arrived on the Continent wearing fur coats.[13]

The first Millicent Sutherland Ambulance was established in a convent in Namur, owned by the Soeurs de Notre Dame. Soon after the unit's arrival, the Germans began to shell the town.[14] Millicent quoted an excerpt from her original diary to describe the events of late August:

> Never shall I forget the afternoon of August 22 … Six motor-cars and as many wagons were at the door, and they were carrying in those unhappy fellows. Some were on stretchers, others were supported by willing Red Cross men. One or two of the stragglers fell up the steps from fatigue and lay there. Many of these men had been for three days without food or sleep in the trenches … So many of the men were in a state of prostration bordering almost on dementia, that I seemed instantly enveloped in the blight of war. I felt stunned – as if I were passing through an endless nightmare.[15]

The bombardment continued, and walking patients took shelter in the cellars of the convent. Millicent's eight nurses, however, were 'most courageous', remaining above ground with those who were helpless and bedfast. Millicent commented that 'no one, until these awful things happen, can conceive the untold value of fully-trained and disciplined British nurses'.[16]

Eventually the Germans entered Namur. A fire – believed to have been started deliberately – spread quickly to engulf a large part of the town. Millicent and her nurses again remained at their posts and reassured their patients. As she describes these events, Millicent recounts how she 'felt as if I were actually *living* some book of adventure, such as I had read in my youth'.[17] Her tendency to recount the whole episode as if it were part of an adventure story is striking, and is typical of this genre of war writing.[18] Following the German occupation, Millicent and her party were escorted on foot to Brussels – a long and difficult journey; but Millicent claims to have shrugged it off as no further than she might walk 'in a day's golfing'. From Brussels they returned home by car and boat via Rotterdam.[19]

By 23 October, Millicent was back on the Continent. The 'Millicent Sutherland Ambulance Car Convoy' landed in Dunkirk and established a 100-bed hospital for Belgian and French soldiers at the Hotel Belle Vue in Malo-les-Bains near Dunkirk.[20] In the summer of 1915, the hospital was transferred to Bourbourg, twelve miles from Dunkirk and outside the range of the enemy's guns. Here, it was famously known as 'the camp in the oat field', and was the subject of a series of paintings by Victor Tardieu.[21] On 15 October that year, the hospital was taken over by the British Red Cross, attached to No. 35 General Hospital near Calais, and began to take in British wounded. Following subsequent moves to Longuenesse, Hazebrouck, and Roublaix, the hospital was finally demobilised on 20 November 1918.[22]

The 'Millicent Sutherland Ambulance' experienced numerous changes of identity, as well as several geographical moves bringing it alternately closer to and further from the front lines. It is Millicent's first 'six weeks at the war', however, that are best known to a modern readership. The pages she wrote so hastily following her return from Belgium in October 1914, incorporating large amounts of text from her personal diary, offer an immediate and, at times, compelling account of the fate of volunteer field hospitals during the earliest weeks of the war.

Escaping the German advance: a war nurse's diary

The establishment of large numbers of ad hoc medical units and temporary field hospitals gave British nurses unexpected opportunities to serve close to the front lines. One nurse, whose anonymous account of her adventures in Belgium was published as *A War Nurse's Diary: Sketches from a Belgian Field Hospital*, describes feelings, at the outset of war, that were typical of a population gripped by 'war fever': 'the great upheaval sent its waves of excitement beating against every shore till it touched the whole world'. The writer was working in a hospital in England. She had joined neither the Reserve of the QAIMNS nor the Territorial Force Nursing Service, and so was forced to watch with 'an almost bitter envy' as many of her colleagues were called away for military service.[23] Enquiries and offers of service to both voluntary and official services yielded only refusals. It was reported that about 30,000 nurses were available, which, at that time, was believed to be 'about one nurse to each soldier' – clearly an estimate that was both inaccurate and inadequate.[24]

Eventually, this nurse author's efforts were rewarded and she was taken on by a volunteer unit bound for Antwerp. Her sense of excitement and adventure, along with her recognition that she was joining an unofficial – and perhaps quite disorganised – expedition are illustrated by her comment on the preparations she and her colleagues made: 'The lady who was the organizer of our hospital had not, I should judge, any previous experience of hospitals or their management. We all felt this, and therefore were quite prepared at an early date to fall into the hands of the Germans, so, as a precaution, we nurses each provided ourselves with a tube of morphia tablets to take in any emergency'.[25] In Antwerp, the nurses established their hospital in a grammar school (formerly a duke's palace) on the Boulevard Leopold. The author offers vivid descriptions of her patients' wounds, commenting that the antiseptic treatment of wounds in a British civilian hospital was very different from 'dealing with mangled and shattered flesh where the wounds are filled with mud, torn clothing and shrapnel'.[26] The bombardment of Antwerp brought with it large numbers of burn victims, some with such severe facial injuries that nurses had to 'force' openings through which to insert tubes to feed their patients.[27]

Like Millicent, the author of *A War Nurse's Diary* was keen to emphasise the courage of nurses under German bombardment. Her situation in Antwerp placed her in a field of great danger, and her description of her experience of shell-fire is particularly vivid:

> a boom far away, immediately followed by a new whistling scream increasing in volume and intensity till it became the roar of a train in a tunnel. It skimmed over our heads, literally raising our hair in its passage. This ended in a large, full explosion. Then all was silence for a breathless second, – when the terrified roar of a wounded animal rent the air, like that of a great bull bellowing. A pistol shot followed, and silence ensued again. I was seized with an uncontrollable ague, whilst my friend reached out her hand and said, 'Remember we are British women, not emotional continentals. We've got to keep our heads.'[28]

This writer chooses to reveal the 'qualities' of British women again when describing the volunteer hospital's departure from Antwerp as part of a mass-evacuation of Belgium. The staff managed to comman-deer five of the London buses that had provided transport for British marines in Belgium. Filling these with patients, they joined a stream of refugees heading for Ostend. Their fourteen-and-a-half-hour jour-ney was both gruelling and hazardous, with nurses taking turns to sit inside the vehicle with the seriously wounded, and outside on the top deck with less dangerously ill cases:

> Just before we started a tall Marine in a navy jersey and sailor's cap was helped in. He sat in the corner next to me. All his ribs were broken down one side, and he had no plaster or support. Opposite me were two Tommies with compound fractures of the leg. I placed both legs on my knees to lessen the jolting. The Marine suffered in silent agony, his lips pressed tightly together, and his white face set. I looked at him helplessly, and he said 'Never mind me, Sister; if I swear don't take any notice.' Fortunately, they had pushed in two bottles of whiskey and some soda-syphons; I just dosed them all around until it was finished. Placing the Marine's arm around my shoulders, I used my right arm as a splint to support his ribs, and so we sat for seven and a half hours without moving.[29]

Following her escape from the German advance, this nurse spent only a few weeks in Britain before returning to the front lines. She travelled with the Duchess of Sutherland Ambulance, but was then placed in a field hospital in Furnes. Attached to her hospital was 'a most interesting body of people': the 'Hector Munro Flying Ambulance Corps'.[30] The eccentric Dr Munro, along with a group of philanthropic British volunteers, had set up a British unit which pro-vided a fleet of ambulances to ferry the wounded directly from the battlefield to a field hospital behind the lines. The ambulance had, only after some persuasion, been recognised and supported by both the Belgian and the British Committees of the Red Cross.[31] Munro, 'the essence of the absent-minded professor',[32] was, in some ways, more forward-thinking than his appearance and manner suggested. He was keen to promote women's rights, and in addition to hiring several female trained nurses, he invited a number of women to work in his ambulance as volunteer nurses or drivers. Among these were Helen Gleason, the American wife of a war correspondent; the aris-tocratic Lady Dorothie Fielding; and novelists Sarah Macnaughtan and May Sinclair.[33] The unit's first ambulance had been established in the first weeks of war at the Flandria Palace Hotel in Ghent,[34] but had been forced, like so many other British units, to escape ahead of the rapid German advance and relocate in a more permanent base in Furnes, well behind the front-line trenches. From here, its drivers went out on nightly missions to rescue the wounded from the Battle of the Yser and the First Battle of Ypres.[35]

The author of *A War Nurse's Diary* offers deliberately graphic descriptions of the war wounds she encountered while working with severely damaged patients in forward field dressing stations. She describes standing by 'grievously stricken men it is impossible to help, to see the death-sweat gathering on young faces, to have no means of easing their last moments', adding: 'this is the nearest to Hell I have yet been'.[36] Munro's unit was broken up in November 1915, when six of its ambulances were placed under the control of the French Service de Santé.[37]

Nurse fighters on the Serbian Front

Among the most unusual accounts produced by volunteer nurses is that of Flora Sandes, who began her wartime career as a volunteer with a British hospital unit and ended it as a fighter with the Serbian army. Angela Smith has suggested that, by actually fighting on the field of battle, Sandes, 'inadvertently, struck a blow for the feminist cause'.[38] After travelling to Salonika, and then into Serbia, Sandes remained behind when other British medical personnel left the country ahead of the Bulgarian advance. Her published diary is a chronicle of her wartime 'adventures'. One episode describes how she is sitting in bed in a small hotel in Prilip, listening to someone attempting to force an entry into her room, and watching, from the window, 'the most villainous-looking Turks squatting about at their supper. These, I tell myself, are the ones who will come in and cut my throat if Prilip is taken to-night, as I don't think any responsible person in the town knows I am here. However, if I live through the night things will probably look more cheery in the morning.'[39] The deliberately casual tone of Sandes's writing is probably intended to convey a sense of her coolness and courage.

Sandes obtained a posting at a mobile field ambulance serving the Second Regiment of the Serbian Army. Her description of her arrival at the ambulance is full of a sense of adventure, and could have come straight from the pages of a Bessie Marchant novel.[40] She – the well-bred Englishwoman – 'roughs it' with the Serbian army:

> It seemed a bit of a problem where I was to sleep, but eventually some of the soldiers turned out of one of their small bivouac tents. These tents are only a sort of little lean-to's [sic], which you crawl into, just the height of a rifle, two of which can be used instead of poles. You seem a bit cramped at first, but after I had lived in one for a couple of months I did not notice it.[41]

The tone of this passage is typical of that of the book as a whole. Even when its heroine is wounded, her account never evokes any real sense of fear. The Serbian soldiers are portrayed as a set of amiable roughnecks, and Sandes's writing sanitises the realities of war. Eventually, Sandes enlisted as a soldier in the Serbian army and rose to the rank of sergeant. Upon returning home to England, she found it almost impossible to tolerate wearing women's clothes and assimilated only with difficulty back into civilian life.[42] And yet an unconscious – and entirely instinctive – sense of herself as a woman who *ought* to be protected comes through in her writing.

Another woman who projected a heroic, masculinised image of herself while clearly retaining a deep-rooted sense of her own femininity was Mabel St Clair Stobart, whose writings were based on her extensive experience of wartime hospital management in both the Balkan War of 1912 and the First World War. Her hard-hitting memoir, *The Flaming Sword in Serbia and Elsewhere*, offers vivid descriptions of the horrors of war.[43] Stobart's deliberate reference to the biblical sword that debarred mankind from the Garden of Eden expressed her sense that warfare was a fall from grace. Her message was clearly stated: human society – controlled by men – had become militaristic and, therefore, dangerously destructive. If women had political influence war might be averted. And yet, society's rationale for debarring women from the exercise of political authority was predicated on the supposed military weakness of the female – the inability of women to endure the hardships of war. Stobart's avowed mission was to overturn society's delusions.[44] She aimed to show, both by example and through her writing, that women were just as capable as men of taking on leadership roles in wartime, and yet that they were also naturally opposed to warfare because of their nurturing and humanitarian qualities.[45] To prove her points, Stobart depicted women participating in the humanitarian efforts of the

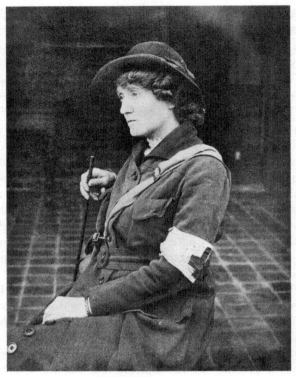

Figure 1 Portrait of Mabel St Clair Stobart

military medical services, and taking on (particularly in her own case) challenging leadership roles.

Mabel St Clair Stobart established her Women's Sick and Wounded Convoy Corps (WSWCC) in 1909, the year in which the VADs were formed.[46] Her purpose was to create an entirely female corps that would be capable of performing humanitarian service, without significant male support, in time of war. The work was deliberately experimental – its purpose to demonstrate that women could exhibit the same level of strategic prowess, courage, and toughness as men. To this end, Stobart's group prepared for a future war by training vigorously on the cliffs above her home at Studland in Dorset. During the Balkan War, in 1912, they spent seven weeks in Serbia offering aid to the sick and wounded, and because of this prior experience, Stobart considered the WSWCC to be ready for action when the First World War began in 1914. She took a group of nurses, doctors, and volunteers to Belgium in August.[47] Their work was short-lived; their unit was overtaken by the rapid German advance and they were forced to return to Britain.

Stobart next decided to take her unit to Serbia, a region with which she was already familiar. The WSWCC undertook humanitarian work among both military and civilian populations until, once again, they were forced to retreat – this time ahead of a joint German and Bulgar advance. But flight itself was an opportunity for publicity, and Stobart's leadership of her unit as it crossed the Albanian Alps in the winter of 1915 became the stuff of legend, as she – 'The Lady of the Black Horse' – forged a path across some of the most rugged and dangerous mountains of Eastern Europe.[48] An image of her on horseback appeared in several daily newspapers, and was (in terms of its power and reach) reminiscent of a much earlier hugely influential image of Florence Nightingale in *The Times* as 'The Lady with the Lamp'.[49] Here, however, the similarities end: Nightingale's image was that of a vulnerable woman in a stark, military environment; Stobart's featured a woman in martial attire seated astride a black horse in a mountain ravine – she was 'A Lady who was made a Major'.[50]

Stobart's writing is at its least convincing when it adopts a didactic, polemical style. It is her story itself that demands attention. Without indulging in any too-obvious self-promotion, she comes across to the reader as a courageous, self-possessed, and commanding personality. Her accounts of the setting-up of her field hospital in Kragujevatz, and of the expansion of her humanitarian work among the Serbian people through a network of dispensaries, impress with evidence of their detailed planning and obvious effectiveness. It is, however, her epic saga of her journey through the Albanian Alps as part of the massive exodus of fleeing refugees that really commands attention. We read of how she insisted upon leading her convoy on horseback; and of how she worked with great patience and determination to keep her unit together, on track, and supplied, during its gruelling trek over the mountains to safety.[51]

Mabel St Clair Stobart's intent was both feminist and pacifist. She insisted that there was an essential correspondence between the two. Towards the end of her account, she adopts a reflective tone:

> This thought came to me vividly one summer night in Serbia. It was during the typhus epidemic, and I stumbled unawares upon an open grave. It was three-quarters full of naked corpses. They were typhus victims. They had been prisoners of war, and the grave would not be closed until there were enough dead to fill it. Heavy rain had fallen, and the bodies were half-submerged in water; but I saw one man above the others. His body, long and strong-limbed, was all uncovered, but his face, fine featured, proudly ignorant of the ignominy, his face was covered with – flies; filthy, bloodsucking flies ... The glamour, the adventure, the chivalry, which of old gilded the horrors of war, have vanished. War is now a bloody business; a business for butchers, not for high-souled gentlemen. Modern militarism involves tortures and extermination, not only of the fighting, but of the non-fighting portion of the population, in a manner which would have shocked even the heroes of the Old Testament.[52]

Stobart, perhaps unwittingly, draws a distinction between modern militarism with its 'tortures and exterminations' and the chivalrous warfare of earlier times. This perhaps undermines her argument that warfare – always a masculine pursuit – has always been a brutal and entirely unnecessary business. Stobart's writings stand alongside those of other female commentators on the war – women such as Catherine Marshall, who argued that the female perspective differed from that of men, because women's natural role in life was to create, rather than to destroy, life,[53] or Sylvia Pankhurst, whose pacifism stemmed from her observations of the impact of war on the most vulnerable members of society: the impoverished women and children of London's East End.[54]

Travelling with Stobart was Olive Aldridge, who described her experiences in Serbia, working at one of the village dispensaries established by the WSWCC. She joined, in November, the retreat through Montenegro and Albania. Like Stobart herself, Aldridge produced an account that focused on the endurance and fortitude of the British women who supported the Serbian campaign.[55] Alongside her account stands that of Ellen Chivers Davies, who commented on the dedication of the British nurses in Serbia during the typhus epidemics of 1915, when 'the Sisters worked as if driven by a fury of pity which could only find expression in work'.[56] In January 1916, the *British Journal of Nursing* produced a column praising the 'British grit' of those nurses who had joined the retreat from Serbia, choosing to present it in rousing propagandist terms as '*the* quality that is going to win the War'.[57]

A quest too far: the death of Sarah Macnaughtan

Some nurse volunteers travelled well beyond Serbia in their determination to serve the war effort. Sarah Macnaughtan's book *A Woman's Diary of the War* reads as an epic travel saga. Macnaughtan appears to have been driven, not only by the wish to help her fellow countrymen, but also by a quest for adventure and a need to prove herself. In this sense, her motivation – and her fate – can be seen as similar to those of many of the combatants she nursed. Macnaughtan, although not a trained nurse, had considerable wartime nursing experience. She was in Antwerp with Mabel St Clair Stobart's unit during the first weeks of the war, and she provides one of the most vivid extant descriptions of the German bombardment of that city. Demonstrating a determined 'stiff upper lip', she refers to the German shelling as 'a little startling' with its 'curious sound of rending, increasing in violence as the missile comes towards one, and giving one plenty of time to wonder, if one feels so disposed, whether it intends to hit one or not'.[58] This deliberate and studied nonchalance belies the intensity of Macnaughtan's feelings, which are revealed in a personal diary, collated after her death by her niece, Betty Salmon, and published as *My War Experiences in Two Continents*.[59]

Macnaughtan appears to have admired what she saw as the peculiarly British qualities of courage and stoicism, and worked hard to display such qualities herself – and to project them in her writing. She comments on how 'The Britisher was born cheery. Even when they were "gassed" they called out, "All right, Allemands, put another penny in the meter!" '[60] It was probably the desire to imitate such extraordinary and openly eccentric courage that led Macnaughtan to take risks that led to her eventual death from infectious disease following an abortive expedition to the East.

Following the retreat and capture of Mabel St Clair Stobart's unit in Belgium, Macnaughtan served for several months with Hector Munro's Flying Ambulance Corps in Furnes, and it was during this time that she wrote *A Woman's Diary of the War*. The book reads as a treatise on British courage and endurance. Not only does it dwell upon the 'unfailing pluck' of the stalwart British nurse, it also philosophises upon how combatants viewed death:

> And the reality lies also in the extraordinary sense of freedom which war brings ... Soldiers know this, although they can never explain it. They have been terrified. They have been more terrified than their own mothers will ever know, and their very spines have melted under the shrieking sounds of shells. And then comes the day when they 'don't mind'. Death stalks just as near as ever, but his face, quite suddenly, has a friendly air.[61]

These words hold a tragic irony for the reader who views them alongside Macnaughtan's later diary entries. After serving for several months with the Hector Munro Flying Ambulance Corps and then running a soup kitchen at Furnes station, Macnaughtan travelled to Russia in October 1915. Deciding that her services could be most effective on the 'Persian Front', she travelled deep into Armenia, where she contracted a serious infectious disease. Helpless, without support, and unable to travel home, she wrote in her diary of how she had 'lost count of time' – how she was just waiting, 'hoping someone will come and take me away, though I am now getting so weak I don't suppose I can travel'.[62] The 'friendly air' of death was no longer near when Macnaughtan wrote sadly: 'One wonders whether there can be a Providence in all this disappointment. I think not. I just made a great mistake coming out here, and I have suffered for it. Ye gods, what a winter it has been – disillusioning, dull, hideously and achingly disappointing!' On a separate page, which she headed 'Memories of Home', she wrote:

> It is too odd to think that until the war came I was the happiest woman in the world ... I can hardly believe now in my crowds of friends, my devoted servants, my pleasant walk, the daily budget of letters and invitations, and the press notices in their pink slips ... The joy, almost the intoxication of life that has been mine. Of course, I ought to have turned back at Petrograd! But I thought all my work was before me ... And now I have reached the end – *Persia! And there is no earthly use for us, and there are no roads*.[63]

Macnaughtan did eventually obtain help, and reached home in the early summer of 1916. A few weeks before her death, she accepted the award of 'Lady Grace of the Order of St John of Jerusalem'. On her gravestone at Chart Sutton are carved the words:

In the Great War, by Word and Deed, at Home and Abroad.
She served her Country even unto Death.[64]

Conclusion: heroines on Western and Eastern Fronts

Some of the earliest published accounts of wartime hospital work were written by wealthy women belonging to Britain's social elite. Very few were trained nurses, but all were fascinated by what they saw as the power of nursing to act as a vehicle through which women might make important contributions to the allied war effort. For some writers, such contributions made an important political point: they demonstrated that women, as well as men, were capable of being actors on a world stage and, therefore, had the right to participate in political decision-making. For women such as Mabel St Clair Stobart, wartime hospital service would win women the right to vote. For a few – and for Stobart in particular – their motivations went beyond merely proving that women could take on significant wartime roles. Offering humanitarian service actually demonstrated their commitment to peace. Yet few were as determinedly pacifist as Stobart. Indeed, some – notably Flora Sandes – seem to have been driven by a personal desire to participate in military action. Sandes clearly took pride in her service with the Serbian army. At no point in her book does she pause from her narrative to make a political point. Her 'blow' for female emancipation was, as Angela Smith asserts, an inadvertent one.[65] Few women wrote treatises that were so obviously political as Stobart's. Many – notably Millicent, Duchess of Sutherland – appear to have had a sense that their experiences and contributions were so extraordinary that they must set them down for others to read. Doing so was, in some ways, an act of self-promotion. It was also a means of revealing both the intensity and significance of nursing work and the strength of character of the nurse herself.

Notes

1 Margaret Deland, *Small Things* (New York: D. Appleton, 1919): 57.

2 On the wartime propaganda that helped evoke and strengthen these sympathies, see Cate Haste, *Keep the Home Fires Burning: Propaganda in the First World War* (London: Allen Lane, 1977); Peter Buitenhuis, *The Great War of Words: Literature as Propaganda, 1914–18 and After* (London: B. T. Batsford, 1989 [1987]): 10–12; Trudi Tate, *Modernism, History and the First World War* (Manchester: Manchester University Press, 1998): 41–63; Alan Kramer, *Dynamic of Destruction: Culture and Mass Killing in the First World War* (Oxford: Oxford University Press, 2007).

3 Elsie Inglis, 'The Tragedy of Serbia', *The Englishwoman*, 30 (1916): 166; Lady Leila Paget, *With Our Serbian Allies* (printed for private circulation, 1916), 34602, Imperial War Museum, London; Leah Leneman, *In the Service of Life: The Story of Elsie Inglis and the Scottish Women's Hospitals* (Edinburgh: Mercat Press, 1994). On the work of the Scottish Women's Hospitals, see also: Jane McDermid, 'What's in a Name? The Scottish Women's Hospitals in the First World War', *Minerva: Women and War*, 1.1 (2007): 102–14; Costel Coroban, 'The Scottish Women's Hospitals in Romania during World War I', *Valahian Journal of Historical Studies*, 14 (2010): 53–68. On the fate of those units that remained in Serbia, see: Angela K. Smith, ' "Beacons of Britishness": British Nurses and Female Doctors as Prisoners of War', in Alison S. Fell and Christine E. Hallett (eds), *First World War Nursing: New Perspectives* (London: Routledge, 2013): 35–50.

4 Millicent, Duchess of Sutherland, *Six Weeks at the War* (London: The Times, 1914).

5 Millicent, Duchess of Sutherland, *Six Weeks at the War*, xiii.

6 Millicent, Duchess of Sutherland, *Six Weeks at the War*, xiii–xiv.

7 Denis Stuart, *Dear Duchess: Millicent Duchess of Sutherland (1867–1955)* (Newton Abbot: David and Charles, 1982).

8 Millicent, Duchess of Sutherland, *Six Weeks at the War*: 10. On Depage see also: Baroness de T'Serclaes, *Flanders and Other Fields* (London: George G. Harrap, 1964): 69–79.

9 T'Serclaes, *Flanders and Other Fields*: 36, 70. There were numerous similarly 'freelance' expeditions to France. See, for example: Dorothy Cator, *In a French Military Hospital* (New York: Longmans, Green, 1915). See also: Christine E. Hallett, *Veiled Warriors: Allied Nurses of the First World War* (Oxford: Oxford University Press, 2014): Chapter 1.

10 Paul Fussell, *The Great War and Modern Memory* (Oxford: Oxford University Press, 2000 [1975]): 19.

11 Margaret Darrow, 'French Volunteer Nursing and the Myth of War Experience in World War I', *American Historical Review*, 101.1 (1996): 80–106; Margaret Darrow, *French Women and the First World War: War Stories from the Home*

Front (New York: Berg, 2000); Katrin Schultheiss, *Bodies and Souls: Politics and the Professionalization of Nursing in France, 1880–1922* (Cambridge, MA: Harvard University Press, 2001).

12 See, for example: T'Serclaes, *Flanders and Other Fields*: 36; Anon., *A War Nurse's Diary: Sketches from a Belgian Field Hospital* (New York: Macmillan, 1918): 1–54; Sarah Macnaughtan, *A Woman's Diary of the War* (London: Thomas Nelson and Sons, 1915): *passim*.

13 Janet Lee, *War Girls: The First Aid Nursing Yeomanry in the First World War* (Manchester: Manchester University Press, 2005).

14 Millicent, Duchess of Sutherland, *Six Weeks at the War*: 21.

15 Millicent, Duchess of Sutherland, *Six Weeks at the War*: 26–8.

16 Millicent, Duchess of Sutherland, *Six Weeks at the War*: 27–8.

17 Millicent, Duchess of Sutherland, *Six Weeks at the War*: 37–8.

18 See also, for example: Violetta Thurstan, *Field Hospital and Flying Column: Being the Journal of an English Nursing Sister in Belgium and Russia* (London: G. P. Putnam's Sons, 1915); Anon., *A War Nurse's Diary*; Helen Dore Boylston, '*Sister*': *The War Diary of a Nurse* (New York: Ives Washburn, 1927).

19 Millicent, Duchess of Sutherland, *Six Weeks at the War*: 78–106.

20 Laurence Binyon, *For Dauntless France: An Account of Britain's Aid to the French Wounded and Victims of the War. Compiled for the British Red Cross Societies and the British Committee of the Red Cross* (London: Hodder and Stoughton, 1918): 48.

21 Natasha McEnroe and Tig Thomas, *The Hospital in the Oatfield* (London: Florence Nightingale Museum, 2014): *passim*.

22 Stuart, *Dear Duchess*: *passim*.

23 Anon., *A War Nurse's Diary*: 3.

24 Anon., *A War Nurse's Diary*: 4.

25 Anon., *A War Nurse's Diary*: 4–5. It may be that this nurse was a part of the unit that was led by Mabel St Clair Stobart, who was to prove herself an able commander and hospital director.

26 Anon., *A War Nurse's Diary*: 19.

27 Anon., *A War Nurse's Diary*: 20.

28 Anon., *A War Nurse's Diary*: 21–2.

29 Anon., *A War Nurse's Diary*: 28–9.

30 T'Serclaes, *Flanders and Other Fields*; Diane Atkinson, *Elsie and Mairi Go to War: Two Extraordinary Women on the Western Front* (London: Preface Publishing, 2009): 39–64.

31 Atkinson, *Elsie and Mairi Go to War*: 1; T'Serclaes, *Flanders and Other Fields*: 36–8.

32 T'Serclaes, *Flanders and Other Fields*: 37.

33 Dorothie Fielding, *Lady under Fire: The Wartime Letters of Lady Dorothie Fielding M.M., 1914–1917*, ed. Andrew Hallam and Nicola Hallam (Barnsley:

Pen and Sword Books, 2010); Macnaughtan, *A Woman's Diary of the War*; Anon., *A War Nurse's Diary*: 54–5; T'Serclaes, *Flanders and Other Fields*: 37.

34 T'Serclaes, *Flanders and Other Fields*: 41.

35 T'Serclaes, *Flanders and Other Fields*: 52–3.

36 Anon., *A War Nurse's Diary*: 67.

37 Binyon, *For Dauntless France*: 46–7.

38 Angela Smith, *The Second Battlefield: Women, Modernism and the First World War* (Manchester: Manchester University Press, 2000): 54.

39 Flora Sandes, *An English Woman-Sergeant in the Serbian Army* (London: Hodder and Stoughton, 1916): 8–9. See also: Flora Sandes, *The Autobiography of a Woman Soldier: A Brief Record of Adventure with the Serbian Army, 1916–1919* (New York: Frederick A. Stokes, n.d.).

40 On the novels of Bessie Marchant, see: Michelle Smith, 'Adventurous Girls of the British Empire: The Pre-War Novels of Bessie Marchant', *The Lion and the Unicorn*, 33.1 (2009): 1–25.

41 Sandes, *An English Woman-Sergeant*: 19–21.

42 Smith, *The Second Battlefield*: 55–6.

43 Mabel St Clair Stobart, *The Flaming Sword in Serbia and Elsewhere* (London: Hodder and Stoughton, 1916): *passim*.

44 Stobart, *Flaming Sword*: 1–4.

45 Stobart, *Flaming Sword*: 1–4. On Mabel St Clair Stobart, see: Angela Smith, 'The Woman who Dared: Major Mabel St Clair Stobart', in Alison S. Fell and Ingrid Sharp (eds), *The Women's Movement in Wartime: International Perspectives 1914–1918* (Basingstoke: Palgrave, 2007): 158–74.

46 On the formation of the WSWCC, see: Smith, *The Second Battlefield*: 50.

47 Stobart's unit travelled to Belgium under the auspices of the St John's Ambulance Association: Stobart, *Flaming Sword*: 5.

48 Stobart, *Flaming Sword*: 123–288. On the journeys made by the WSWCC and other Serbian units, see: Hallett, *Veiled Warriors*: Chapter 3.

49 Mark Bostridge, *Florence Nightingale: The Woman and Her Legend* (London: Viking, 2008): 251–4.

50 Angela Smith has commented on how significant this image was in conveying 'an inversion of expected gender roles': Smith, *The Second Battlefield*: 64–5.

51 Stobart, *Flaming Sword*. The account of the unit's journey across the Albanian Alps is between pp. 153 and 292.

52 Stobart, *Flaming Sword*: 313–14.

53 Catherine Marshall, *Militarism versus Feminism* (London: Virago, 1987 [1915]): *passim*.

54 E. Sylvia Pankhurst, *The Home Front* (London: Hutchinson, 1987 [1932]): *passim*.

55 Olive M. Aldridge, *The Retreat from Serbia through Montenegro and Albania* (London: Minerva, 1916): *passim*.

56 Ellen Chivers Davies, *A Farmer in Serbia* (London: Methuen, n.d.): 121.

57 Anon., Column, *BJN* (8 January 1916): 29.
58 Macnaughtan, *A Woman's Diary of the War*: 41.
59 Sarah Macnaughtan, *My War Experiences in Two Continents*, ed. Mrs Lionel Salmon [Betty Keays-Young] (London: John Murray, 1919).
60 Macnaughtan, *A Woman's Diary of the War*: 52.
61 Macnaughtan, *A Woman's Diary of the War*: 163.
62 Macnaughtan, *My War Experiences*: 256.
63 Macnaughtan, *My War Experiences*: 256–7 (italics as in the original).
64 Macnaughtan, *My War Experiences*: conclusion.
65 Smith, *The Second Battlefield*: 54.

2

Le petit paradis des blessés

Introduction: the little paradise

The majority of British and North American women who cared for the war's wounded were posted to official army medical units. Yet, volunteer hospitals played a significant role in the military medical efforts of all allied nations.[1] 'L'Hôpital Chirurgical Mobile No. 1' was one of the most unusual military hospitals of modern times. The unit – one of the closest to the front lines near Ypres – was donated to the French Service de Santé by American millionaire philanthropist Mary Borden Turner,[2] an enigmatic woman, known by those who read the *British Journal of Nursing* as 'Mrs Turner'; by her own nurses as 'La Directrice'; and, later, by all, as 'Lady Spears'. The name she used as author of her many books was simply her maiden name: 'Mary Borden'.[3] Her hospital, which came to be known amongst the French as 'le petit paradis des blessés', was the result of a remarkable feat of persuasion: she met directly with General Joffre in the spring of 1915 and convinced him that, even though she had worked as a volunteer nurse for only a few months and had no previous nursing training or experience, she was capable of creating and directing a front-line hospital. She opened L'Hôpital Chirurgical Mobile No. 1 – a hutted encampment of about 160 beds – in July 1915, in the small Belgian town of Rousbrugge.[4] Throughout the war, she clung resolutely to the right to direct her hospital, even after such independent, voluntary establishments had been effectively outlawed by the allied military medical services. She also insisted on retaining the right to appoint all of her unit's nurses, many of whom were fully trained British, American, Australian, and Canadian professionals. The hospital's doctors and orderlies operated under the auspices of the French military medical services, but its day-to-day running remained in Borden's own hands.

During the Somme campaign, Borden established a new, much larger hospital at Bray-sur-Somme,[5] but L'Hôpital Chirurgical Mobile No. 1 remained in Belgium, moving two or three times when it came under heavy shelling.[6] In April 1917, Borden established a third hospital behind the Chemin des Dames, to support the Nivelle offensive.[7]

Narratives of L'Hôpital Chirurgical Mobile No. 1

The staffing of L'Hôpital Chirurgical Mobile No. 1 was made possible, in part, by the efforts of Grace Ellison, founder of the 'French Flag Nursing Corps' (FFNC).[8] Ellison had obtained some of her schooling in France, and felt, by her own account, a 'deep love' for the country. Just after the Battle of the Marne she travelled there to offer her services as a 'very willing but amateur nurse'.[9] She quickly realised that France had very few fully qualified professional nurses. Although some care was offered by highly trained and experienced nuns and a small cadre of professional nurses, most was in the hands of untrained orderlies and 'volunteer-ladies'. The work of the latter was coordinated by the French Red Cross, which was a more significant force than its sister-organization across the English Channel.[10] Some French volunteer nurses had passed a series of technical examinations and held the title 'infirmière-major', but most, in the words of Ellison, 'had as diplomas their good intentions only'.[11]

Ellison's response to the shortage of fully trained nurses in France was to offer the French minister of war 'a little army of fully trained British nurses',[12] who might be deployed in French military hospitals to fill the gaps in the existing provision. This and other opportunities for British nurses to travel to France and work close to the front lines coincided with a failure of the British military medical services to make full use of their professional skills and knowledge. Anne Summers has pointed out that, in the decades prior to the First World War, the QAIMNS – whilst fully recognised as an elite nursing corps – had remained small, with the bulk of potential military nurses forming its 'Reserve' or belonging to the Territorial Force Nursing

Service.[13] Although these existing services were rapidly mobilised in August 1914, the British army was slow to make full use of the large numbers of other fully trained nurses who came forward to offer their services to the war effort. In fact, the tendency for the British army to allow untrained volunteers of high social status to establish their own hospitals in Belgium and northern France angered members of the nursing profession, and led many to offer their services to organisations such as the FFNC.[14]

Keen to be close to the front lines, to make use of their skills, and to be part of a great enterprise that they believed would soon be over, trained British nurses travelled to France and Belgium with a number of organisations operating under the auspices either of the Red Cross or of overseas military medical services. 'A curious crowd they were', commented Ellison, 'all suffering from war fever'.[15] Many of those who applied to the FFNC did not hold certificates of training, and Ellison sought the services of campaigner for state registration Ethel Gordon Fenwick to assist in the selection of only the most fully trained.[16] No volunteer nurses were admitted to the ranks of the FFNC. Ellison remarked with pride that 'they were all highly qualified women with the real pioneer spirit'.[17] The FFNC supplied more than half the nurses to L'Hôpital Chirurgical Mobile No 1,[18] the remainder being carefully selected from the ranks of those French nurses who had some form of recognised training. Their work was supported by French male orderlies.

Much has been written about L'Hôpital Chirurgical Mobile No. 1, most of it fragmentary and vague.[19] Much can be unearthed by the diligent researcher, yet, even when carefully pieced together, the fragments provide only a half-formed image, full of lacunae, half-truths, and highly interpreted narratives. The historical record, although fairly voluminous, thus leaves the frustrated researcher with an insoluble puzzle. At least three published memoirs of women's wartime nursing experiences are reminiscences of L'Hôpital Chirurgical Mobile No. 1, and a fourth text appears to be a disguised account of the same hospital, in which names and details have been deliberately changed.

Mary Borden's *The Forbidden Zone* offers a series of vivid narratives.[20] Highly allegorical and infused with its author's powerful sense of spirituality, Borden's text offers the reader 'fragments of a great

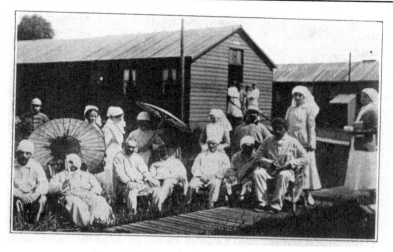

Figure 2 L'Hôpital Chirurgical Mobile No. 1

confusion'.[21] Written in a very similar style and yet with an entirely different tone, Ellen La Motte's *The Backwash of War* is shocking in its clarity and simplicity, horrifyingly successful in penetrating the reader's consciousness with its author's dark and disturbing vision of the war.[22] Totally different from either of these is the writing of Canadian nurse Agnes Warner, who became Borden's 'Head Nurse' at Rousbrugge, and continued to direct the nursing care there following Borden's departure for Bray-sur-Somme in September 1916. Her letters home to her mother and sisters, published in New Brunswick without her knowledge as *My Beloved Poilus*, offer a homely and sympathetic perspective on the heroism of the hospital's French patients – patients about whom Borden is pitying and La Motte scathing.[23]

A fourth text, although it never states which hospital it relates to, appears to be an account of L'Hôpital Chirurgical Mobile No. 1. *A Green Tent in Flanders*, authored by American volunteer nurse Maud Mortimer, describes a field hospital located in Belgium, donated to the French by its American 'Directress', who is an 'artist'. A number of vivid and colourful characters work at this hospital, among whom are a cynical nurse writer collecting material for a book, and a deeply compassionate and highly experienced Canadian nurse.[24]

One of the most intriguing images in these texts is the metaphor of the First World War as a vast sea, from which the wounded are washed up. Mary Borden's patients are 'lost men, wrecked men, survivors from that other world that was here before the flood passed this way, washed up against the shore of this world again by the great backwash'.[25] For Maud Mortimer, the waves of the war's ocean crash against a shore close to the hospital, and the patients are the 'spindrift of [a] shattered endeavour'.[26] For both writers, the war is filled with heroic effort. La Motte too conveys a watery metaphor; but hers carries a totally different meaning. In her introduction, she writes that: 'There are many little lives foaming up in the backwash. They are loosened by the sweeping current, and float to the surface, detached from their environment, and one glimpses them, weak, hideous, repellent.'[27] For La Motte, the sea of war is a turgid and relentless one, and the patients in the field hospital are the tiny, helpless, and essentially ugly life-forms that are disturbed by its movement.

In this chapter, the writings of Borden and Warner will be examined closely. Each was a significant figure within the hospital: Borden was its 'Directrice', Warner her 'Head Nurse'. But where Borden wore her authority with an air of glamour, Warner cloaked her more authentic clinical and professional leadership in a homely and dutiful demeanour.

Mary Borden's *Forbidden Zone*

In one sense, Mary Borden could be said to have been a chameleon. Changing not only her appearance, clothing, and manner, but apparently her entire personality, to fit into a range of backgrounds, she excelled as society hostess, successful novelist, and 'Directrice' of a French field hospital. Yet, this capacity for moulding her talents did not mean that, chameleon-like, she blended into the background. In her own writings, she refers to a French First World War nurse (possibly reflecting on her own appearance) as a 'white peacock', and it was, perhaps, her capacity for standing out from a crowd, exciting attention, and forming a striking impression on the mind that was her strongest characteristic. Born into a wealthy Chicago family, Borden enjoyed an expensive boarding-school education; married first a missionary and then a British staff officer; and moved in literary circles, enjoying relationships with members of the intelligentsia, such as Ford Madox Ford and Percy Wyndham Lewis. The extraordinary qualities of her writing owe much to her range of experiences and acquaintances.[28]

Born on 15 May 1886, Borden was one of four surviving siblings, and spent much of her time accompanying her brothers on expeditions, fishing trips, and games with other boys. Although something of a tomboy, she was also said to have been feminine in appearance and behaviour, and was reputed to have been a 'stylish and original dresser'.[29] The family home was a large house in a fashionable area by the shore of Lake Michigan. Her mother was devoutly Christian, and underwent an 'evangelical' conversion in the 1890s – an event that had a profound influence on the entire Borden household.[30] Borden's education, first at Rye Seminary on Long Island and then at the prestigious Vassar College, nurtured her desire to be a writer and offered her both the classical education and the training in self-possession and independence of mind that would support her work.[31]

On her father's death in 1906, she inherited a share of his fortune. When she graduated from Vassar in 1907, she was persuaded by her mother to use some of her wealth to travel the world, visiting Christian mission stations. In Lahore she met Douglas Turner, the man who would become her first husband. Engaged to him within a week of their first meeting, she appears to have had doubts about the relationship, but married him in Lausanne, on 28 August 1908.[32] Moving to London in 1913, Borden began to publish novels under the pseudonym Bridget Maclagan, and became closely involved in the suffragette movement – even to the point of being arrested in the autumn of that year for throwing a stone at a window of the Treasury building in Whitehall.[33]

Borden's life in London consisted of lavish parties and the writing of novels about her experience in India. These pre-war novels set the trend for her writing, which always closely mirrored her own experiences. It was said that she was 'using her inheritance to buy her way into the London literary scene', and that her parties and soirées were among the most lavish and entertaining in the capital.[34]

When Britain entered the First World War in August 1914, Borden was pregnant with her third daughter, Mary. She volunteered her services to the London Committee of the French Red Cross, and, soon after Mary's birth, travelled to Malo-les-Bains near Dunkirk to nurse typhoid patients. Her first posting was to a makeshift hospital in a converted casino and she was appalled by its lack of equipment and trained staff. She herself had undergone no formal nurse training at all and was obliged to learn from better experienced British colleagues and from her own mistakes.[35] As she gained experience, she became openly critical of the poor care received by the casino's patients. Eventually, she decided to write to General Joseph Joffre, Commander in Chief of the French forces, offering to fund, staff, and run her own field hospital.[36] This audacious move resulted in the establishment of L'Hôpital Chirurgical Mobile No. 1, on the road from Dunkirk to Ypres, just seven miles behind the front-line trenches. Doctors, transport, and supplies were provided by the French military medical services, but nursing staff and running costs were funded by Borden herself.[37] Joffre permitted her to exercise complete control over the nursing work of the hospital, as its 'Directrice'.[38]

Borden's earliest unit served the Thirty-Sixth Corps of the French Eighth Army and was composed of long wooden huts that acted as hospital wards, each with twenty beds. One was set up as an operating theatre, with X-ray and dressing rooms; another was a kitchen and store. There was also a 'reception hut', to which wounded men were brought from ambulances to be triaged. Here, decisions were made about how urgent each case was, and from here patients were sent either straight to the operating theatre; to X-ray; to a ward to await treatment; or, for the worst cases, to the moribund ward where only palliative care was given. Borden spend much of her time in the reception hut during the great 'rushes' of casualties that followed unsuccessful assaults on the Western Front. The model of this first reception hut was copied at L'Hôpital d'Evacuation on the Somme Front in 1916, about which Borden wrote one of her most vivid short essays, 'Blind'.[39] Borden's belief that she had acquired expert clinical observational skills is made clear by this text, in which she explains, in highly poetic terms, the ways in which she assessed her patients and made decisions about their treatment needs.[40] She also dwells on the joy she felt in knowing that her field hospital had the lowest mortality rate on the French Front. In its first six months, L'Hôpital d'Evacuation treated over 800 cases, with only 68 deaths.[41]

Borden moved her children and household from London to 21 Bois de Boulogne in Paris.[42] She appears to have held evening parties here. Although wartime stringency meant that these in no way resembled the lavish soirées she had held in pre-war London, it was noted by writer Gertrude Stein that Borden's house was one of the few where there was enough fuel to keep warm during the terrible winter of 1915.[43] It is not clear how well Borden and Stein knew each other, but references in Stein's *Autobiography of Alice Toklas* suggest that they were fairly close acquaintances, and that Borden visited Stein's salon at the rue de Fleurus on several occasions.[44] It may have been here that Borden met writer Ellen La Motte, although it is also possible that Stein, Borden, and La Motte already knew each other; all had attended Vassar College at the turn of the century.

Borden's second unit – on the Somme Front – was offered to the French Service de Santé in the autumn of 1916, when it became clear that the fiercest fighting was taking place far to the south of Rousbrugge. By this time, the French military medical services had taken a decision to staff their hospitals only with French nurses, and Borden had great difficulty in persuading the authorities to permit her to establish her second unit, L'Hôpital d'Evacuation, five kilometres behind the front-line trenches, at Bray-sur-Somme.[45]

At L'Hôpital d'Evacuation, Borden had only 12 nurses for 2,000 patients, and was forced to use these to staff wards reserved for the most seriously wounded. The hospital was heavily dependent on the work of orderlies.[46] It was whilst running L'Hôpital d'Evacuation that Borden met Captain Edward Louis Spears, a liaison officer with the British Expeditionary Force. From the spring of 1917 they were exchanging frequent letters, which show that they had embarked on a passionate and secret love affair.[47]

At the beginning of 1917, Borden's medical team was moved to Villers-sur-Condon, between Soissons and Rheims, in preparation for the Aisne campaign. Here, during the Nivelle offensive, her hospital was damaged by shell-fire. Soon after this, she returned to her original unit at Rousbrugge, which was, in turn, bombarded on 5 June. Several orderlies, one patient, and one nurse were wounded.[48] The next day, gas shells reached the hospital. Borden had already been awarded the Croix de Guerre in March, and now a 'palm' was added, and was conferred on her by General Pétain in person. A few days after this, she was rushed to hospital in Dunkirk – an event that is shrouded in secrecy, but appears to have been due to a miscarriage. A long period of ill health followed, which was complicated by severe pneumonia. Borden attempted to continue working but was obliged to take frequent breaks to rest and convalesce. In February 1918, she suffered another miscarriage.[49]

In the summer of 1917, Borden published some short journal articles; these were later incorporated into her book *The Forbidden Zone*.[50] In August, she submitted the full manuscript to Collins, but was instructed by the censor to edit the work, and decided not to go ahead with publication.[51] During this time, her life was extremely turbulent. Not only was she involved in the running of her field hospitals, and attempting to get her work published; she was also suing her husband for divorce. Proceedings began on 18 December 1917, but led to a prolonged and bitter battle over the custody of the couple's three daughters.[52]

During 1917 Borden's writing for *The Forbidden Zone* began to take clearer shape. Although the book recounts experiences from both Rousbrugge and Bray-sur-Somme, it is clear that some of the metaphors adopted in the section of the book entitled 'The North' were being developed during Borden's time on the Somme. One in particular offers a complex metaphorical representation of pain as a demonic lover. She also describes pain as a harlot who is 'holding the damp greenish bodies of the gangrene cases in her arms'.[53] The nurse, in the face of such suffering, loses her humanity and her womanhood and becomes 'really dead, past resurrection'.[54] At around the time she was writing these vignettes, Borden enclosed a poem in a letter to Edward Spears, in which a different metaphor is developed – this time pain is a powerful and overwhelming male lover, who claims her as his mistress:

> Leave me to this hungry lust
> Of monstrous pain. I am his mistress now
> These are the frantic beds of his delight
> Here I succumb to him, anew, each night.[55]

Borden and Spears married at the British consulate in Paris on 30 March 1918, just days after the commencement of the German offensive.[56] Following the allied victory, the couple continued to live in Paris, keeping 'open house' during the Peace Conference; and

Borden gave birth to a son, Michael, on 2 March 1921.[57] Throughout the 1920s, Borden pursued her writing career, publishing a succession of novels.[58]

Mary Borden was a significant female modernist whose work offered a profound insight into the realities of the First World War.[59] She wrote obsessively, and Jane Conway has attributed to her the statement that writing a book was like having 'an attack of typhoid fever with headaches and fits of depression'.[60] Among her books none is more extraordinary than her semi-fictionalised account of her work at Rousbrugge and Bray-sur-Somme. Having been obliged to shelve *The Forbidden Zone* in 1917, Borden returned to it at the end of the 1920s – probably for financial reasons,[61] believing that it would match the public mood that was receiving books such as Erich Maria Remarque's *All Quiet on the Western Front*, and Ernest Hemingway's *A Farewell to Arms*, with acclaim.[62] Her confidence was somewhat misplaced; many critics were shocked that a woman should write so frankly about the realities of war.[63]

Borden's main purpose appears to have been to expose the spiritual truths that lay behind the horrors of war. This is not, however, to deny the obviously pacifist intentions of her work. The vignettes she offers are clearly intended also to illustrate the debasing qualities of warfare and the damage it inflicts on human beings. Perhaps one of the best-known excerpts from her book is one in which she depicts the hospital as a laundry where men, like packages of clothes, are processed and returned to the front:

> You say that these bundles are the citizens of the town? What do you mean? Those heavy brown packages that are carried back and forth, up and down, from shed to shed, those inert lumps cannot be men. They are delivered to this place in closed vans and are unloaded like sacks and are laid out in rows on the ground and are sorted out by the labels pinned to their covers. They lie perfectly still while they are carried back and forth, up and down, shoved into sheds and pulled out again. What do you mean by telling me that they are men?[64]

Borden adopts a subtly erotic tone as she writes of how the medical staff 'conspire' against a patient's 'right to die'.[65] His purpose has not yet been fulfilled. He must be repaired and sent back to the front line, where he can still be of use against the enemy. He is a passive victim into whose 'innocent wounds' the nurses and doctors stare. The final insult comes when the medical staff 'dig into the yawning mouths of his wounds. Helpless openings, they let us into the secret places of his body. To the shame of the havoc of his limbs we add the insult of our curiosity and the curse of our purpose, the purpose to remake him.'[66] The scenario is not only reminiscent of rape – full of what Trudi Tate refers to as 'eroticised horror'[67] – it is also an affront against humanity 'en masse': the repair of one small element of a larger war machine, the purpose of which is not to restore a human being but, rather, to remake a component. What is most disturbing is the patients' gratitude: 'When we hurt them they try not to cry out, not wishing to hurt our feelings. And often they apologise for dying.'[68]

Hazel Hutchison has commented on how 'profoundly troubled' Borden was by the 'ironies of nursing in wartime'.[69] These feelings are brought out clearly in writing that is ironic in tone – mocking the ignorance of those who have remained safely at home, away from the realities of the battlefield. Borden possessed remarkable capacity for portraying trauma, in both its physical and its emotional guises.[70] And yet she was also exhilarated by war service. In the reception hut of her field hospital on the Somme, her hospital 'throbbed and hummed … like a dynamo' and her emotions were fired by 'a sense of great power, exhilaration and excitement'.[71] Her work is a powerful depiction of what Santanu Das refers to as 'the precipice between the exhilaration of service and the trauma of witnessing'.[72]

Soon after publishing *The Forbidden Zone*, Borden returned to novel-writing.[73] As always, she poured her personal experience, feelings, and opinions into her writing and, as always, her books provoked controversy. A further book, designed to promote and support a greater emotional and sexual freedom for women, *The Technique of Marriage*, was published in 1933.[74]

At the outbreak of the Second World War, Borden was approached by Lady Hadfield to run a mobile field hospital. The so-called 'Hadfield–Spears Unit' served in North Africa, winning both official recognition and public acclaim.[75] After her experiences of desert war, Borden, by this time over fifty, returned home to England, where she continued writing both fiction and semi-fictionalised autobiographical work.[76]

Mary Borden died on 2 December 1968 at the age of eighty-two.[77] She had experienced at first hand some of the most dramatic events of the twentieth century and had engaged deeply and personally with one of the most revolutionary social and cultural trends of her time: the emancipation of women. She had claimed the right to perform the work she considered important, divorced her first husband, and fought for custody of her children. In her writings – as in her actions – she claimed a freedom that must, at times, have created discomfort and distress for those around her, yet she won the respect and admiration of many who knew her. Mary Borden seems to have wanted to be a woman of truth rather than compromise, and her truth can be read most forcibly through her astounding record of two of her First World War field hospitals. *The Forbidden Zone* confronts its readers with some of the most shocking realities of war.

Agnes Warner: devoted professional

In the winter of 1915/16 there were four Canadian nurses at L'Hôpital Chirurgical Mobile No. 1. Three were Army Nursing Sisters, who had been placed with the hospital by the FFNC. The other was a former probationer of the New York Presbyterian Hospital, who had travelled to France as a private nurse and become involved in the French war effort. This fourth nurse, Agnes Warner, is still remembered in the twenty-first century in her home town of Saint John, New Brunswick. She was, in the second decade of the twentieth century, one of its most celebrated daughters.[78] The town's small library and archive has a file on her, and local historians incorporate her story into their guides. Daughter of a famous father, Warner won the respect and admiration of her own contemporaries, largely because of the way in which her wartime work (which was actually not so different from the work of thousands of other nurses) was celebrated in the local press as a succession of 'deeds' and 'exploits'.[79]

Agnes Warner's father, Darius, had been a general in the Union Army during the American Civil War. Having been seriously wounded, he retired from military service and was made American Consul to the strategically important Canadian town of Saint John.[80] He won the respect of the townspeople for his authoritative and compassionate handling of the great fire of 1877,[81] and it is quite possible that his second daughter, Agnes, was drawn to nursing, and ultimately to the nursing of wounded soldiers, by her upbringing in a

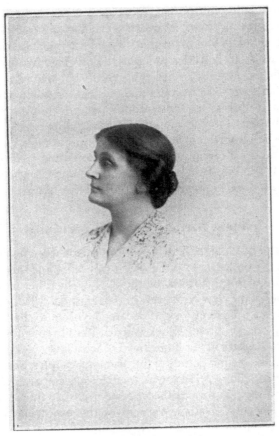

Figure 3 Portrait of Agnes Warner

family in which public service was highly valued, and where doing 'great deeds' was something to be lived out rather than read about in novels.[82] As she lived her own 'great adventure', she wrote letters home describing her experiences and feelings as a Canadian-born, American-trained nurse caring for the French wounded, first in a temporary hospital in the Alsatian town of Divonne-les-Bains, and secondly at L'Hôpital Chirurgical Mobile No. 1 in Rousbrugge and at other locations in Belgium. Warner's letters home were collected by her mother and sisters, and passed, without her knowledge, to a local Saint John publisher, N. B. Barnes. *My Beloved Poilus*, a collection of these letters – offering tantalising glimpses of her life and work – was published in 1917, while she was still serving as head nurse at L'Hôpital Chirurgical Mobile No. 1.[83]

Warner's letters were widely read, highly celebrated, and, ultimately, were published because of the social circle in which she moved. As members of one of New Brunswick's most prominent families, she and her sisters attended parties and events organized by other upper-middle-class ladies of their own 'set', and joined one of the most prominent chapters of the influential 'Independent Order of the Daughters of the Empire', an elite patriotic society that flourished at the turn of the century and operated as a significant promoter of the Canadian war effort.[84] In Saint John alone, there were six chapters of the Daughters of the Empire; Warner's work gained particular financial and practical support from the Demonts Chapter. One local newspaper article, which reported on her wartime work, offered a somewhat hyperbolic account of the patriotic feeling with which the Order was infused: 'As broad as the empire upon which the sun never sets – as deep as the great oceans which girdle it – as high as the aspirations of the heroic sons who have laid down their lives in its defence stands the order of the Daughters of Empire.'[85]

Agnes Warner, unlike the other female members of her family, appears never to have intended to remain at home in Saint John. She attended McGill University, Montreal, graduating in natural sciences in 1894 and giving a valedictory lecture to her year group, in which she commented that 'the day was past when women were laughed at for their ignorance and yet denied the right of a good education.'[86] After graduating, in 1902, from the renowned New York Presbyterian Hospital School of Nursing, she became private nurse and companion to a wealthy, elderly Long Island couple, Mr and Mrs Roswell Eldridge, and spent much of the early part of the twentieth century travelling with them through Europe.[87] At the beginning of August, she was with her employers in the southern French spa town of Divonne-les-Bains. She wrote to her mother: 'August 2, 1914: the awful war we have all been dreading is upon us – *France is mobilizing* … We have started teaching the women and girls to make bandages, sponges, etc., for the hospital which will be needed here.'[88] On 23 August, she wrote of her admiration for the French people and of her decision to help in the Red Cross hospital that was being created.[89]

Warner travelled back to New York with the Eldridges and spent Christmas 1914 in Saint John with her family. She then returned to France, and spent a few months working at the American Ambulance in Paris.[90] This may have been where she met Mary Borden, and was invited to consider joining the ranks of L'Hôpital Chirurgical Mobile No 1.

On 19 February 1915, she was back again in Divonne-les-Bains, and was writing to her mother: 'I have thirteen patients, nine in bed all the time, and the others up part of the day. One of the women of the village helps me in the morning, two others help with the cleaning up and serving meals; everything has to be carried up three flights of stairs, so you can imagine the work.'[91] The workload was, indeed, onerous for a woman of Warner's age,[92] yet a close reading of her letters reveals how convinced she was of the justice of the allied cause and how deep and genuine was her desire to help the French people. On 25 April she commented: 'We have been very busy all week, new patients coming every day till now we have forty. Most of them are not wounded. Poor fellows, they are utterly done out; some have pneumonia, others rheumatism, one paralyzed and all sorts of other things.'[93]

In May, following another visit to Paris, Warner returned to find 'two new patients, one with a leg as big as an elephant and the other out of his head'.[94] Soon after this, in early June the French military authorities decided to enlarge the hospital, make it a semi-military institution of 400 beds, and invite Warner to take charge. Days later, she heard that Canadian troops had left Saint John – her own nephew among them – and expressed mixed feelings: patriotic pleasure that her countrymen were assisting the war effort; and fear at their likely fate.[95]

Within months, Warner was writing of her impending move to join L'Hôpital Chirurgical Mobile No. 1 in Belgium, expressing pleasure at the prospect of being so close to the firing line, and, in particular, 'nearer the Canadian boys'.[96] In September, she wrote:

Mobile No.1, France, 1915. I am really not in France but Belgium. I cannot tell you just where, but it is within ten miles of the firing line, and not far from the place where so many of our boys from home have been sent ... The first night I arrived I did not sleep, for the guns roared all night long, and we could see the flashes from the shells quite plainly; the whole sky was aglow. The French and English guns sounded like a continuous roar of thunder; but when the shells from the German guns landed on this side we could feel a distinct shock, and everything in our little shanty rattled ... There are about one hundred and fifty beds in all here.[97]

Life at L'Hôpital Chirurgical Mobile No. 1 was not easy. On 5 December, Warner was writing that: 'last night we had the most awful wind storm. I thought our little hut would be carried over into the German lines. It rained in torrents and the roof leaked, and I could not get my bed away from the drips, so I put up my umbrella.'[98] Later, in March 1916, she recounted: 'another awful storm ... wind and rain. Windows blew off and doors blew in, and one poor little night nurse was blown off the sidewalk and nearly lost in the mud.'[99]

Warner's phlegmatic indifference to discomfort seems to have been an integral part of her psyche. Stoicism and determined good cheer are typical of nurses who adopted a traditional style of writing.[100] In Warner's case, there can be little doubt that the positive gloss she places on her experiences – the sense that, really, the discomfort is all part of a 'great adventure' – is heavily influenced by the anticipated primary reader of her letters: her mother. During the war, many 'letters home' by both combatants and nurses were written in full recognition that they were likely to find their way into multiple hands and be read by a large circle of family and friends.[101] In the days before technology, the writing and reading of letters was seen as an aesthetic pleasure to be shared, and letters from war participants were particularly highly prized. Still, Warner probably never anticipated that letters intended for a close family audience would be published and distributed throughout her province. A clue to her feelings when she heard of their publication may be found in an unidentified newspaper clipping, dated 28 April 1917, which has been pasted into a fourth-edition copy of *My Beloved Poilus* and which quotes one of Warner's later letters:

It was awfully good to take so much trouble to have my stupid letters published and I am more than delighted to get the money for My Beloved Poilus (soldier) [sic] ... I must say it was an awful shock when I first received it, but if the people are interested, in spite of the appalling English, and it sells well, I must not mind. You know I did not even have time to read over my letters and they are rather a disgrace to a graduate of McGill.[102]

Warner's book attracted great attention in her own province of New Brunswick,[103] bringing not only funds from sales, but also donations of many kinds, ranging from 'yarn for French peasants to make into socks for the soldiers',[104] to boxes of surgical supplies.[105] Warner's hut at L'Hôpital Chirurgical Mobile No. 1 came to be known as the 'high class bazaar', as she amassed a range of useful objects for the hospital.[106]

It is easy for a modern readership, steeped in later perspectives on the futility of the First World War, to condemn the apparently propagandist nature of Warner's writing. The lectures and journalistic interviews she gave on her brief visit home in December 1914 clearly highlighted stories of German atrocities that had been circulating in France during the early months of the war, and offered a poignant image of the beleaguered heroism of the French people. Whether such outputs were deliberately intended to encourage young Canadian men to enlist is doubtful. It is more likely that Warner's passionate involvement with the French people compelled her to write and speak as she did.

In February, 1916 Warner commented:

> We are so busy here that we scarcely know where to turn. It is just a procession of wounded coming and going all the time, for we have to send them off as quickly as possible in order to make room for the new arrivals. Thirty-eight went off last Tuesday and fifteen on Friday, but the beds are filled up again. The last ones we have been getting are so badly wounded that I wonder who can be moved on Tuesday.[107]

On 20 March 1916, Warner commented that she had been left in charge of the field hospital, adding that supervising an entire staff composed of French, English, American, Canadian, and Australian nurses was making her nervous.[108] Later that summer, she announced that 'Mrs T is going to organize another hospital on the Somme and is going to keep this one as well', adding, 'She certainly has done a splendid work.'[109]

It was not only their patients who were delighted with the nurses at 'le petit paradis'. Their French doctor colleagues commented on the 'dedication' of these professional co-workers. Their letters were hungrily collected and avidly reported by Ethel Gordon Fenwick, editor of the *British Journal of Nursing* – a keen campaigner for nurses' professional status. In January 1917 a letter received by Grace Ellison was published in the journal:

> I cannot refrain from writing to thank you for the English nurses who have been sent here. From the technical point of view it would be impossible not to appreciate them, the only thing one can say is that, thoroughly understanding and loving their work as they do, they have been able to replace the doctor in so many ways ... And added to this, I have found in the Sisters a frank, simple gaiety which greatly helps towards recovery of the poor wounded.[110]

In April 1917, in a dramatic incident, the hospital was subjected to bombardment from the air, and one of its Canadian nurses, Madeleine Jaffray, was severely wounded. Both Jaffray, and colleague Hilda Gill, who came to her rescue, were awarded the Croix de Guerre, a decoration normally reserved for French combatants. As Jaffray recovered in a Belgian field hospital, she received a visit from Violetta Thurstan, matron at the nearby Hôpital de l'Océan, who reported back to Ethel Gordon Fenwick: 'I have just been to see your wounded French Flag Nurse, Miss Jaffray ... I am glad to say she is as well as can be expected and is suffering a good deal less today.'[111] Jaffray was, eventually, transferred to the American Ambulance in Paris, where bone-grafting surgery was performed on a wounded foot.[112] For their loyalty and fortitude during this air raid, all the nursing staff of the hospital received the French *Insigne*, an accolade that was also enthusiastically reported by the *British Journal of Nursing*.[113]

In the spring of 1918, during the rapid German advance, the hospital's position became even more hazardous, and – for their own safety – its nursing personnel were moved back to Forge-les-Eaux, well behind the lines. While there, Warner received a letter from a former surgeon colleague, now working close to the front without any nursing staff:

> We worked all night hoping some rest for the day after, but the arrivage [*sic*] was about 2,000 and every day like that during ten days. For five days Messr R. (chief surgeon) and I were alone. We asked for you the first day. No compresses, no towels for the operations, amputations or debridgements [*sic*]. Extractions of projectiles were made on the brancards (stretchers) often without an anaesthetic. How many poor chaps died without care! How many would not be dead if you had been here![114]

A small group of five nurses – Warner among them – campaigned to be posted back to the front lines with their hard-pressed medical colleagues. After several weeks of waiting and working at the American Ambulance in Paris, their request was granted and they were placed with Ambulance 16/21, a unit serving the Thirty-Sixth Corps of the French army.[115] As part of this unit, Warner and her colleagues followed the allied advance into the occupied zones. They established makeshift hospitals in tents, ruined chateaux, and schools, and cared for military casualties, former prisoners- of-war, and civilian patients. On one occasion, they salvaged a stove on which to do their cooking, only to find that it had been filled with hand grenades.[116] One of the nurses, in a letter to the *British Journal of Nursing*, commented on the plight of former prisoners: 'their condition is truly pitiful. Covered with vermin, just skin and bone. Their joy at being with us and having decent food to eat was enough to reduce one to tears.'[117] Ambulance 16/21 was said to have been one of the first hospital units to cross the Hindenburg Line and to follow the advancing allied armies into Germany.[118]

On 21 December 1918, four sisters of Ambulance 16/21 were decorated with the Croix de Guerre. Warner, who had already been awarded the Medaille des Epidémies and the Medaille d'Honneur en Bronze,[119] received the following citation:

> Miss Warner (Agnes Louise) Infirmière Major, Ambulance 16.21, has been in the 'formations sanitaires' of the French Armies for four years, where she is well known as a model of enduring energy, of disinterestedness and of devotion. Spent day and night attending to gassed and severely wounded cases, regardless of fatigue and bombardments. Has commanded the admiration of all.[120]

Agnes Warner returned to her home town of Saint John in March 1919 to a heroine's welcome.[121] Invited by every significant female institution in the town – from her former high school to the Women's Canadian Club – to give public lectures on her wartime experiences, Warner was feted and showered with flowers and gifts. She became, for a short time, a focal point for Saint John's outpouring of post-war patriotism; flags were displayed; national anthems played; and red, white, and blue bouquets presented.[122] And Warner embraced her role at the heart of this nationalist fervour. At one reception, given by the Royal Standard Chapter of the Daughters of Empire, she spoke of how 'she had seen her wounded Poilus suffer such unbelievable things with courage, fortitude, endurance and resignation in order that freedom and liberty might prevail'.[123] A *Daily Telegraph* reporter who heard her speak at a Canadian Club special luncheon believed that 'she must indeed have been an angel of mercy to the wounded', commenting on how 'many of her hearers were scarcely able to restrain their tears'.[124] Warner's lectures were infused with anti-German propaganda. One reporter who heard her 'address' at the Baptist Institute referred to 'the devlish cruelty of the Germans'.[125] The sincerity of this message and its heartfelt emotionalism were clearly its most powerful traits.

Agnes Warner died of breast cancer at the New York Presbyterian Hospital on 23 April 1926 at the age of fifty-four. A lengthy obituary in the *Saint John Globe* emphasised her war service and her medals and honours, quoting the citation for her Croix de Guerre: 'a fait l'admiration de tous'. It reads like so many outpourings of the early inter-war period, finding meaning in patriotic duty and service:

> Miss Warner, the quiet beauty of whose life and whose fine scholarship were in themselves notable contributions to the community in which she lived and to those with whom she was daily associated. Her name lives in France: her services are recorded in its military records and her story as told in My Beloved Poilu [sic] is among the French Archives. On the Roll of Honour [sic] in the Saint John High School, on that of McGill University and of the New York Presbyterian Hospital her name is among those that will live forever because she heard and always answered when and wherever duty called.[126]

Conclusion: the 'Directrice' and the head nurse

Although celebrated in her home town of Saint John and well known in her own time, Agnes Warner has not survived well in the historical record. Whilst much has been written about the wealthy philanthropist Mary Borden – founder of L'Hôpital Chirurgical Mobile No. 1 – less is known about the astute head nurse who kept her extraordinary hospital alive. Borden's memory survives because of the artistry of her own writing. Renowned as a literary modernist, her work has achieved scholarly acclaim.[127] Warner's simple letters to her mother delighted a parochial readership in her own time, but had little impact on a wider academic audience and failed to find a significant place in the historical record. In her *Journey down a Blind Alley*, Mary Borden referred fleetingly to 'frail Miss Warner with her eye-glasses and grey hair'[128] – a vague and passing mention of a woman to whom she probably owed much of her own wartime success. Such are the vagaries of the historical record.

Notes

1 For a list of volunteer units that formed part of the British Army Medical Establishment on the Western Front, see: Iain Gordon, *Lifeline: A British Casualty Clearing Station on the Western Front, 1918* (Stroud: History Press, 2013).

2 Mary Borden, *Journey down a Blind Alley* (London: Hutchinson, 1947 [1946]): 9; Margaret Higonnet, *Nurses at the Front: Writing the Wounds of the Great War* (Boston, MA: Northeastern University Press, 2001): x; Hazel Hutchison, 'The Theater of Pain: Observing Mary Borden in *The Forbidden Zone*', in Alison S. Fell and Christine E. Hallett (eds), *First World War Nursing: New Perspectives* (New York: Routledge, 2013): 139–55; Shawna Quinn, *Agnes Warner and the Nursing Sisters of the Great War* (Fredericton, NB: Goose Lane Editions with New Brunswick Military Heritage Project, 2010): 51.

3 Borden was a prolific writer. Her earliest novels had been written under the pseudonym Bridget Maclagan. See, for example: Bridget Maclagan, *The Mistress of Kingdoms; or, Smoking Flax: A Novel* (London: Duckworth, 1912); Bridget Maclagan, *Collision* (London: Duckworth, 1913); Mary Borden, *The Romantic Woman: By Bridget Maclagan – Mary Borden Turner* (London: Constable, 1924 [1916]); Mary Borden, *Jane – Our Stranger: A Novel* (London: William Heinemann, 1923).

4 Laurence Binyon, *For Dauntless France: An Account of Britain's Aid to the French Wounded and Victims of the War. Compiled for the British Red Cross Societies and the British Committee of the Red Cross* (London: Hodder and Stoughton, 1918): 156–7.

5 Borden, *Journey down a Blind Alley*: 9; Anon., 'Nursing and the War', *BJN* (30 September 1916): 269.

6 It appears that the hospital's first move was in April 1917, and that this took it closer to the French lines. Subsequent moves – as a result of direct hits by enemy shelling – took place later in 1917, and in 1918. Anon., Column, *BJN* (14 April 1917): 254; Anon., Column, *BJN* (6 April 1918): 241; Binyon, *For Dauntless France*: 156–7.

7 Borden, *Journey down a Blind Alley*: 9.

8 Grace Ellison, 'Nursing at the French Front', in Gilbert Stone (ed.), *Women War Workers: Accounts Contributed by Representative Workers of the Work Done by Women in the More Important Branches of War Employment* (London: George G. Harrap, 1917): 155–80.

9 Ellison, 'Nursing at the French Front': 162.

10 The French Red Cross was composed of three societies: the Société de Secours aux Blessés Militaires, the Union des Femmes de France, and the Association des Dames Françaises: Ellison, 'Nursing at the French Front': 159.

11 Ellison, 'Nursing at the French Front': 159–60.

12 Ellison, 'Nursing at the French Front': 162.

13 Anne Summers, *Angels and Citizens: British Women as Military Nurses, 1854–1914*, rev. edn (Newbury: Threshold Press, 2000).

14 Anon., 'Is It Just?', in 'Letters to the Editor', *BJN* (4 July 1914): 22; Anon., 'Letters to the Editor', *BJN* (19 December 1914): 497; Anon., 'The Nursing Outlook: War Fever and the War Spirit', *The Nursing Mirror and Midwives Journal* 19 (22 August 1914): 397. On the FFNC, see: Christine E. Hallett, *Veiled Warriors: Allied Nurses of the First World War* (Oxford: Oxford University Press, 2014): Chapter 1.

15 Ellison, 'Nursing at the French Front': 163.

16 Ethel Gordon Fenwick, as owner and editor of the *BJN*, used the columns of her journal to promote the work of the FFNC. A regular column on the work of the corps appeared throughout the war from 24 October 1914 onwards. For examples of references to the work of FFNC nurses at L'Hôpital Chirurgical Mobile No. 1, see: Anon., 'Nursing and the War' (30 September 1916); Anon., 'French Flag Nursing Corps', *BJN* (14 April 1917): 254; Anon., 'French Flag Nursing Corps', *BJN* (23 June 1917): 434; Anon., 'Decorations for Nurses', *BJN* (30 June 1917): 452; Anon., 'French Flag Nursing Corps', *BJN* (16 February 1918): 113.

17 Ellison, 'Nursing at the French Front': 164.

18 These included trained nurses from the British dominions, particularly Canada and Australia. American volunteers were also recruited – though not through the FFNC. On the recruitment of FFNC nurses to L'Hôpital Chirurgical Mobile No. 1, see: Anon., 'French Flag Nursing Corps', *BJN* (26 May 1917): 361, 362. Jane Conway reports that the hospital initially had seventeen staff, composed of nurses, doctors, and orderlies: Jane Conway, *Mary Borden: A Woman of Two Wars* (Chippenham: Munday Books, 2010): 47.

19 There is a description of the hospital (sixteen huts, composed of wards, a 'salle des entrées', a 'salle des opérations', a 'salle de pansements', kitchen, laundry, and linen room), in: Anon., 'Hôpital Mobile No. 1', *BJN* (16 September 1916): 232–3. For references to certain aspects of work at the hospital, see: Higonnet, *Nurses at the Front*: Introduction; Ariela Freedman, 'Mary Borden's *Forbidden Zone*: Women's Writing from No-Man's Land', *Modernism/Modernity*, 9.1 (2002), 109–24; Quinn, *Agnes Warner*.

20 Mary Borden, *The Forbidden Zone* (London: William Heinemann, 1929).

21 Borden, *The Forbidden Zone*: preface.

22 Ellen N. La Motte, *The Backwash of War: The Human Wreckage of the Battlefield as Witnessed by an American Hospital Nurse* (New York: G. P. Putnam's Sons and The Knickerbocker Press, 1916).

23 Anon., *My Beloved Poilus* (Saint John, NB: Barnes, 1917).

24 Maud Mortimer, *A Green Tent in Flanders* (New York: Doubleday, Page, 1918). On the 'Golden Godmother and Directress' of the hospital, see pp. 60 and 68; on the nursing staff, see pp. 67 and 69–71; on the cynical nurse writer she refers to as 'Organization', see pp. 156–8. One of the most compelling pieces of evidence for the likelihood that Mortimer's book refers to L'Hôpital Chirurgical Mobile No. 1 is her recounting of an incident in which the nurses of the hospital care for a young woman in the neighbouring village who has severe burns (pp. 199–210). The same incident is recounted by Agnes Warner in: Anon., *My Beloved Poilus*: 91. The details of the incident are remarkably similar, and both accounts place it towards the end of February 1916.

25 Borden, *The Forbidden Zone*: 115.

26 Mortimer, *A Green Tent in Flanders*: 198.

27 La Motte, *The Backwash of War*: vi.

28 Jane Conway suggests that Borden had an affair with Percy Wyndham Lewis in the spring of 1914, and it is likely that her own writing – particularly in *The Forbidden Zone* – was heavily influenced by Wyndham Lewis: Conway, *Mary Borden*: 32–6. Angela Smith locates Borden's writing with the 'post-war culture of despair' that characterised the modernists, particularly Wyndham Lewis: Angela Smith, *The Second Battlefield: Women, Modernism and the First World War* (Manchester: Manchester University Press, 2000): 84.

29 Conway, *Mary Borden*: 11.

30 In her early and largely biographical novel *The Romantic Woman*, Borden explores these early influences on her life: Borden, *The Romantic Woman*: 25–6.

31 Conway, *Mary Borden*: 15–22.

32 Conway, *Mary Borden*: 23–7.

33 Conway, *Mary Borden*: 29–30.

34 Conway, *Mary Borden*: 31. Conway is citing, though not directly quoting, E. M. Forster.

35 It may have been because of this experience that, when she later formed her own field hospital, she insisted that the nursing must be done only by fully trained nurses. On Borden's experience in the typhoid hospital, see: Conway, *Mary Borden*: 39–41.

36 Borden, *Journey down a Blind Alley*: 9.

37 Because a unit of the FFNC was based at Borden's field hospital, several articles in the *BJN* refer to it. See, for example: Anon., 'French Flag Nursing Corps', *BJN* (29 April 1916): 378; Anon., 'French Flag Nursing Corps', *BJN* (27 May 1916): 458; Anon., 'Hôpital Mobile No. 1'; Anon., Column, *BJN* (20

January 1917): 41; Anon., Column, *BJN* (14 April 1917); Anon., 'French Flag Nursing Corps' (26 May 1917): 361. See also: Conway, *Mary Borden*: 45.

38 Conway, *Mary Borden*: 41–2.
39 This essay was incorporated into Borden, *The Forbidden Zone*: 136–59.
40 Christine Hallett, *Containing Trauma: Nursing Work in the First World War* (Manchester: Manchester University Press, 2009): 28.
41 Conway, *Mary Borden*: 47.
42 Conway, *Mary Borden*: 43.
43 Gertrude Stein, *The Autobiography of Alice B. Toklas* (London: Penguin, 2001 [1933]): 185. See also: James R. Mellow, *Charmed Circle: Gertrude Stein and Company* (London: Phaidon Press, 1974).
44 Stein, *The Autobiography of Alice B. Toklas*: 185.
45 Anon., Column, *BJN* (30 September 1916): 269.
46 Conway, *Mary Borden*: 53–5.
47 On her meeting with Louis Spears, see: Borden, *Journey down a Blind Alley*: 9. See also: Conway, *Mary Borden*: 65.
48 See the report in *BJN*: Anon., 'Croix de Guerre for Sister Jaffray', *BJN* (16 June 1917): 416.
49 Conway, *Mary Borden*: 71–3, 89.
50 Several sections of the book appeared in *The English Review* in August 1917: Mary Borden-Turner, 'At the Somme', *The English Review* (August 1917): 97–102. On Mary Borden's writing in *The Forbidden Zone*, see: Hutchison, 'The Theater of Pain'; Margaret Higonnet, 'Cubist Vision in Nursing Accounts', in Fell and Hallett, *First World War Nursing*: 156–72.
51 Conway, *Mary Borden*: 77.
52 Conway, *Mary Borden*: 80–8, 102.
53 Borden, *The Forbidden Zone*: 59.
54 Borden, *The Forbidden Zone*: 59.
55 Mary Borden, letter to Edward Spears, Churchill Archives, Churchill College, Cambridge, SPRS files 1–3, SPRS 11/1/1.
56 Anon., Column, *BJN* (6 April 1918): 241.
57 Conway, *Mary Borden*: 94, 104.
58 Mary Borden, *Jericho Sands: A Novel* (London: William Heinemann, 1925); *Four O'Clock and Other Stories* (London: William Heinemann, 1926); *Flamingo; or, The American Tower* (London: William Heinemann, 1927); *Jehovah's Day* (London: William Heinemann, 1928); *The Woman with White Eyes* (London: William Heinemann, 1930); *Action for Slander: A Novel* (London: William Heinemann, 1936); *The Black Virgin: A Novel* (London: William Heinemann, 1937); *Passport for a Girl* (London: William Heinemann, 1939).
59 Smith, *The Second Battlefield*; Higonnet, *Nurses at the Front*; Margaret Higonnet, 'Authenticity and Art in Trauma Narratives of World War I', *Modernism/Modernity*, 9.1 (2002): 91–107; Freedman, 'Mary Borden's *Forbidden Zone*'.

60 Conway, *Mary Borden*: 140.

61 Conway, *Mary Borden*: 149–50.

62 Erich Maria Remarque, *All Quiet on the Western Front*, trans. Brian Murdoch (London: Vintage, 1996 [1929]); Ernest Hemingway, *A Farewell to Arms* (London: Arrow, 1994 [1929]).

63 Laurie Kaplan, 'Deformities of the Great War: The Narratives of Mary Borden and Helen Zenna Smith', *Women and Language*, 27.2 (2004): 35–43.

64 Borden, *The Forbidden Zone*: 114.

65 Borden, *The Forbidden Zone*: 119.

66 Borden, *The Forbidden Zone*: 120.

67 Trudi Tate, *Modernism, History and the First World War* (Manchester: Manchester University Press, 1998): 84. Angela Smith also comments on the 'metaphoric rape' in this passage: Smith, *The Second Battlefield*: 90.

68 Borden, *The Forbidden Zone*: 121.

69 Mary Borden, *The Forbidden Zone*, ed. Hazel Hutchison (London: Hesperus Press, 2008 [1929]): xiii.

70 Freedman, 'Mary Borden's *Forbidden Zone*'; Higonnet, 'Authenticity and Art'; Hallett, *Containing Trauma*: 28, 40, 66, 68, 93, 103, 162, 183–5.

71 Borden, *The Forbidden Zone*: 146.

72 Santanu Das, *Touch and Intimacy in First World War Literature* (Cambridge: Cambridge University Press, 2005): 221.

73 Mary Borden, *Sarah Gay* (London: William Heinemann, 1931); *Mary of Nazareth* (London: William Heinemann, 1933); *The King of the Jews* (London: William Heinemann, 1935).

74 Mary Borden, *The Technique of Marriage* (London: William Heinemann, 1933).

75 Borden, *Journey down a Blind Alley*; Conway, *Mary Borden*: 213–78.

76 Borden wrote several commercially successful novels after the Second World War: Mary Borden, *No. 2 Shovel Street: A Novel* (London: William Heinemann, 1949); *For the Record* (London: William Heinemann, 1950); *Martin Merriedew* (London: William Heinemann, 1952); *Margin of Error* (London: William Heinemann, 1954); *The Hungry Leopard* (London: William Heinemann, 1956).

77 Conway, *Mary Borden*: 312.

78 On Agnes Warner, see: Quinn, *Agnes Warner*.

79 Three local Saint John newspapers each published articles on Warner's work in France, based on her letters, and on a series of public addresses she gave following her return from the war: the *Saint John Globe*, the *Saint John Standard*, and the *Daily Telegraph*. All are available at the Saint John Archives, Saint John, New Brunswick, Canada.

80 Anon., 'General Warner', *Saint John Globe* (27 February 1917: 4); Anon., 'General D. B. Warner, War Veteran', *Saint John Globe* (27 February 1917): 10; Anon., obituary for General Darius B. Warner, *Daily Telegraph* (28 February 1917): 7.

81 Quinn, *Agnes Warner*: 41.
82 Agnes Warner was the third of six siblings: one older brother died in infancy before she was born; one younger brother died in early childhood in 1877. Quinn, *Agnes Warner*: 41.
83 Anon., *My Beloved Poilus*.
84 Katie Pickles, *Female Imperialism and National Identity: Imperial Order of the Daughters of the Empire* (Manchester: Manchester University Press, 2002).
85 Anon., Article, *Daily Telegraph* (23 December 1916): 9.
86 Anon., Announcement, *Saint John Globe* (2 May 1894). Warner appears to have had a great interest in botany – an interest that was probably nurtured during her schooling at the Victoria High School for Girls, Saint John. George Upham Hay, the school principal, was a prime mover in the New Brunswick Natural History Society. Warner amassed a large collection of plants, which are stored at the Herbarium of the New Brunswick Museum, Saint John, New Brunswick. I am indebted to Stephen Clayden, curator of the museum, for numerous insights into Warner's early life. See: Stephen R Clayden, 'Hay, George Upham', in George Williams Brown, David M. Hayne, Francess G. Halpenny, and Ramsay Cook (eds), *Dictionary of Canadian Biography*, Vol. XIV (Toronto: Toronto University Press, 1998).
87 The *Alumni Quarterly* of the New York Presbyterian Hospital School of Nursing placed Agnes Warner in Paris on a number of occasions, including 1906 and 1907. It is likely that she travelled frequently to France during the first decade of the twentieth century: Anon., Notation, *New York Presbyterian Hospital Alumni Quarterly*, 1 (July 1906). I am indebted to Shawna Quinn for drawing my attention to this volume. See also: Quinn, *Agnes Warner*: 43–5.
88 Anon., *My Beloved Poilus*: 5.
89 Anon., *My Beloved Poilus*: 7–8. On her return to Canada in December 1914, Warner gave a talk to the townspeople of Saint John emphasising the heroism and endurance of the French people: Anon., 'Red Cross Nurse from Front on Visit Here Tells of War's Horrors', *Daily Telegraph* (26 December 1914): 12. See also: Anon., Society Page, *Daily Telegraph* (26 December 1914): 6; Anon., 'Miss Warner on Her Way Back to the Front', *Daily Telegraph* (14 January 1915): 10; Anon., Society Page, *Daily Telegraph* (16 January 1915): 10.
90 Anon., *My Beloved Poilus*: 9–13.
91 Anon., *My Beloved Poilus*: 14.
92 Warner was forty-two at the outbreak of war and forty-seven by the time she returned home to Saint John.
93 Anon., *My Beloved Poilus*: 24.
94 Anon., *My Beloved Poilus*: 31.
95 Warner's nephew, Bayard Coster, survived the war.
96 Anon., *My Beloved Poilus*: 56.

97 Anon., *My Beloved Poilus*: 59–61. Another Canadian nurse, Margaret Hare, based in Poperinghe, wrote of having met Warner: Anon., Article, *Saint John Globe* (12 July 1916): 3.

98 Anon., *My Beloved Poilus*: 74.

99 Anon., *My Beloved Poilus*: 95.

100 Many unpublished nurses' accounts have this determinedly cheerful tone. See, for example: Miss Bickmore, MS essay, 3814; 85/51/1, Imperial War Museum, London; H. M. Harpin, MS letters, 3051 Con Shelf, Imperial War Museum, London; Mrs I. Edgar (née Layng), letters and diary, P211, Imperial War Museum, London.

101 Christine Hallett, 'The Personal Writings of First World War Nurses: A Study of the Interplay of Authorial Intention and Scholarly Interpretation', *Nursing Inquiry*, 14.4 (2007): 320–9; Christine Hallett, 'Portrayals of Suffering: Perceptions of Trauma in the Writings of First World War Nurses and Volunteers', *Canadian Bulletin of Medical History*, 27.1 (2010): 65–84.

102 I am indebted to Shawna Quinn for forwarding me this quotation. See also the frontispiece to Anon., *My Beloved Poilus*, which states that Warner's letters were 'published by her friends without her knowledge, simply and solely to raise money to aid her in her work'.

103 Anon., Society Page article about *My Beloved Poilus*, *Daily Telegraph* (24 February 1917): 9; Anon., Society Page note, *Daily Telegraph* (10 March 1917): 12.

104 Anon., Society Page note, *Daily Telegraph* (7 October 1916): 12.

105 Anon., Society Page note, *Daily Telegraph* (16 January 1915): 10; Anon., Article, *Daily Telegraph* (19 January 1915): 3; Anon., Note, *Daily Telegraph* (6 February 1919): 7.

106 Anon., *My Beloved Poilus*.

107 Anon., *My Beloved Poilus*: 86.

108 Anon., *My Beloved Poilus*: 93.

109 Anon., *My Beloved Poilus*: 112.

110 Anon., Column, *BJN* (20 January 1917). See also: Anon., 'Praise for Unit 16/21', *BJN* (1 February 1919): 66.

111 Anon., 'Croix de Guerre for Sister Jaffray'.

112 Anon., 'French Flag Nursing Corps' (23 June 1917).

113 Anon., 'Decorations for Nurses'; Anon., 'French Flag Nursing Corps', *BJN* (16 February 1918): 113.

114 Anon., 'Miss Warner Speaks at Reception'.

115 Anon., 'French Flag Nursing Corps', *BJN* (3 August 1918): 80–81; Anon., 'French Flag Nursing Corps', *BJN* (19 October 1918): 234.

116 Anon., 'Miss Warner Speaks at Reception'.

117 Anon., 'French Flag Nursing Corps: En Avant', *BJN* (14 December 1918): 363.

118 Anon., 'First Nursing Unit over Hindenburg Line', *Saint John Globe* (7 December 1918): 5.

119 On Warner's decorations, see: Anon., 'War's Lessons Should Not Soon Be Forgotten', *Daily Telegraph* (11 April 1919): 3; Anon., 'Obituary', *Saint John Globe* (26 April 1926: 3); Anon., 'Spent Five Years of Nursing among the French Soldiers', *Saint John Standard* (31 March 1919): 3.

120 Sister Hilda Gill, who had already been decorated with the Croix de Guerre for her rescue of Sister Jaffray in 1917, was also recognised with a further decoration: Anon., 'French Flag Nursing Corps', *BJN* (4 January 1919): 6–7. See also: Anon., 'Miss Warner Gets Croix de Guerre', *Saint John Globe* (11 January 1919): 12.

121 Anon., Column, *Daily Telegraph* (1 March 1919): 2; Anon., 'Miss Agnes Warner Is Expected Soon', *Daily Telegraph* (3 March 1919): 4.

122 Anon., Society Page, *Daily Telegraph* (12 April 1919): 12; Anon., Column, *Daily Telegraph* (25 April 1919): 3; Anon., 'Nursing Sister Agnes Warner Was Entertained', *Saint John Standard* (5 April 1919); Anon., 'Returned Nursing Sister Entertained at Luncheon', *Saint John Standard* (8 April 1919).

123 Anon., 'Nursing Sister Agnes Warner Highly Honoured', *Daily Telegraph* (5 April 1919): 5.

124 Anon., 'Miss Warner Speaks at Reception'.

125 Anon., 'War's Lessons Should Not Soon be Forgotten'. See also: Anon., 'Returned Nursing Sister Entertained at Luncheon'.

126 Anon., 'Obituary', *Saint John Globe*. See also: Anon., 'Death Notice', *Saint John Globe* (23 April 1926): 10; Anon., 'Agnes Warner Death Notice and Obituary', *Telegraph Journal* (24 April 1926).

127 Higonnet, *Nurses at the Front*; Higonnet, 'Authenticity and Art'; Freedman, 'Mary Borden's *Forbidden Zone*'.

128 Borden, *Journey down a Blind Alley*: 7.

3

The hell at the heart of paradise

Introduction: more writings from L'Hôpital Chirurgical Mobile No. 1

Mary Borden published *The Forbidden Zone* in 1929, more than ten years after the armistice.[1] Long before this – indeed, even before the war itself had ended – Agnes Warner's *My Beloved Poilus* had appeared in her home town of Saint John, New Brunswick.[2] But it was one of Borden's trained nurses, Ellen La Motte, who produced the earliest memoir of L'Hôpital Chirurgical Mobile No. 1. *The Backwash of War* was published by Putnam's in New York in 1916.[3] The book bears remarkable stylistic similarities to Borden's *The Forbidden Zone*. The two women almost certainly knew each other, and historian Margaret Higonnet has suggested that they observed each other closely.[4] La Motte refers directly to Borden as 'La Directrice' and offers her patron a dedication in the frontispiece to her book.[5] By contrast, Borden (although she makes several interesting observations about trained nurses) never mentions La Motte directly. Some of *The Forbidden Zone*'s chapters were published as journal articles long before its release as a full-length book; but the lapse of eleven years before its publication suggests that it might have been influenced by a reading of *The Backwash of War*. A fourth writer – Maud Mortimer – describes a hospital that bears such remarkable similarities to the field hospital described by Borden, Warner, and La Motte that it seems highly likely that she, too, is writing of L'Hôpital Chirurgical Mobile No. 1.

Agnes Warner commented: 'They call the hospital "le petit paradis des blessés" and are so glad to be sent here.'[6] La Motte, by contrast, adopts a relentlessly cynical tone, and opens her book with an episode in which a man who has attempted suicide is dragged to the hospital against his will, to be saved so that he can be shot as a deserter.

War's backwash

If Mary Borden can be likened to a chameleon, her contemporary and colleague at L'Hôpital Chirurgical Mobile No. 1, Ellen La Motte, was surely more of a rhinoceros. On 3 December 1951, in an article published in the *Greensburg Morning Review*, a journalist reported that:

> On the walls of her red frame house in Washington's old Georgetown section Miss Ellen La Motte has pictures of rhinoceroses. In her living room she has a parrot called Albert. The rhinoceros is a favourite [*sic*] animal of Miss La Motte. She liked the idea of its making its own way through the jungle, something she fancies she herself has done in her lifetime.[7]

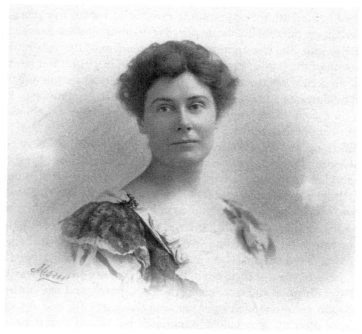

Figure 4 Portrait of Ellen La Motte

77

Born in Louisville, Kentucky in 1873, La Motte was probably one of the most highly trained nurses of her generation. She entered the respected John's Hopkins Training School for Nurses in Baltimore at the turn of the century, graduating in 1902.[8] Yet she appears to have been dissatisfied with her hospital experience. Almost half a century later, in October 1951, now living in Washington DC, she completed a questionnaire for May Ermer McNeill, secretary of the Johns Hopkins Hospital Nurses Alumnae Association, in which she responded tersely to a question about her experience as a student nurse: 'Nothing to evaluate. Did not like it'; and even more tersely to a similar question about her experience as a graduate nurse: 'Ditto.'[9]

La Motte appears to have had an itinerant childhood, spending part of her time with relatives in Wilmington, Delaware, before attending a fashionable boarding school in Arlington, Virginia.[10] She enjoyed a highly successful career, working as a supervising nurse at the Johns Hopkins Hospital for two years, before moving to St Luke's Hospital in St Louis, as assistant superintendent. In 1905 she turned her attention to community nursing and spent five years as a tuberculosis nurse with the Instructive Visiting Nurses Association in Baltimore. She was appointed Superintendent of the Tuberculosis Division of the Baltimore Health Department in 1910.[11] But her success masked a controversial approach to tuberculosis nursing, and Keiko Sugiyama has suggested that her departure for France in 1915 was an escape from 'minority status in the controversies about the treatment of tuberculosis'.[12]

Ellen La Motte's dispute with senior figures in the US nursing profession is revealing of her personality. It appears to have revolved around her adoption of a hard-line approach to the control of tuberculosis. Her philosophy was set down in a textbook, *The Tuberculosis Nurse*, which was published soon after her departure for France. In it, she advised that, 'tuberculosis is largely a disease of the poor – of those on or below the poverty line. We must further realize that there are two sorts of poor people – not only those financially handicapped and so unable to control their environment, but those who are mentally and morally poor, and lack intelligence, will-power and self-control.'[13] La Motte recommended open communication with, and the careful education of, tuberculosis sufferers,[14] but added that if patients did not comply with preventive measures they must be segregated from the rest of society. This rather harsh approach was at odds with the more overtly nurturing attitudes of nurse leaders, such as Lillian Wald and Lavinia Dock.[15] La Motte also risked alienating her physician colleagues by virtually accusing them of exploiting their patients by withholding information.[16] In his introduction to her book, Louis Hamman, physician in charge of the Phipps Tuberculosis Dispensary, commented diplomatically: 'one is impressed by the honesty and enthusiasm of the book, but some may wish that certain of the statements, and particularly some strictures had been a little mollified'.[17]

During her training at Johns Hopkins La Motte may have become acquainted with Gertrude Stein (who was, at that time, a medical student at the hospital). Stein, one of the most remarkable intellects of her time, did not complete her medical training, but went on, instead, to study psychology with William James, and then to pursue a career as a writer. She developed an extraordinary style that was later to be viewed as an important strand in the development of twentieth-century literary modernism.[18] It was probably she who introduced La Motte to Mary Borden. Stein's 'salon' at the rue de Fleurus in Paris was a recognised avant-garde centre of art and literature. Although their emphases were different, Borden and La Motte wrote in similar styles, drawing upon their personal experiences to produce terse and harrowing accounts of the war.[19]

La Motte – a descendent of influential French Huguenots – was probably motivated, at least in part, by a desire to support her ancestral homeland.[20] When she first arrived in Paris, she nursed at the American Hospital at Neuilly, finding it a profoundly unsatisfying place to work. Not only was it under-equipped and marred in its operation by an unwieldy bureaucracy, it was also over-staffed with volunteers.[21] La Motte realised that the most essential and effective wartime nursing work could only be done close to the front lines. According to Stein, La Motte was 'gun-shy'.[22] Nevertheless, she wanted to nurse in a field hospital, where her expertise could be of use, and, in the summer of 1915, she accepted an invitation to work for Mary Borden at the newly formed Hôpital Chirurgical Mobile No. 1.[23]

In June 1915, La Motte found herself under bombardment at Dunkirk whilst en route from Paris to Rousbrugge. She decided to 'kill time' by writing an account of her experiences for the popular American journal *The Atlantic Monthly*. Her writing is vivid and immediate; she informs the reader that she is describing events as they unfold, in an attempt to calm her nerves, adding that 'as each shell strikes I spring back to the window, and my chair falls backwards, while the others laugh'.[24] Her article was published five months later. In its opening paragraphs, she focuses on how her arrival in the 'zone of the armies' made her feel that 'individual liberty was gone', adding: 'the longer one stays in the military areas, the more this sense of being a prisoner at large weighs upon one'.[25]

La Motte's description of bombardment brings the reader close to the emotions of those trapped within Dunkirk's walls, waiting for each high-explosive shell. The day she is there, the town is steadily bombarded: approximately every forty minutes four shells fall, before the guns are left to cool. At first, watching from the balcony of her hotel, La Motte finds the bombing 'overwhelmingly interesting and exciting'.[26] But later that morning, an ill-advised journey into the centre of the town results in a much closer encounter with bombardment. La Motte describes how she begins to feel 'cold terror', as she realises that, while smaller shells can tear holes in buildings, 'these monster *obus*, dropping from the sky, crush buildings to the earth'.[27] As the shells begin to fall again, La Motte experiences a moment of paralysing fear, and far from 'walking slowly through the bombardment' like the nurses in Antwerp described by Sarah Macnaughtan,[28] she stands bewildered:

> Never for a second was there any fear of death, but an agonizing fear of the concussion, of a jaw torn off, of a nose smashed in … In that fearful moment, there was not one intellectual faculty I could call upon. There was nothing in past experience, nothing of will-power, of judgement, of intuition, that could serve me. I was beyond and outside and apart from the accumulated experience of my lifetime. My intelligence was worthless in this moment of supreme need. Every decision would be wrong, every movement would be in the wrong direction, and it was also wrong to stand still.[29]

Eventually, La Motte finds shelter in the cellar of a private house. Here, she is impressed by the calm fatalism of Dunkirk's residents, and feels moved to record the striking contrast between their 'dignified acceptance' of their position in the front line of war and 'the hysterical sobbing of the London press, raving over "baby-killers" and "slayers of women" '.[30] Such deliberate and open critique of British propaganda is rare in La Motte's writing. Her more usual approach is to confront the reader with the realities of war; this is the strategy she uses in a succession of articles for US journals, later drawn together into her book, *The Backwash of War*.

La Motte opens *The Backwash of War* with an introduction in which she makes it clear what her intentions are. She is, she informs the reader, about to relate her experiences in a French military hospital, about ten kilometres behind the front lines, in Belgium. Here 'months of boredom' are 'punctuated by moments of intense fright'.[31] In the 'zone of the armies', although there may at times be 'glorious deeds of valour, courage, devotion, and nobility' there is also 'a stagnant place',[32] where

> much ugliness is churned up in the wake of mighty, moving forces. We are witnessing a phase in the evolution of humanity, a phase called War – and the slow, onward progress stirs up the slime in the shallows, and this is the Backwash of War. It is very ugly. There are many little lives foaming up in the backwash. They are loosened by the sweeping current, and float to the surface, detached from their environment, and one glimpses them, weak, hideous, repellent. After the war, they will consolidate again into the condition called Peace.[33]

La Motte's world view is an intensely bleak one: although human nature has the capacity to be good, it is also often repulsive and disgusting. She will, she says, reveal this ugly side of humankind.

The short stories that follow, drawn from La Motte's own experience at L'Hôpital Chirurgical Mobile No. 1, are powerful. They repel even as they fascinate, compelling the reader to encounter what La Motte views as the truth. Her purpose is undoubtedly pacifist, yet her writing feels like an aggressive assault on the reader's consciousness. The opening sequence to her first story, which is ironically entitled 'Heroes', begins with an attempted suicide:

> When he could stand it no longer, he fired a revolver up through the roof of his mouth, but he made a mess of it. The ball tore out his left eye, and then lodged somewhere under his skull, so they bundled him, cursing and screaming, to the nearest field hospital. The journey was made in double-quick time, over rough Belgian roads. To save his life, he must reach the hospital without delay, and if he was bounced to death, jolting along at breakneck speed, it did not matter. That was understood. He was a deserter, and discipline must be maintained. Since he had failed in the job, his life must be saved, he must be nursed back to health, until he was well enough

to be stood up against a wall and shot. This is War. Things like this also happen in peace time, but not so obviously.[34]

'Heroes' had first been published in August 1916 in *The Atlantic Monthly*.[35] It is probably the most powerful of the thirteen vignettes that make up *The Backwash of War*. The short sentences, the staccato feel to the text, and the insistent repetition of ugly truths assault the reader, who is compelled to watch, to see, to listen. And it is this insistence on forcing the reader to confront truth that gives La Motte's writing its power.

The Backwash of War had a difficult reception. First published in the USA in the autumn of 1916, it was suppressed by the censor in 1918, several months after America's entry into the war.[36] Its publication had been permitted neither in Britain nor in France. In a new introduction, written for a 1934 reprint of her book, La Motte describes how she had only realised that the book had been banned in the USA when an issue of the journal *The Liberator* appeared with a recommendation for *The Backwash of War* inked out.[37] In the mid-1930s, as another European war seemed imminent, La Motte warned 'there can be no war without this backwash'.[38] Her book was rediscovered in the late twentieth century by feminist historians and critical theorists, excited by its uncompromising attitude to warfare and the beauty of its literary style.[39]

For Ellen La Motte, L'Hôpital Chirurgical Mobile No. 1 – which others had named 'le petit paradis des blessés' – was a place of horror and degradation. The importance of perspective and the power of interpretation become clear when one compares the narratives of Agnes Warner, for whom every French soldier is a hero; Mary Borden, who seems to be searching for a spiritual reality beyond individual suffering; and Ellen La Motte, who sees only human weakness and a monumental waste. In her article 'A Joy Ride', La Motte refers to Borden as 'the Directrice, who is my friend',[40] and she dedicates *The Backwash of War* to 'Mary Borden-Turner[,] "The Little Boss" to whom I owe my experiences in the zone of the armies';[41] but in her fifth chapter, 'A Belgian Civilian', she seems to satirise the way in which Borden scolds a Belgian mother for not remaining with her dying child, when Borden herself has left three children at home in England to pursue 'the life and adventures of the Front'.[42]

One of the truths that La Motte is anxious to convey is that, in fact, life in the zone of the armies is not exciting and adventurous:

> At times, at the front, it gets frightfully dull. When there is an attack and in consequence, plenty of work to do, it is all right in a field hospital. But when there are no attacks, when there are no new patients and all the old ones become convalescent, when there is practically no work, it becomes insupportable. Nothing but the green hedge on all sides of us, shutting us into ourselves, into our little, gossiping enclosure, with no newspapers, with no aeroplane to fly overhead, with nothing to do but walk down to the little pond and sail boats.[43]

In 'A Joy Ride', La Motte recounts how, at one time of such maddening boredom, her 'friend', the 'Directrice', gives her a *laissez passer* permitting her to take a trip with a Canadian colleague who is going to look for her nephew stationed at a rest camp near Poperinghe. The narrative that unfolds is both poignant and humorous – and very different from the harsh realities of *The Backwash of War*. La Motte is frank about her fear, inviting the reader to laugh not only at her two companions – an eccentric English chauffeur and a Canadian nurse who insists on going too close to the front lines – but also at herself: the gun-shy American who is searching for a lamb to bring back to the hospital as a pet. She openly confesses: 'I am not naturally what one would call brave, and since last summer, after our fourteen-hour bombardment in Dunkirk, the sight of a shelled town makes me feel quite sick.'[44]

As the trio pass the observation balloons that mark the proximity of the front lines, and turn down a dirt track towards the Canadian camp, La Motte's anxiety increases. They pass horses with rope fringes over their eyes to protect them from shrapnel, and drive through a camp, in which Canadian troops are living in primitive 'conical wooden huts' and 'shacks' – 'just like animal pens, in which animals wait to be slaughtered'.[45] Suddenly, several shells burst in a field near to the road along which they are travelling, and the three begin to argue about whether to go on:

> MacAlister wanted to see Donald. I had no wish whatever to see Donald, especially under these circumstance … 'Go back quick!' I commanded. 'Can't you see they're shelling the road?' 'Eh?' said Williamson; while MacAlister kept repeating, 'I want to see Donald.' Between that slow-witted parson-chauffeur and that devoted girl, I got exasperated. I hate shells and am desperately afraid of them. It is so refreshing to admit the truth.[46]

At this point, La Motte gets out of the car, telling the others to drive on without her, and stands in a field in Flanders, 'surrounded by half-a-dozen grinning Canadian soldiers' – a situation that she finds 'a little unusual'.[47] Unfortunately, she is the one who is subjected to further danger – from anti-aircraft fire as a *Taube* flies overhead. She takes refuge in a 'flimsy' shelter, in which she is offered a very British-Canadian afternoon tea and a shell-casing to take home as a souvenir, while her colleague continues on her journey, successfully locating 'a grateful, dirty little nephew … overjoyed to see his aunt'.[48] La Motte's writing offers a satirical insight into the irrationality of war. The identity of the Canadian nurse who was searching for her nephew is unknown, but on 28 August 1916, Canadian nurse Agnes Warner wrote home to her family: 'I have met our boy B – at his rest camp not very far from here. It was a joy to find him looking so well, and big and brown.'[49] Agnes Warner's nephew, Bayard Coster, was serving with the Canadian forces on the Ypres front.[50] It is tempting to wonder whether he was the 'Donald' of La Motte's story, and Warner herself 'that devoted girl', 'MacAlister'. But humour – even of the self-effacing variety – is rare in La Motte's writings.

La Motte was based at Borden's field hospital in Rousbrugge for over a year, from summer 1915 to autumn 1916. Towards the end of 1916, with *The Backwash of War* just published, she escaped the 'zone of the armies' and chose to put thousands of miles between herself and war-torn Europe, travelling to China with longstanding friend and companion Emily Chadbourne, and remaining there for two years, visiting Japan, French Indo-China, Siam, and the Straits Settlements. She spent much of her time writing and campaigning against the exploitation of colonised people, and most particularly against the opium trade.[51] For her efforts, she was awarded the Lun Tse Hsu Memorial Medal by the Chinese Nationalist Government and the Order of Merit by the Japanese Red Cross.[52] Keiko Sugiyama has commented on how La Motte exposed the hypocrisy of western men and women who, 'under the banner of civilization and Christianity, were taking advantage of the natives and victimizing them'.[53] La Motte does, nevertheless, still portray 'native' people as stereotypically uncivilised, just as she portrays the suffering French *poilu* as stereotypically weak and self-indulgent, and the American immigrant tuberculosis patient as ignorant and wilful. Her attack on western imperialism was highly unusual for her time, but even more unusual was her attack on the weakness and immorality of the western male.[54]

La Motte's efforts to fight the opium trade also took her to London, where she lived for twenty years, travelling to Geneva for anti-opium meetings of the League of Nations.[55] She continued to write extensively for journals and magazines.[56] One of her more whimsical pieces, 'A Desert Owl', relates the story of an elderly lady living in a garret in Westminster, who purchases a desert owl, and accidentally takes home the wrong box – containing two wild exotic birds. As always, her piece shows the slightly contemptible side of human nature; yet it is also gentle and humorous, evocative of London life in the late 1920s.[57]

Towards the end of her life, in her interview for the *Greensburg Morning Review*, La Motte observed that during the Great Depression she had moved to Washington 'to get on as best she could'. She had bought and 'fixed up' old Georgetown houses, commenting that she could get them 'awfully cheap'. It was clear that, by 1951, La Motte was 'getting on' rather well. She commented to her interviewer that 'Albert [her parrot], my friends and the stock market keep me interested.' She died – no doubt, still interested – ten years later in 1961.[58]

Not all of La Motte's writings are hard-hitting exposés or satirical commentaries on the double standards of imperialism. One of her short stories – 'Under a Wine Glass' – tells the strange and whimsical tale of a talented man who has lost his creativity and his sense of self. In it La Motte asks the question: 'Do you think people ever recover themselves? When the precious thing in them, the spirit of them, has been overlaid and overlaid, covered deep with artificial layers?'[59] For La Motte, it seems, her own sense of self was most intact – her spirit most free – when she had a mission to fulfil. But her clarity of expression was twinned with a sharpness of tone that exposed her to criticism and censure. Much of her writing is biting in its critique of the destructiveness of human society – as if she felt that any tone of conciliation would have compromised the truth of her message.

Maud Mortimer: witnessing nursing

When Maud Mortimer arrived at an unnamed field hospital in Flanders, she commented on its isolation. Within eight kilometres of the front-line trenches, and hence almost in the thick of the 'action', the field hospital was nevertheless so closed – the passage through its perimeter hedge so restricted in either direction – that its inhabitants knew less about the progress of the war than their relatives at home. Their busyness and their isolation were such that any war news that reached them was both delayed and distorted.[60]

The hospital consisted of 'sixteen wooden shacks', supplemented by tents, of which eight were wards, caring for about 140 patients in total. There was an operating room, also containing a 'radiographic cabinet'; a pharmacy; a *salle d'attente*, or reception room; a wash-house and linen room; and staff quarters. Mortimer adds that 'all the shacks and tents are connected by narrow walks or *trottoirs* which thread quite picturesquely back and forth across our muddy enclosure'. In her own small corner of the nurses' accommodation hut, 'everything blows, creaks, and flaps together. One feels much as a spider might in a tight crevice of bark with leaves for curtains.'[61]

One of Mortimer's most compelling pen-portraits is of the Canadian-trained nurse who loves night duty and who has given herself the nickname 'The Night Hawk':

> The Night Hawk loves poetry and quiet. She is Canadian and of the gold one bends in one's hands, out of which primitive peoples fashion their ornaments and their gods. She is all disinterestedness, all devotion and self-forgetfulness; a thoroughly trained nurse with a heart that never loses the freshness of its sympathy nor its willingness to be spent in the service of these men whose pluck is so amazing, whose rare lack of it, so pitiful. I have the happiest time in the world flitting through the night at her heels.[62]

A similar account of the night nurse 'flitting' into hutted wards carrying a lantern finds its way into Borden's *The Forbidden Zone*. The white-clad nurse moves silently across the hospital compound, carrying a glowing lantern. She encounters and fights pain – but this is a losing battle. She enters the hut reserved for gas gangrene cases. 'Pain is lying in there waiting for her', remarks Borden: 'It is holding the damp greenish bodies of the gangrene cases in her arms'.[63] In Mortimer's account:

> We carry our lanterns flickering over mud and snow and put them down at the door of each ward we visit ... While on her rounds she glides through darkened ward after darkened ward. Death – mysterious, spasmodic breathing-out of life which our instinct so curiously shrinks from – is here,

is there, is everywhere. The beautifying touch of his obliterating finger dis-
arms her fear. It is not so with pain, in whose wry, haunted environment is
neither life nor death, but a grimly barriered and bounded No Man's Land
where the bravest lose their bearings.[64]

Not only are these writers' descriptions strikingly similar;
the detail of their narratives corresponds as well. At L'Hôpital
Chirurgical Mobile No. 1, the same events may be recounted by two
or three consummate story-tellers from totally different perspectives. Ellen La Motte's 'At the Telephone' offers a stark and bleak
insight into the death of a young telephone operator who dies during surgery.[65] Maud Mortimer recounts a similar story of a death
from typhoid:

> For six lagging weeks the sympathy and science of the hospital clung to the
> chance of saving him … But death held on hungrily to him. In his delirium
> he was back in the trenches again, the receiver in his hand, feverishly active
> as message after message reached him and had to be sent on.
> Suddenly his excitement grew. He was in the fury of bursting shells
> … The pause was strained with the agony of attention. Then the muscles
> relaxed into a creeping smile and the lips moved again:
> 'Ah, ça y est, maintenant. Le bon Dieu est à l'appareil.'
> The boy was dead.[66]

On her return to her hometown of Saint John, New Brunswick at
the end of the war, Agnes Warner inspired her audience by recounting, as part of a public lecture, the story of 'a boy of nineteen who died
of typhoid. He was delirious and thought he was at his telephone in
the field. He gave orders all day, but at last turned to the Sister with a
smile and said, "It's alright now. It is God at the telephone." '[67]

Borden, La Motte, and Mortimer all recount stories of the famous
'Bataillon d'Afrique', France's punishment battalion for convicted
criminals.[68] Mortimer writes of 'one of the pets of the hospital and the
pride of the doctors – not because of any show of health he made, poor
lamb, but because he was still alive after all they had been allowed to
do to him, and out of gratitude to him for all they thought they had
learned to do against another time'.[69] She describes the patient's fate:

> Our Le Groux then, 'Light Breeze' or 'Joyous One' – a bullet through the
> spleen and kidney, half-flayed, with stomach, liver, and part of his intestines
> laid impudically [sic] bare, drains in the abdominal cavity and in his back –
> was one of the pets of the hospital and of the medical staff. If the doctors

cherished him and cherished themselves in him, he no less cherished the doctors ... And not only did he adore his doctor, but he also adored his faithful friend the nurse – his nurse, the Night Hawk – to whom alone, by virtue of her skill and devotion, was entrusted the ceremony of his terrible dressings, and whose care came nearer to a true mother's than anything this boy had ever known.[70]

As Le Groux died, 'he stretched out his hands to his nurse who folded him in her arms, her hot tears falling on the white face'. Twenty minutes later the general arrived to award Le Groux a medal, only to be told that the patient had died. Mortimer describes how, 'without a word, his head bent, the General turned and left the ward, two little unopened boxes in his hand, his sheathed sword hanging impotently at his side'.[71]

In La Motte's version of a similar (or, perhaps, the same) event, the 'Directrice' (Borden), who wants to enhance the reputation of her hospital, is seen as, effectively, conspiring with a surgeon, 'who was bent on making a reputation for himself', to prolong the man's life, even though he is in agony and there is no hope of a cure.[72] Yet, it is also the 'Directrice' who notices the man's courage in the face of such treatment and campaigns to have him decorated with the highest French military honour: the Croix de Guerre. The general is sceptical and delays for so long that he arrives too late. We are told that the patient 'held on as long as he could', but 'died, finally, after a long pull, just twenty minutes before the General arrived with his medals'.[73]

The differences in emphasis between the narratives is striking. In Mortimer's version, the focus is on the importance of the relationship between the patient and his doctors and nurses. The clinicians really believe they may have a chance of saving the patient. And when the general arrives too late with his medals, he is despondent. In La Motte's recounting of the same (or a similar) story, the doctors are merely cynical scientists who experiment on their patient for their own ends; and the general arrives too late because it takes the hospital staff so long to convince him that a member of the Bataillon d'Afrique deserves to be decorated.[74]

A similar – possibly the same – patient appears in Agnes Warner's *My Beloved Poilus*, where he is referred to as 'Le Roux', a name remarkably similar to Mortimer's 'Le Groux'. La Motte's description is cynical, Mortimer's emotional. Warner's is characteristically matter-of-fact:

January 16, 1916 ... Le Roux, the boy who has been here so long and who has been so terribly ill, died on Tuesday. I had great hopes of him up till the last day. Half an hour after he died the General came up to decorate him. I hope they will send the medals to his people, it seems hard that they should have been just too late to give them to him.[75]

In spite of its apparent casualness, Warner's writing is pervaded by affection for her young patient. She describes how she attended his funeral the next day, adding: 'the ward seems very empty without Le Roux, but I am glad that the poor boy is at rest for he has suffered so long'. And at this point – one of the few in a long series of letters – Warner betrays her own despair: 'I am beginning to think that death is the only good thing that can come to many of us.'[76]

Another story of death in L'Hôpital Chirurgical Mobile No. 1 relates to a patient who expires in the moment he is decorated by the general. Mortimer's account is deliberately poignant:

The sound of rapid footsteps comes down the long ward. The General stands at the foot of the bed. Lamplight glints on his drawn sword and on the Croix de Guerre hanging from the ribbon which he holds in his hand.
'In the name of the Republic – to you, Jean Magnard' – familiar words and oft repeated in these shacks anchored too near the breaking end of the turbulent waves of human strife not to catch the spindrift of their shattered endeavour – 'In the name of the Republic ...' The erect old soldier leans forward, gently pushes back the damp wisps of hair and kisses the dying man. Then with a hand on one of the relaxed cold ones he murmurs, 'Merci, l'ami.'[77]

In La Motte's version of the same – or a similar – story, the patient, who dreads death, accepts that he is dying only after the general awards him his medal: 'We all knew what it meant. So did the man. When he got the medal, he knew too. He knew there wasn't any hope. I held the medal before him, after the General had gone, in its red plush case. It looked cheap, somehow. The exchange didn't seem even. He pushed it aside with a contemptuous hand sweep, a disgusted shrug.'[78] For La Motte, the general is merely a symbol of the harsh regime that sends men to their deaths, according them the empty, meaningless trappings of a spurious heroism.

Both La Motte and Mortimer also tell the story of a patient who dies alone while two orderlies neglect him. In Mortimer's version, we hear that 'one of the night nurses is still up and wishes to remain with him through the luncheon hour. But the nurse of Salle I will not hear of it …When his nurse comes back from her midday rest, Methurin lies dead, alone. The orderlies are playing cards in the pantry.'[79] La Motte's version is altogether harsher: 'After a short time [the nurse] came back from lunch, and hurried to see Rochard, hurried behind the flamboyant, red, cheerful screens that shut him off from the rest of the ward. Rochard was dead. At the other end of the ward sat the two orderlies, drinking wine.'[80]

Maud Mortimer describes an interesting character at her anonymous French field hospital – a character to whom she gives the nickname 'Organization' – a fascinating American nurse who appears to be using her experience in the hospital to collect data that can be used to formulate some truth about the war:

> She is almost cubistic in her dire simplifications. When she is not harassed by the tortuous complexities of other people's minds – of latin minds in particular – she has the pleasantest ways and a witty good-fellowship which plays seductively over her relentless absolutism. She adores uniformity and in all that does not touch America, she is pacifist and neutral to the backbone, though not without a weakness for politics. A fully trained and excellent nurse, she yet has done with nursing. She is not here now to probe physical weakness but to cut deeper – for the purification of art and sentiment – down to the unquestionable depravity of the human heart.[81]

'Organization' believes that 'there is nothing so simple as truth and that it is always ugly'.[82] She seems to be using the hospital quite deliberately as a field of enquiry, and Mortimer employs the metaphor of the 'vacuum cleaner' to illustrate the way in which she 'makes one buzzing round, then settles down to choose from her bag'.[83] 'Organization' comes across to the reader of *A Green Tent in Flanders*, as a detached spectator who 'turns and turns the chewing gum of her inquiry',[84] rather than engaging deeply in the life of the hospital. When she leaves, 'her attaché case bulges with the documentary evidence of the obliquity of human nature especially as observed under torture in a field hospital'.[85] Maud Mortimer's book was published in 1918, more than a year after La Motte's. In the character of 'Organization', Mortimer may be painting a carefully anonymised portrait of Ellen La Motte: turning a soft irony against the soft ironist herself, producing a mysterious message whose code could only be broken by those who had been present at L'Hôpital Chirurgical Mobile No. 1.

Conclusion: the power of interpretation

In the small world of the field hospital, a number of nurses were caring for the same patients, observing the same events, and yet experiencing and writing about them in very different ways. Was Warner the nurse who begged a patient to eat and who took him in her arms as he died, only to describe his fate in such gently sympathetic, yet matter of fact, terms to her mother? Or was she, herself, observing one of her Canadian colleagues, of whom she later writes: 'May 3, 1916 ... The two Canadian nurses are a joy to work with, for they have had splendid training and are the kind that will go till they drop.'[86] And was the dying patient 'Le Roux' the same man as Mortimer's 'Le Groux', and La Motte's anonymous patient who dies 'after a long pull'?

These authors' visions of their patients are very different. For La Motte, they are 'weak, hideous, repellent'.[87] For Mortimer, they are suffering human beings to be pitied. For Warner and Borden, they are admirable men who have been stripped of their identities by modern warfare, and yet are able to behave with the utmost courtesy and patience. Borden describes the patients who are carried into the reception hut of her field hospital on the Somme: 'They were all so courteous voiced, using such beautiful phrases, as if they were in my drawing room. They apologized gravely in their exhaustion for the dirt, the blood, the ugly wounds.'[88]

A woman such as Agnes Warner – infused with patriotic fervour, and steeped in the values of her own time – provides a vivid illustration of the power of a pervasive imperialist ideology. The perspectives she and women like her took with them into the First World War paralleled the perspectives of combatants, whose consciously heroic willingness to go 'over the top' has astounded later generations. For Warner's close colleagues and associates, American volunteer nurses Mary Borden and Maud Mortimer, the courage and endurance of such women were both an inspiration and an education. They extolled the healing work of the professional nurse; yet they also recognised the destructiveness of the ideological forces that made her work so necessary. Agnes Warner herself never questioned the authority that drew her patients into the most destructive war that had ever been fought. She merely poured her compassion and expertise into the repair of her damaged 'poilus', and her thoughts and feelings into her letters home.

Another member of L'Hôpital Chirurgical Mobile No. 1 wrote with the deliberate intention of destroying the false heroic myths of the First World War and revealing what she saw as its squalid and horrific truths.[89] Ellen La Motte, one of the most biting and cynical of wartime writers, was a professional nurse, who had undergone additional training and experience as a tuberculosis specialist – one of the most dangerous occupations of the early twentieth century – and who was later to travel to China as a campaigner against the opium trade.[90] She was clearly not afraid of danger; yet she was referred to by Gertrude Stein as 'gun-shy' and wrote with self-denigrating wit of her encounters with bombardment.

Four nurses observed the work of one small hospital – L'Hôpital Chirurgical Mobile No. 1 – and spoke with four very different voices. Maud Mortimer's narrative was, perhaps, the most complete. In her *A Green Tent in Flanders*, characters are given pseudonyms, yet events are recorded vividly. Mortimer herself was not a trained nurse but, in common with that of many volunteers, her writing is redolent with a sense of her fascination for nursing work, and admiration for those who could do it well and with compassion. Her heroine was the 'Night Hawk', an unnamed Canadian nurse at whose light heels she 'flitted' through the dense darkness of the field hospital.

Notes

1 Mary Borden, *The Forbidden Zone* (London: William Heinemann, 1929).
2 Anon., *My Beloved Poilus* (Saint John, NB: Barnes, 1917).
3 Ellen N. La Motte, *The Backwash of War: The Human Wreckage of the Battlefield as Witnessed by an American Hospital Nurse* (New York: G. P. Putnam's Sons and The Knickerbocker Press, 1916).
4 Margaret Higonnet, *Nurses at the Front: Writing the Wounds of the Great War* (Boston, MA: Northeastern University Press, 2001): xvii–xx.
5 La Motte, *The Backwash of War*: frontispiece.
6 Anon., *My Beloved Poilus*: 118.
7 Transcript of an article taken from the *Greensburg Morning Review*, Pennsylvania (3 December 1951), Ellen La Motte, biographical file, The Alan Mason Chesney Medical Archives, The Johns Hopkins Medical Institutions, Baltimore, Maryland, USA.
8 Shortly after graduation, La Motte became a member of the Johns Hopkins Nurses Alumnae. See frequent references to her work for the Alumnae

Committee in: Anon., *The Johns Hopkins Nurses Alumnae Magazine*, 7 (1908), *passim*.

9 Ellen La Motte, biographical file, The Alan Mason Chesney Medical Archives, The Johns Hopkins Medical Institutions, Baltimore, Maryland, USA, questionnaire.

10 La Motte, biographical file.

11 La Motte, biographical file.

12 Keiko Sugiyama, 'Ellen La Motte, 1873–1961: Gender and Race in Nursing', *The Japanese Journal of American Studies*, 17 (2006): 129–141 (133).

13 Ellen N. La Motte, *The Tuberculosis Nurse: Her Function and Her Qualifications. A Handbook for Practical Workers in the Tuberculosis Campaign. By Ellen N. La Motte, R.N., Graduate of Johns Hopkins Hospital; Former Nurse-in-Chief of the Tuberculosis Division, Health Department of Baltimore*, introduction by Louis Hamman, M.D., Physician in Charge, Phipps Tuberculosis Dispensary, Johns Hopkins University (New York and London: G.P. Putnam's Sons and The Knickerbocker Press, 1915): 3.

14 La Motte, *The Tuberculosis Nurse*: 285.

15 Sugiyama, 'Ellen La Motte': 131–3. On the late-nineteenth-century disputes over the control of tuberculosis, see also: Jessica M. Robbins, 'Class Struggles in the Tubercular World: Nurses, Patients, and Physicians, 1903–1915', *Bulletin of the History of Medicine*, 71.3 (1997): 412–34.

16 La Motte, *The Tuberculosis Nurse*: 103.

17 La Motte, *The Tuberculosis Nurse*: introduction.

18 Higonnet, *Nurses at the Front*; Margaret Higonnet, 'Authenticity and Art in Trauma Narratives of World War I', *Modernism/Modernity*, 9.1 (2002): 91–107; Ariela Freedman, 'Mary Borden's *Forbidden Zone*: Women's Writing from No-Man's Land' *Modernism/Modernity*, 9.1 (2002): 109–24.

19 Gertrude Stein writes of her meetings with Ellen La Motte and Mary Borden in her autobiographical account: Gertrude Stein, *The Autobiography of Alice B. Toklas* (London: Penguin, 2001 [1933]): 172, 184–5. On the deliberately challenging nature of Stein's writing, see: Sidonie Smith and Julia Watson, *Reading Autobiography: A Guide for Interpreting Life Narratives* (Minneapolis: University of Minnesota Press, 2010): 36. On the nature of early-twentieth-century literary modernism, see: Lawrence Rainey, *Modernism: An Anthology* (Oxford: Blackwell Publishing, 2005): xix–xxix; Howard Booth and Nigel Rigby (eds), *Modernism and Empire* (Manchester: Manchester University Press, 2000). On the links between modernism and the First World War, see: Allyson Booth, *Postcards from the Trenches: Negotiating the Space between Modernism and the First World War* (Oxford: Oxford University Press, 1996); Trudi Tate, *Modernism, History and the First World War* (Manchester: Manchester University Press, 1998).

20 She was a member of the Huguenot Society of America: La Motte, biographical file.

21 Ellen N. La Motte, 'An American Nurse in Paris', *The Survey*, 34 (10 July 1915): 333–6.

22 Stein, *The Autobiography of Alice B. Toklas*: 184.

23 On La Motte's arrival in Paris, see: Higonnet, *Nurses at the Front*: xi; Angela Smith, *Women's Writings of the First World War: An Anthology* (Manchester: Manchester University Press, 2000): 330.

24 Ellen La Motte, 'Under Shell-Fire at Dunkirk', *The Atlantic Monthly*, 116 (November 1915): 692–700 (700).

25 La Motte, 'Under Shell-Fire': 692.

26 La Motte, 'Under Shell-Fire': 695.

27 La Motte, 'Under Shell-Fire': 697.

28 Sarah Macnaughtan, *A Woman's Diary of the War* (London: Thomas Nelson and Sons, 1915).

29 La Motte, 'Under Shell-Fire': 698.

30 La Motte, 'Under Shell-Fire': 699.

31 La Motte, *The Backwash of War*: v.

32 La Motte, *The Backwash of War*: v.

33 La Motte, *The Backwash of War*: vi.

34 La Motte, *The Backwash of War*: 3–4.

35 Ellen N. La Motte, 'Heroes', *The Atlantic Monthly*, 118 (August 1916): 208–10.

36 On the suppression of *The Backwash of War*, see: Angela Smith, *The Second Battlefield: Women, Modernism and the First World War* (Manchester: Manchester University Press, 2000): 77–8; Claire Tylee, *The Great War and Women's Consciousness: Images of Militarism and Womanhood in Women's Writings, 1914–64* (Houndmills and London: Macmillan, 1990): 94.

37 Ellen N. La Motte, *The Backwash of War: The Human Wreckage of the Battlefield as Witnessed by An American Hospital Nurse* (New York: G. P. Putnam's Sons, 1934), introduction.

38 La Motte, *The Backwash of War* (1934): introduction.

39 Smith, *The Second Battlefield*; Higonnet, *Nurses at the Front*; Higonnet, 'Authenticity and Art': 91–107; Freedman, 'Mary Borden's *Forbidden Zone*': 109–24.

40 Ellen N. La Motte, 'A Joy Ride', *The Atlantic Monthly*, 118 (October 1916): 481–90 (481).

41 La Motte, *The Backwash of War* (1916): frontispiece dedication.

42 La Motte, *The Backwash of War* (1916): 70.

43 La Motte, 'A Joy Ride': 481.

44 La Motte, 'A Joy Ride': 484.

45 La Motte, 'A Joy Ride': 485.

46 La Motte, 'A Joy Ride': 486.

47 La Motte, 'A Joy Ride': 486.

48 La Motte, 'A Joy Ride': 489.

49 Anon., *My Beloved Poilus*: 111.

50 I am indebted to Shawna Quinn for drawing my attention to the parallels between Warner's letter and La Motte's narrative, and also for sending me, amongst many other sources, an electronic link to Bayard Coster's attestation papers: www.collectionscanada.gc.ca/databases/cef/001042-119.01-e.php?7id_nbr-118774&interval-20&&PHPSESSID-c7db3klk2va2d63c6e9hiek717 (accessed June 2011).

51 While in Asia and then later in London, La Motte wrote extensively on the latter topic. See, for example: Ellen N. La Motte, *Civilization: Tales of the Orient* (New York: Books for Libraries Press, 1919); *Peking Dust* (New York: Century, 1919); *The Opium Monopoly* (New York: Macmillan, 1920); *The Ethics of Opium* (New York: Century, 1924); *'Snuffs and Butters' and Other Stories* (New York: Century, 1925); *Opium at Geneva; or, How the Opium Problem Is Handled by the League of Nations* (New York: The Nation, 1929). For a comment on La Motte's work in Asia, see: Sugiyama, 'Ellen La Motte', 135–8.

52 La Motte, biographical file.

53 Sugiyama, 'Ellen La Motte': 136.

54 Sugiyama, 'Ellen La Motte': 129–41.

55 La Motte, biographical file, questionnaire.

56 La Motte herself commented, in 1951, that her publications were 'too numerous to recall', and included contributions to *Harper's Magazine*, *The Atlantic Monthly*, *The Nation*, and *Foreign Affairs*: La Motte, biographical file.

57 Ellen N. La Motte, 'A Desert Owl', *The Atlantic Monthly* (January 1927): 81–6, available in La Motte, biographical file. In the same collection, see also: Ellen N. La Motte, 'The Three Widows: The True Story of an International Crisis', *Harper's Magazine* (March 1931): 428–35.

58 Sugiyama, 'Ellen La Motte': 129–41.

59 Ellen N. La Motte, 'Under a Wine Glass', *The Century Magazine* (December 1918): 150–4.

60 Maud Mortimer, *A Green Tent in Flanders* (New York: Doubleday, Page, 1918): 49.

61 Mortimer, *A Green Tent in Flanders*: 57–8.

62 Mortimer, *A Green Tent in Flanders*: 165.

63 Borden, *The Forbidden Zone*: 59.

64 Mortimer, *A Green Tent in Flanders*: 167–8.

65 La Motte, *The Backwash of War* (1916): 159–64.

66 Mortimer, *A Green Tent in Flanders*: 76–7.

67 This quotation appears in a local New Brunswick daily newspaper: Anon., 'Miss Warner Gave Splendid Lecture', *Saint John Standard* (11 April 1919). See also another account of the same lecture: Anon., 'War's Lessons Should Not Soon Be Forgotten: Miss Warner Tells New Phases of Her Work in France', *Daily Telegraph* (11 April 1919): 3, available at Saint John Archives, New Brunswick, Canada.

68 Borden's narrative, 'Enfant de malheur', focuses on a relationship between a disturbed – almost demonic – patient, his staid British nurse, and the French Catholic priest who gives him the last rites: Borden, *The Forbidden Zone*: 66–92.
69 Mortimer, *A Green Tent in Flanders*: 146.
70 Mortimer, *A Green Tent in Flanders*: 147–51.
71 Mortimer, *A Green Tent in Flanders*: 153.
72 La Motte, *The Backwash of War* (1916): 168.
73 La Motte, *The Backwash of War* (1916): 178.
74 The details in these two narrations of the same story are remarkably similar – even to the point that each states that the general arrived only twenty minutes after the patient's death: La Motte, *The Backwash of War* (1916): 167–78.
75 Anon., *My Beloved Poilus*: 81.
76 Anon., *My Beloved Poilus*: 83.
77 Mortimer, *A Green Tent in Flanders*: 196–8.
78 La Motte, *The Backwash of War* (1916): 119–20.
79 Mortimer, *A Green Tent in Flanders*: 212.
80 La Motte, *The Backwash of War* (1916): 59.
81 Mortimer, *A Green Tent in Flanders*: 157.
82 Mortimer, *A Green Tent in Flanders*: 158.
83 Mortimer, *A Green Tent in Flanders*: 158.
84 Mortimer, *A Green Tent in Flanders*: 159.
85 Mortimer, *A Green Tent in Flanders*: 183.
86 Anon., *My Beloved Poilus*: 102. The two Canadian nurses being referred to here are members of the Canadian Unit of the FFNC. One, Helen McMurrich, spent several years working closely with Warner, and travelled home with her in 1919. See: Anon., 'French Flag Nursing Corps' *BJN* (29 April 1916): 378; Anon., 'French Flag Nursing Corps', *BJN* (27 May 1916): 458.
87 La Motte, *The Backwash of War* (1916): vi.
88 Borden, *The Forbidden Zone*: 168.
89 On the creation of heroic myths of warfare, see: Michael Paris, *Warrior Nation: Images of War in British Popular Culture, 1850–2000* (London: Reaktion Books, 2000), *passim*; Graham Dawson, *Soldier Heroes: British Adventure, Empire and the Imagining of Masculinities* (London: Routledge, 1994), *passim*.
90 On Ellen La Motte's career, see: Higonnet, *Nurses at the Front*: ix–xv; Sugiyama, 'Ellen La Motte': 129–41.

Part II

Professional women

In August 1914, at the outbreak of the First World War, British women volunteered in their thousands to participate in what most people thought would be a short-term conflict with a clear, decisive end. Members of the QAIMNS and its Reserve were among the first to travel to France as part of the British Expeditionary Force (BEF). Nurses of the British Dominions followed, with Canadian, Australian, and New Zealand nurses reaching Europe by late 1914 or early 1915.[1] The American Army Nurse Corps was not mobilised until the entry of the United States of America into the war in April 1917, although numerous trained American nurses offered their services to the French and Belgian Red Cross Societies and were engaged in 'front-line nursing' from 1914 onwards, and a small number of 'official' American units also travelled to France.

Members of the army nursing corps of allied nations saw themselves as belonging to elite units. Trained in the most prestigious nursing schools of their day, they carried with them a remarkable degree of confidence and self-belief, and their achievements were eagerly reported by professional nursing journals in their native countries.[2] Although they were not always fully accepted by the army medical services to which they were attached, and though they experienced, at times, a certain degree of prejudice and opposition, they came to be recognised as vital components of the organisations that offered life-saving services close to the front lines.

Notes

1 The New Zealand Army Nursing Service was the latest to organise, the first fifty nursing staff not embarking for Europe until April 1915. See Anna Rogers, *While You're Away: New Zealand Nurses at War 1899–1948* (Auckland: Auckland University Press, 2003): 55.

2 The most influential of these were: in Britain the *BJN*, *The Nursing Mirror and Midwives Journal*, and *The Nursing Times*; in Australia *Una: The Journal of the Victorian Trained Nurses Association*; in New Zealand *Kai Tiaki*; and in the USA the *American Journal of Nursing*, although it should be noted that the pacifist convictions of Lavinia Dock, Head of the International Office of the *American Journal of Nursing*, meant that the early years of the war were not reported in that journal.

4

In France with the British Expeditionary Force

Introduction: the power of professional nursing

In the second decade of the twentieth century, a British nursing reform movement, which had begun more than seventy years previously, was reaching its zenith. In the 1840s, small and isolated groups of British nurses, inspired by Continental examples and working under the patronage of the Church, had begun to demonstrate the value of a disciplined nursing workforce. Their achievements had been catapulted into the public consciousness by Florence Nightingale's highly publicised mission to the Crimea in the 1850s.[1] By raising the profile of the lady-nurse who acted as both compassionate carer and 'sanitary missioner', Nightingale had opened up nursing work as a field for women from the higher social echelons on both sides of the Atlantic. In the USA, the message that significant work could be performed in military settings by female nurses was further emphasised by the achievements of Civil War 'nurses' such as Clara Barton, Harriet Eaton, and Mary Chesnut.[2] The high-profile nursing achievements of elite women encouraged the development of professional nursing schools on both sides of the Atlantic.

By 1914, such schools, in both Britain and the USA, were well established, and had a clear sense of the distinctness of nursing care from medical practice. They produced nurses who were secure in their knowledge and confident in their skills. In the American context, Patricia D'Antonio has suggested that the development of professional nursing was driven forward because some women's desire for medical knowledge coincided with physicians' needs for more educated and knowledgeable assistance in their increasingly techno-logical work.[3] In elite schools, such as those of London, Edinburgh, New York, Philadelphia, and Baltimore, nurses were given theoretical instruction by doctors, and were then assisted by nurse tutors and head nurses in developing the art of translating such knowledge into expert practice. This process resulted in an increasing sense of auton-omy among nurses, who saw their role as something that went well beyond that of doctor's assistant.

Two highly trained nurses, one British, the other American, wrote significant memoirs of their war experiences. British nurse writer Kate Luard, a veteran of the Second Anglo-Boer War (1899–1902) began the First World War as a sister with the QAIMNS Reserve and rose to the position of Head Sister to one of the most signif-icant British advanced casualty clearing stations. American Alice Fitzgerald, a prominent member of the nursing profession in the USA, joined the QAIMNS Reserve as a sister in 1916, but left to take up a senior role with the American Red Cross following the USA's entry into the war.

The quintessential British nurse: Kate Luard

Katherine Evelyn Luard (known to her colleagues as 'Kate') might be viewed as a typical member of the early-twentieth-century British nursing elite.[4] Born into the Victorian gentry, her upbringing imbued her with a sense of an inextricable link between privilege and ser-vice. Her father, the Revd Bixby Garnham Luard, was a member of the Anglican clergy, and in 1872, the year of Kate's birth, the family was living in Aveley Vicarage in Essex. Kate was the tenth of thirteen children and, while still young, she moved with her family to Birch Rectory, a large and comfortable living near Colchester.[5]

The Luard family was, perhaps, typical of the British gentry in the last decades of the nineteenth century. While there were ample means to provide a good standard of living for all, and an expensive public school education for the boys, the girls' education was not consid-ered a high priority.[6] Girls were expected to marry and be supported by their husbands. In the Luard family, though, this expectation was

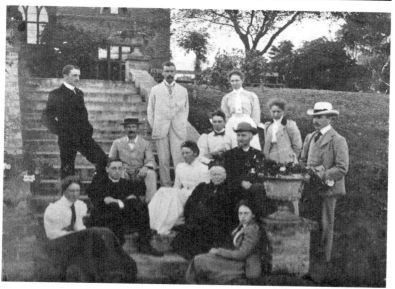

Figure 5 The Luard family at Birch Rectory, Essex. Kate is on the back row, right-hand side.

confounded: only one of the six Luard girls – Helen Lucy – ever did marry. All were educated at home by governesses, and some, Kate among them, also attended Croydon High School in their late teens.[7] Yet, in spite of its apparent limitations, the Luard sisters' education was clearly effective. Two of the girls, Clara Georgina and Rose Mary, went on to graduate from Lady Margaret Hall, Oxford, while Kate herself enjoyed a successful career as a nurse, rising quickly through the ranks of the nascent profession to become matron of a sanatorium in the decade just prior to the First World War.

Luard's life could hardly be seen as one of impoverished gentility, and yet, her early adulthood was characterised by self-sufficiency and obligation. She worked as a governess for about a year in order to earn sufficient funds to pay her way through her probationary nursing years,[8] first at the East London Hospital for Children and Dispensary for Women, then at the prestigious King's College Hospital, London.[9] In the last four decades of the nineteenth century, a nurse probationer could choose whether to apprentice herself to the hospital, thus gaining board and lodgings and free training, or to pay her own way by becoming a 'paying' or 'special' probationer.[10] At a time when identifying oneself as a 'lady' was seen as incompatible with any kind of paid work, the decision to become a special probationer was probably an automatic one for someone such as Luard.[11] This genteel identity was soon to become part of her persona as a professional military nurse: a member of an elite corps of female experts who combined a moral and sanitary mission with membership in a social elite.[12]

When Britain declared war on Germany in August 1914, Luard already had experience of military work. She had spent two years, from 9 June 1900 to 19 August 1902, as a member of the Army Nursing Service, caring for British casualties of the Second Anglo-Boer War in South Africa.[13] She had, subsequently, chosen to work as a civilian nurse, but she enlisted for service as part of the QAIMNS Reserve on 6 August 1914.[14] As a Reserve sister of the QAIMNS, Luard was in an enviable position. The 'war fever' of summer 1914 meant that a large proportion of the young female population of Britain were desperately anxious to join their brothers on 'active service' and play their part in Britain's war effort. Even fully trained nurses found it difficult to persuade the Army Medical Services to accept their offers of help. Yet Luard was one of the first nurses to travel overseas with the BEF.[15]

Several of Luard's brothers were already members of – or were soon to join – Britain's armed forces, and this may have had an important influence on her writing. One brother, Frederick, was a captain with a West Indian Regiment; another, Hugh, was an army surgeon; and Frank and Trant were Royal Marines. Alexander had died in an accident on board ship before the war; Frank was killed at Gallipoli in 1915.[16]

On first mobilisation on 9 September 1914, Luard was posted to No. 1 British General Hospital. She subsequently moved several times: her War Office file indicates that she spent time at various general hospitals, stationary hospitals, and casualty clearing stations (CCSs).[17] One posting does not appear in her file: the ambulance train that provides the subject-matter for her first – anonymously published – book, *Diary of a Nursing Sister on the Western Front*.[18] The absence of this posting in the official record is an indication of the chaos of the war's opening months. At this time the front was moving rapidly and unpredictably, and forces were experiencing bloody battles at the River Marne and at Mons, before the so-called 'race to the sea'. Eventually, a system of entrenchments stretching from the North Sea to the Swiss border, which came to be known as the 'Western Front', would form. In its earliest phase, no-one understood that what they were eventually to term the 'Great War' had no precedents. As historian Paul Fussell points out, terms such as 'the race to the sea' had 'the advantage of a familiar sportsmanlike Explorer Club overtone, suggesting that what was happening was not too far distant from playing games, running races, and competing in a thoroughly decent way'.[19] This 'sportsmanlike' tone also pervades Luard's early writings. Women's historian Claire Tylee has commented on the susceptibility of British women to war propaganda.[20] It is difficult to see Luard – a woman with a strong and resolute character – as the victim of propaganda; and yet, like other members of her class, she was steeped in the values of her time – values that emphasised valour, self-sacrifice, and service to the British Empire.[21]

In 1915, when the First World War was still in its early stages, Luard published her first memoir. Her book was compiled from a series of 'journal' entries written for her family, and mailed home to Birch Rectory. Luard had been an avid letter-writer since first leaving home, addressing her frequent letters sometimes to individual siblings, sometimes to an 'inner circle' of close family members, and sometimes to a wider audience of family and friends. In 1915, her siblings persuaded her to have her 'journal' letters compiled into book form and submitted to a publisher. The result is one of the most authentic 'voices' of the First World War.[22] *Diary of a Nursing Sister on the Western Front*, published when the war was only a year old, won glowing reviews. It begins by recounting the thrill of travelling to France from Dublin on a troopship,[23] followed by the tedium of establishing a general hospital in a boggy hay-field. On Sunday 20 September, Luard wrote of how the latest fighting had produced an 'enormous' number of casualties. She had been posted to a railway station, where she offered urgent care to wounded men who were being transported from the front in cattle trucks. They were lying on straw and had only the first field dressings on their wounds. Most were malnourished and dehydrated. Luard, who, as we have seen, was a veteran of the Second Anglo-Boer War, declared that their infected wounds were 'more ghastly than anything I have ever seen or smelt'.[24]

Seven days later she was reporting that she had been appointed to a fully equipped ambulance train and described her feelings in her diary: 'It was worth waiting five weeks to get this; every man or woman stuck at the Base has dreams of getting to the Front, but only one in a hundred gets the dream fulfilled.'[25] But by 25 October, her mood was shifting. Her continuing enthusiasm for hospital train work was being moderated by the horror of what she saw, and she was describing the war as 'carnage'. On its most recent journey, the train had transported 368 wounded men, of whom 200 were dangerously ill. Medical officers were working under enormous pressure in regimental aid posts, and there were, as yet, very few CCSs. Some of the wounded had received treatment only from stretcher-bearers or their own comrades. Equipment was inadequate, and many of those with fractures had only makeshift splints created out of rifles and pick-handles. One had a tourniquet made from a piece of string and a bullet. Luard's *Diary* describes how:

> They were bleeding faster than we could cope with it; and the agony of getting them off the stretchers on to the top bunks is a thing to forget ... All night and without a break till we got back to Boulogne at 4pm next day (yesterday) we grappled with them, and some were not dressed when we got into B—. The head cases were delirious, and trying to get out of the window, and we were giving strychnine and morphia all round. Two were put off dying at St Omer, but we kept the rest alive to Boulogne. The outstanding shining thing that hit you in the eye all through was the universal silent pluck of the men; they stuck it all without a whine or complaint or even a comment: it was 'Would you mind moving my leg when you get time', and 'Thank you very much', or 'That's absolutely glorious', as one boy said of having his bootlace cut, or 'That's grand', when you struck a lucky position for a wound in the back.[26]

In similar vein, she writes of 'one extraordinarily sporting boy' with a neck wound, who had to be fed through a rubber tube, and 'stuck it, smiling all the time',[27] or of a stretcher-bearer with severe leg wounds who nearly died of shock but was 'pulled round somehow', and who, when Luard asked him how he was feeling, replied: 'Quite well, delightfully warm, thank you!'[28]

Such narratives offer a clue as to the purpose of Luard's writing. Its tone is both resolutely positive and hauntingly poignant. Her motivation appears to be to convey to her readership a sense of the courage, tenacity, and fortitude of her patients. In doing so, she is, perhaps

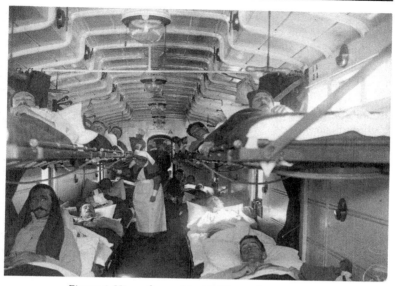

Figure 6 View of a ward inside Hospital Train No. 18

unconsciously, promoting the myth of a 'good war', which later writers such as Vera Brittain and Mary Borden would, with hindsight, deplore.[29] Luard's anxiety was, undoubtedly, to let people 'at home' know of what she saw as the heroism and sacrifice of their brothers and sons. Her writing places a remarkably positive gloss on the sufferings of those sent into battle – not because she wanted to hide the true horror of war, but because she wished her readers to admire the courage and fortitude of the wounded. All around her, as she was writing her *Diary*, were severely – and often irreparably – damaged human beings; yet she chose to interpret their damage as the life-affirming actions of those who were fighting for a better world. It may have been impossible for her to see the war in any other way; and, yet, towards the end of her *Diary*, there is a recognition of the danger of propaganda. In a field hospital close to the front lines in May 1915, she comments on how 'awfully sick' her patients got when they read the newspaper headlines: ' "The Hill 60 Thrill"! "Thrill indeed! There's nothing thrilling about ploughing over parapets into a machine gun, with high explosives bursting round you, – it's merely beastly," said a boy this evening, who is all over shrapnel splinters.'[30] And yet, this boy, like so many others, was valued by Luard for a quality that is so often mentioned by those who nursed the wounded of the First World War – the ability to 'stick it', to overcome fear and remain at their posts until carried away on a stretcher. In similar ways, too, they 'stuck' their treatments, often suffering the agonies of having complex dressing-changes, or minor surgery without anaesthetic.[31]

Luard's later book, *Unknown Warriors*, was published in 1930, and hence might be expected to convey that sense of hindsight that is a feature of many memoirs of the late 1920s and early 1930s.[32] Surprisingly, although the book has more polish, and is clearly more thoroughly edited than Luard's earlier work, and although, this time, she chooses to name herself as its author, *Unknown Warriors* has very much the same tone as *Diary of a Nursing Sister on the Western Front*, and contains similar content. Luard chooses, once again, to quote directly from her diary and letters, resulting in a text that has a compelling sense of immediacy. Perhaps the success of *Diary of a Nursing Sister* induced her to retain the same style for her later book, or perhaps it was a matter of conviction for her to relate her diary entries as they stood, with apparently very little alteration, in the belief that they contained a 'truer' account of events than any later reminiscences would be able to convey. Again, Luard's intention seems to be to convey the heroism of the wounded. The title of the book itself provides a clue to her desire to bear witness to what she sees as the remarkable qualities of those who fought, were injured, and died in the Great War.

One of the most poignant features of *Unknown Warriors* is the way in which it allows the reader to follow the progress or deterioration of individual, named, patients. A sequence of entries that begins on 29 May 1915 follows the fortunes of a 'rush of in-extremis cases' to the CCS. Three die within hours of their arrival. Luard reports that 'there seems to be an unusual number of charming boys, who have joined in tremendous keenness and are now filling the cemetery'.[33] This sentence is typical of her writing, which is both succinct and purposeful. The men who have died are both 'charming' and 'keen'; actually, though, they are so youthful that they are not men at all – only boys. The phrase 'filling the cemetery' is a deliberate exaggeration. The 'boys' who arrived that morning did not literally 'fill' the cemetery – yet Luard's words fed a post-war generation's vision of the iconic rows of white gravestones that formed the orderly and crowded war cemeteries created by the War Graves Commission in the 1920s. Luard's vision of slaughter and sacrifice merges with the perceptions of survivors, which, themselves, merge myth with reality.[34]

Having reported on the rush of cases received that morning, Luard's 'entry' for 29 May continues:

> One called Reggie something, who talks like a gentleman, is slowly losing the fight with a lung wound. And another called Jack is paralysed from a fractured spine. He says wonderingly, 'What is it, Sister? I can't move my legs – will it be alright?'
>
> My two gas gangrene boys side by side with continuous drips on their arm and leg stumps have never once lost their mental balance or fussed or cried or fretted. Their chief anxiety is to say 'thank you' and to smile and to say 'What should we do without you?'

Two days later, Luard's diary describes how she has been able to 'slip away' from the hospital for a walk to a nearby slag heap. From its summit, she is able to sit on the grass among ox-eye daisies and survey the British Front. Yet tonight she is back with her patient 'Jack'. Her writing conveys a vivid impression of immediacy – the work of a night nurse writing at a desk in the centre of a quiet surgical ward, full of severely wounded and acutely ill patients:

> Jack is dying to-night, paralysed from a wound in the spine. He doesn't know what is the matter with him and can't feel anything, so he goes on smiling and making polite little jokes, and thanking and apologizing till we could all cry. Reggie is worse to-night. He holds out his small hand and says, 'Will you come and sit by me for a little while and hold my hand – it encourages me.' A boy who has lost one eye and can't see out of the other said this evening, 'I do feel bad, will you come and talk to me?' and you hardly ever can.[35]

Luard's fragments are more moving than any studied account of the men's injuries would have been. She opens a window onto a scene of suffering and endurance – but only momentarily – and she juxtaposes the scene where she is able to escape (to a slag heap) and see the ox-eye daisies, before returning the reader to the relentless reality of 'Jack's' slow death: 'Jack is alive still but very weak and wandering, asking us all day to take off his boots; we scrabble about with his bare feet and he is happy for a moment, and then begins again.' In the same entry, the reader is offered a brief 'other-worldly' vision of the garden at home in England, as Luard comments on the letters she has received from her sisters. Her commitment to the war effort is then revealed as she declares, tersely, 'we have got to take the top of this Vimy Ridge', before returning to descriptions of her wounded patients: '*Friday, June 2nd* … Jack died at half-past ten last night, and three abdominals: this time they have been about the most appalling shell wounds I've ever seen – how they get here alive I don't know.'[36]

Other stories emerge, such as a narrative of 'Walter', who says, when Luard is washing him: 'Mother thinks the world o' me. I'm the eldest, I'm glad she can't see me now.' She adds: 'There's a worn-out Newcastle man with a wound in his liver who when he is uncomfortable wails, "I can't find a resting place. I shouldn't mind nothin' if I could find a resting place."'[37] Luard's use of the men's voices to develop her narrative is probably a deliberate attempt to make these patients real for her readership – to bring home the realities of their suffering and to give them voice. The tendency to use colloquialisms and convey a variety of accents may be due to a desire to make these voices as authentic as possible. For Luard's 1930s audience, they may have made the men more real and their plight more pitiable. And yet the distinction between Luard's own commentary, offered in cultured 'King's English', and the accents of her patients conveys a sense of class distinction. It also suggests that Luard felt maternal towards her patients – her voice is a fully adult one, whist theirs are often childlike. Indeed, one 'little Lancashire lad in the big ward … calls out "Howd on Mother" when you are going to touch him. He calls us all Mother – "Give over, Mother" is his favourite way of saying he's had enough. His name is Joe.'[38]

On 6 June, Luard records that 'Reggie is going to be put on the train to-morrow. His mother will cry when she sees the little panting skeleton who was a marching soldier when she last saw him. But it's a wonder that she sees him at all: it didn't seem possible he could live with such holes in his lung.'[39] Luard's ability to juxtapose hope with horror is one of the most powerful elements of her writing. The way in which she traces 'Reggie's' progress from 'dangerously ill' patient who is 'slowly losing the fight with a lung wound', to 'panting skeleton' on his way home to his mother, offers her readers a glimpse of what she sees as the true rewards of her nursing work.

Kate Luard's war record was one of dedicated service, characterised by extraordinary courage and commitment. She clearly believed that her own courage must match that of her patients, and was mentioned in dispatches on 1 January 1916 and 24 December 1917.[40] In January 1916 she was awarded the Royal Red Cross (First Class),[41] a decoration that had been created by Royal Warrant in 1883 to ensure that distinguished service by nurses would be recognised.[42] Her War Office file contains glowing references from matrons of various military hospitals on the Western Front. Sister Wrage, assistant matron of No. 16 General Hospital, reported that 'Miss Luard has an extremely good influence on every round her [sic], and is a most clever, capable sister.'[43] In similar style, G. A. Howe, the matron of No. 47 General Hospital, 'found her a most capable ward sister, and a good disciplinarian', adding that 'she exerted a very good influence on all her staff'.[44]

One of the most challenging periods for the medical and nursing services on the Western Front was the spring of 1918, following the German counter-attack. During this time, Luard was sister in charge of No. 41 CCS, close to a volatile and rapidly moving front line. The medical officer in charge of the CCS, Lieut. Col. S. B. Evans, reported that she had 'performed her duties in an eminently capable manner: showing at all times, tact, sound judgement, patience and marked administration powers'. He ends by commenting that 'no one could have shown more zeal and untiring energy'.[45]

After more than four years of service with the BEF, Kate Luard's military service came to a premature and rather sad end. On 23 November 1918, she wrote to her matron at No. 10 General Hospital requesting permission to terminate her service. Her father was very ill and was said to be 'constantly asking for her'. Her resignation was accepted in a letter dated 16 December.[46]

Kate Luard surfaces again in the historical record on 20 March 1919, in a letter written by her to Maud McCarthy, former matron-in-chief of the BEF in France. Luard comments that her age is preventing her from obtaining work (she was, by this time, in her late forties) and requests a testimonial. McCarthy's response is to write both a brief testimonial, stating that Luard was 'a splendid woman – capable of any amount of work and strong', and a more lengthy statement of support, mirroring the comments of Luard's wartime colleagues:

> She is capable of doing a great deal of work. She has performed charge duties at the front almost continuously since May 1915 under the most trying and distressing conditions. She was constantly in areas where bombing

raids were taking place. Her health is excellent. She is a devoted nurse and has the gift of getting on well with all under whom she serves.[47]

Luard's last professional appointment was as 'Lady Matron' of Bradfield College, a private boys' school, where she was clearly very popular with both staff and pupils. An obituary in the alumni magazine, written by an 'old boy' of the school, alludes to her 'essential humanity underlying a determined character', commenting that: 'to be brought to her shocked after some accident was to know all the reassurance given by devotion, gentleness and efficiency'.[48]

The words of this 'old boy' leave the reader with a sense that Luard had never lost the staunch and sympathetic manner she had shown towards her earlier 'boys': those young men – many of them barely out of school – to whom she had devoted four years of her life during the Great War. For Kate Luard, the war was a simple matter. In her writings she rarely judged, rarely commented on the political or strategic decisions that brought patients in their thousands to the doors of her general hospitals and CCSs. She appears to have accepted warfare as something inevitable. Perhaps this is understandable in a woman from a middle-class English family, several of whose brothers fought in the conflict. She comes across as a highly intelligent and articulate woman, yet also as one who never questioned the norms of her time, or the decisions of those in authority. This is unsurprising when one considers how steeped in the traditions of both clergy and army her background was. In this sense she was the perfect military nurse. Her character, whilst far from simple, was astonishingly pure and unsullied for someone who had clearly encountered some of the worst horrors of the First World War.

Kate Luard worked as 'Lady Matron' of Bradfield College for several years before being forced to retire by a back problem, the nature of which is unknown, though it is difficult to avoid speculation on its possible origins in her onerous and heavy nursing work. In old age, she lived with two sisters in Wickham Bishops, Essex. She became increasingly disabled and eventually found herself dependent on others, a situation that was 'trying to someone of such energetic and independent character'.[49] Katherine Evelyn Luard died on 18 August 1962 at the age of ninety.

In Talbot House, Poperinghe, east of Ypres in Belgium, there is a sepia photograph on display. It captures the moment when a nurse bends over a patient lying on a wooden bed. Beside the photograph is a quotation from *Unknown Warriors*:

> When I comforted the boy, he said: 'You're the best sister in the world – I know I'm a nuisance, but I can't help it – I've been out there and I am so young – will you give me a sleeping draft and a drop of champagne to make me strong?' He had both and slept like a lamb, but he died today.[50]

Alice Fitzgerald: entrapped nurse

American nurse Alice Fitzgerald volunteered to work with the British QAIMNS in 1916. She nursed British and Dominion troops in France until the winter of 1917, when she moved to take up a senior position with the American Red Cross. She was 'gifted' to the British by a committee of Boston philanthropists, who funded her travel and living expenses and named her 'The Edith Cavell Nurse from Massachusetts'.[51] The offer of assistance to the allies was intended as a mark of respect and remembrance for the sacrifice of British nurse Edith Cavell, who had been executed by the Germans on 12 October 1915.[52]

Alice Fitzgerald wrote a memoir of her life as a wealthy society lady who entered formal nurse training, and then volunteered for war service. She added to this an edited version of her 'War Diary'. Her ladylike background and her enthusiasm and capacity for nurse leadership made Fitzgerald an obvious choice to be the Boston social elite's 'Edith Cavell Nurse'. Her 'Diary' begins on the day she left New York in February 1916. The last entry is dated 15 December 1917, and recounts her decision to leave the British Expeditionary Force (BEF) and join the American Red Cross.[53] Twenty years later, in 1936, Fitzgerald added twenty-two pages of 'memoirs' to a typescript of the diary. In this brief prologue she wrote of her childhood in various parts of Europe, her privileged upbringing, her determination to become a nurse, and her training. This introductory 'Memoir', which ends with her journey to London to join the BEF, is written as if she is sitting in a chair before a fire in her London lodgings, dreaming of her former life and of the adventure to come. It is impossible to tell whether the text was actually written on that night in London, or composed later and 'placed' in the London blackout for artistic reasons.[54]

Fitzgerald later went on to write a full memoir of her life, incorporating lengthy excerpts from her war diary into the chapters relating to her war service. Of her purpose in keeping a diary Fitzgerald writes very self-consciously, apparently intending her record of the war to be read by future generations. Although she made a number of attempts to find a publisher, the memoir remained unpublished and is now lodged in the Maryland Historical Society Archives in Baltimore, USA.[55] The only extant, published writings belonging to her consist of a set of letters to her Boston committee, published by committee members in 1917, as *The Edith Cavell Nurse from Massachusetts*, in an obvious attempt to gain support for the war effort.[56]

Fitzgerald lists the locations in which she wrote her diary: 'in London, at 13 General Hospital in Boulogne, at a hospital in St Pol near Bethune in the north, and at a casualty clearing station buried in mud along the Somme Front, where the Germans surrounded us on three sides, and the guns belched, and the shells whined and Death held a festival day and night'.[57] She adds an intriguing disclaimer:

> My diary was not written with any idea of propaganda or even of publication. It was the day by day account of events in a war-mad world set down as they were actually happening, chiefly as an outlet for my pent-up feelings. It is far too long to quote in full and many of the entries, especially those made near the battle front, are but daily narrations of the same theme of suffering, death, destruction and human endurance beyond belief, of waste and futility and useless sacrifice which is war at close quarters.[58]

Alice Fitzgerald's time with the British military nursing services was an intensely stressful one, and her problems appear to have been compounded by her status as an 'outsider' from a neutral country. Her Boston committee's offer of her services to Britain was made 'in the hope that it may be this nurse's high fortune to serve not only the Allies' heroic wounded but their prisoners'.[59] Fitzgerald's work with the BEF was, from the first, affected by the ambivalence of her position. Although the humanitarian nature of her work, and the strong similarities between British and American nursing techniques and training, gave her much in common with her British colleagues, her political neutrality, combined with her age (forty-two at the time of her departure for France) and the fact that, as a guest, she was provided with her own, rather than shared, accommodation, threatened to isolated her. Her powerful personality and diplomatic skill appear to have done much to ameliorate her situation.[60] Her diary resonates with anxiety and conveys a sense of an individual who is attempting to cover her unhappiness with a determinedly positive spirit.

Fitzgerald chose to train at one of the most prestigious nurse training schools of her day: the Johns Hopkins Hospital Training School in Baltimore, whose superintendent was the formidable Adelaide Nutting.[61] In 1908, she had her first experience of humanitarian work overseas, when she travelled to Messina, Italy, to assist the Red Cross relief effort following an earthquake.[62] In the first decades of the twentieth century, she held prestigious positions at the Johns Hopkins Hospital; the Bellevue Hospital, New York; the General Hospital, Wilkes-Barre, Pennsylvania; the Robert W. Long Hospital, Indianapolis, Indiana; and Dana Hall School, Wellesley, Massachusetts.[63] Her service in France with the BEF returned her to the role of 'nursing sister' – one that she appears to have embraced.

Her early nursing career had been remarkable for the way in which it opened up opportunities to travel and seek out promotion in the vast and expanding field that was late-nineteenth-century America. Such mobility was not unusual for a successful nurse. In this sense, her training, initially, gave Fitzgerald freedom to travel, to seek both adventure and promotion, and to attain the highest level of clinical and managerial skill of which she was capable. It was only after she accepted the invitation of the Edith Cavell Memorial Committee and joined the BEF that her life became constrained and her freedom curtailed. At first this seemed a small price to pay, and one of Fitzgerald's early letters home refers to her feeling 'very deeply the strength of my mission'.[64] The book of her letters is an intriguing and clearly highly selective account of Fitzgerald's experiences, opinions, and feelings. Although the letters were probably published largely unabridged and unedited, they reveal a remarkable degree of self-censorship. Fitzgerald's sense of adventure, her belief in the importance of her work, and her assertive determination to experience life close to the front lines can be read through the letters. Yet, her relentless cheerfulness and insistently positive tone strike a false note – as when she comments that 'I am right in the thick of it now; and the shells whizz by our ears in great style. It is queer that, where there is such real danger, one does not think of it.'[65] This enforced cheerfulness becomes more clearly false when one compares the letters against her manuscript diary, in which she reflects: 'the more I see of these terrible cases the more I worry about every man caught in this awful war.'[66]

Alice Fitzgerald offers contrasting perspectives on her wartime experience. While it is difficult to know which is the most revealing of her true perspectives – the cheerful 'letters home', or the more reflective diary entries – it seems likely that the unpublished account is the 'truer' of the two: more revealing of her actual experiences and feelings. Her earliest letters resonate with a sense of adventure, which is heightened as she moves closer to the front lines, from No. 13 General Hospital in Boulogne, via No. 12 Stationary Hospital at St Pol, to the battered and muddy Second London CCS (given the ironic nickname 'Grovetown') at Meaulte, within sight and sound of shelling.[67] Following her first two months in Boulogne, she comments that 'the English Tommies are the most wonderful men – never a grumble, never a loud word, and they stand pain like super-human beings. It is best not to stop and think too much; one could never do the work.'[68] In April 1916 she recounts her experience of nursing several horrific 'cases', among them Jones, with a 'wound of buttocks and rectum', who 'was taken to the operating room where a large piece of shell was removed and wound packed; he suffered agonies and died two hours later'. Of another, similar case, she comments that she had 'never seen a live man with so much dead flesh on him'.[69]

By the time Fitzgerald reached 'Grovetown' her mood had been further modified by her encounters with other horrific results of industrial warfare. Eventually, a tone of deep anxiety becomes unmistakable in her writing – one, however, that is still heavily and deliberately masked by the forced cheerfulness of her letters. She writes, for example, of a 'beautiful air fight' that took place over her camp.[70] Later, she comments that 'if noises could kill, we should all be corpses. It is roar, roar, roar, day and night – guns nearer by with their louder reports, air craft fights, anti-air-craft guns, bombs exploding, German shells whizzing over our camp. And with it all, it is a blessing to be busy.'[71] But in the personal diary, she allows herself to reveal her fear, as she becomes fully aware of the damage that war could do – indeed, in many ways, is already doing – to her. She comments that 'the exploding of bombs and the pounding of heavy field artillery helped to fill in the pages in the dreadful story of War of which I had read only the outlines in Boulogne'. She becomes aware that 'lying down is the only safe position as the shells burst upward after striking and the fragments pass over you'.[72]

In the late summer and autumn of 1916, even Fitzgerald's cheerful letters home to her committee begin to take on a more serious tone: 'I have come to the conclusion that even in the very small part that I play, each day makes me a week older. I cannot quite explain it. It is not only the hard work, but the whole situation and atmosphere in which we live.[73]

In late September 1916, as the numbers of casualties from the Battle of the Somme began to abate slightly, Fitzgerald did obtain some respite from her relentless work at 'Grovetown'. To her committee in Boston, she wrote: 'I suppose you have read about the "Tanks"? I went into one the other day – pure cheek! Every one laughs, and says, "Trust USA to get there!"'[74] In her memoir, she offers a much more detailed description of her excursion 'out of bounds', and of her discovery of three tanks, which are 'like some sort of gigantic beast … I can readily understand how they could strike terror into anyone.[75]

On 23 September Fitzgerald experienced a 'terrifying night':

> I had already gone to sleep when I was awakened by unusually loud reports and I was just thinking how queer it was to bring back the big guns and place them near to us when suddenly the earth shook to the accompaniment of a terrific crash which I can only compare to the sudden collapse of a thousand buildings with the crumbling of stone and the shattering of glass and metal.[76]

A high-explosive bomb had been dropped from a German *Taube* just outside 'Grovetown'. Another such night came on 10 October, and in early November things become even worse, when an ammunition dump nearby was struck by German bombing. In her diary, Fitzgerald describes 'the concussion felt after an explosion … the horrible sinking feeling that grips you as you wait for the next jolt which you know is bound to come'.[77] She began to take a sedative before going to bed each night, and on 10 November, recorded that her fear of facial injury had become so acute that she had borrowed a steel helmet from one of the sergeants; this she placed over her face every night as soon as the bombing began.[78]

In addition to constant fear, Fitzgerald and her British colleagues experienced real hardship. In some of the tents of the CCS there was no flooring, and nurses were obliged to 'slip and slop around in great style'. 'What is nursing here?', Fitzgerald writes in her diary, after a day in which she has knelt in mud between stretchers to care for, dress, and feed her patients, with insufficient time to provide for anything but their most basic and essential needs. She could 'more readily understand what terrible hardships the men are suffering in the trenches in this kind of weather with never a chance to dry out'.[79] In September she began to experience a series of minor ailments, which gradually worsened – first colitis (caused, she believed, by the dampness of her quarters); next exhaustion; and then chilblains, which, in November, began to spread across the whole of both feet. The situation was made worse by an autocratic commanding officer who refused to allow her (or any of the other nurses) to travel to Amiens for new shoes.[80]

As the winter weather became colder, Fitzgerald found that the only way of keeping warm was to sleep in woollen pyjamas, bed socks, and a dressing gown, inside a sleeping bag, covered by two rugs, a fur-lined coat, and a rubber sheet. In stormy weather, she was obliged to go out and re-peg her tent every few hours throughout the night, aware that, 'no matter how bad things might be, they would be much worse if my tent fell down on me'. On 14 December she wrote:

> The last few days have been like a nightmare to look back upon. I have had a touch of influenza and my feet have grown worse and are agonizingly painful all the time day and night. At times in the ward, I could have screamed from the pain, yet I cannot get permission to go to Amiens to get shoes … In addition to these two very personal troubles, the work has been simply overwhelming and I just could not give in.[81]

Yet her letters to her Boston committee are still pervaded by her attempts to retain her sense of humour. In a letter despatched towards the end of the year, she writes: 'I am in the thick of it, as this is the nearest Casualty Clearing Station to the Front. I assure you I am all but in the trenches!'. She adds that it is impossible to get leave, 'unless I am taken in a "box", which is perfectly possible'.[82] A glance at Fitzgerald's personal memoir reveals that she did manage to obtain 'leave' on 31 December. Upon her arrival in London, she consulted a doctor who promptly prescribed a sedative for 'shell shock'.[83]

In Fitzgerald's unpublished memoir, the reader comes face-to-face with the full reality of a war in which men endure extreme hardship and are irrecoverably maimed. On 25 September 1916, she writes:

> The rush is on. I have never spent such a day. Two wards full with 120 patients and as fast as we could get them dressed they were taken to the evacuation tent and others took their places. I never worked harder nor more hopelessly in my life as we only had time for the barest of care for each … At times I feel completely hopeless and do not know where to turn next so as not to leave anything important undone … Blood is thick over the uniforms and flies settle on the bloody spots. It is ghastly … The only consolation I can think of is that they might still be lying on the battle field.[84]

So many of her patients came to the CCS already suffering from gas gangrene infections that she felt she could not get away from 'the awful smell of it' – even in her own tent. In October 1917, Fitzgerald resigned her posting with the QAIMNS and accepted a senior position with the American Red Cross. Although onerous, this allowed her to take a more supervisory and less physically demanding role.

On Armistice Day, when 'the sorrow and anxiety of four hideous years were suddenly transformed into irrepressible joy', Fitzgerald had been on active service almost constantly for over two years. She continued to work for the Red Cross, arranging relief for former prisoners-of-war. During one trip through the aptly named 'devastated zone', she passed the site of the CCS in which she had spent the last four months of 1916. Her memoir records how 'a flood of memories of days with the B.E.F. overwhelmed me; memories of mud and blood and horrible nights; of thundering guns and dropping bombs; of super human courage and useless sacrifice'.[85]

Conclusion: professional nurses in military hospitals

Not all nurses in Britain and the USA came from wealthy and elite social backgrounds. The majority were still drawn from the lower social classes. Some belonged to impoverished 'gentry' families, while others were working-class women seeking social advancement.[86] Yet women such as Kate Luard and Alice Fitzgerald may be viewed as part of a 'professional vanguard' that aimed to demonstrate to both medical practitioners and hospital governors that a disciplined nursing service was essential to good patient care. This lesson was translated only with difficulty into military practice. The harsh challenges faced by Fitzgerald within the somewhat chauvinistic scenario of 'Grovetown' contrast with the ease and collegiality with which she had worked with senior surgeons such as William Osler and Harvey Cushing in Baltimore.

The position of elite professional nurses such as Luard and Fitzgerald was an inherently ambiguous one: their contribution to the care of sick and injured men was recognised, but their presence close to the front lines of battle was still regarded with suspicion. By the time they were nursing the wounded of the First World War, theirs had become a respectable 'profession' for women of high social status. Nevertheless, its lingering taint as work for women of poor reputation meant that Fitzgerald's parents had had serious reservations about its suitability for their daughter. And these reservations appear to have been shared by many within the military medical establishment. Such ambivalence does not appear to have had any great impact on the thinking of either Luard or Fitzgerald. Both wrote with confidence and, although at times they experienced great stress, the role ambiguities they faced do not seem to have detracted from their certainties about the value and significance of their work.

Notes

1 Mark Bostridge, *Florence Nightingale: The Woman and Her Legend* (London: Viking, 2008).

2 Mary Boykin Chesnut, *Mary Chesnut's Diary*, with introduction by Catherine Clinton (New York: Penguin, 2011); Harriet Eaton, *This Birth Place of Souls: The Civil War Nursing Diary of Harriet Eaton*, ed. Jane E. Schultz (Oxford: Oxford University Press, 2010); Jane E. Schultz, *Women at the Front: Hospital Workers in Civil War America* (Chapel Hill: University of North Carolina Press, 2004).

3 Patricia D'Antonio, *American Nursing: A History of Knowledge, Authority, and the Meaning of Work* (Baltimore: John's Hopkins University Press, 2010).

4 Midori Yamaguchi states that Luard's given names were Katherine Evelyn, in that order. Her pen-name, for her book *Unknown Warriors*, was 'Kate Luard'. Her family is said to have referred to her as 'Evelyn' or 'Evie'. Midori Yamaguchi, '"Unselfish" Desires: Daughters of the Anglican Clergy, 1830–1914' (unpublished Ph.D. thesis, University of Essex, 2001). I am indebted to Kate Luard's great nephew, Tim Luard, with whom I worked on an introduction for a new edition of *Unknown Warriors*; and to her great nieces: Caroline Stevens, who

edited the new edition, and Catherine Fry, who provided valuable material and insights into her great aunt's life. See: Kate Luard, *Unknown Warriors: The Letters of Kate Luard, R.R.C. and Bar., Nursing Sister in France 1914–1918*, ed. John Stevens and Caroline Stevens (Stroud: History Press, 2014).

5 Yamaguchi, '"Unselfish" Desires', Chapter 8, 'Writing a Family of a Clergy Daughter': 281–325 (284). See also: Leonore Davidoff and Catherine Hall, *Family Fortunes: Men and Women of the English Middle Class, 1780–1850*, rev. edn (London: Routledge, 2002 [1987]).

6 John Lawson and Harold Silver, *A Social History of Education in England* (London: Methuen, 1973): 341–4.

7 Kate attended for three years from 1887 until 1890: Yamaguchi, '"Unselfish" Desires': 306–7.

8 Yamaguchi, '"Unselfish" Desires': 315–16.

9 'Kate Evelyn Luard' is entered into the Register for Nurses for 1923 as registrant no. 1495. It is stated that she trained at King's College Hospital, London, between 1897 and 1900: Register for Nurses, 1923, General Part, Archive of the Nursing and Midwifery Council, London.

10 Jane Brooks, 'Structured by Class, Bound by Gender: Nursing and Special Probationer Schemes, 1860–1939', *International History of Nursing Journal*, 6.2 (2001): 13–21.

11 Many of the earliest 'specials' – famous nurses such as Eva Luckes and Isla Stewart – became matrons of prestigious institutions in their mid-twenties. See Susan McGann, *The Battle of the Nurses: A Study of Eight Women who Influenced the Development of Professional Nursing, 1880–1930* (London: Scutari Press, 1992): 9–34, 35–57; Winifred Hector, *The Work of Mrs Bedford Fenwick and the Rise of Professional Nursing* (London: Royal College of Nursing, 1973): 2.

12 On the gentrification of nursing, see: Brian Abel-Smith, *A History of the Nursing Profession* (London: Heinemann, 1960): 17–35; Christopher Maggs, *The Origins of General Nursing* (London: Croom Helm, 1983): 63–87; Anne Simnett, 'The Pursuit of Respectability: Women and the Nursing Profession', in Rosemary White (ed.), *Political Issues in Nursing: Past, Present and Future*, 3 vols (Chichester: John Wiley and Sons, 1986–88), Vol. II; Robert Dingwall, Anne Marie Rafferty, and Charles Webster, *An Introduction to the Social History of Nursing* (London: Routledge, 1988): 69–70.

13 Kate Luard War Office file, WO 399/5023, record of service in South Africa: register no. 4862/Reserve/3387, The National Archives, Kew, London, UK.

14 The Reserve of the QAIMNS had been created as part of the Haldane reforms in 1908. Luard's signing for service was registered by her brother, the Revd Edwin Percy Luard of Birch Rectory, Colchester: Kate Luard War Office file, WO 399/5023.

15 On 'war fever' amongst nurses, see: Anon., 'The Nursing Outlook: War Fever and War Spirit', *The Nursing Mirror and Midwives Journal*, 19 (22 August 1914): 397. On the eagerness of young men to participate, see: Niall Ferguson,

The Pity of War (London: Allen Lane, 1998); Eric Leed, *No Man's Land: Combat and Identity in World War One* (New York: Cambridge University Press, 1979); Modris Eksteins, *Rites of Spring: The Great War and the Birth of the Modern Age* (Boston, MA: Houghton Mifflin, 1989).

16 Yamaguchi, '"Unselfish" Desires'.

17 Luard's War Office file indicates that she was based at No. 16 General Hospital, No. 32 CCS, No. 12 Stationary Hospital, No. 10 Stationary Hospital, and No. 37 CCS. There is also a reference from the matron of No. 47 General Hospital: Kate Luard War Office file, WO 399/5023.

18 Anon., *Diary of a Nursing Sister on the Western Front 1914–1915* (Edinburgh and London: William Blackwood and Sons, 1915).

19 Paul Fussell, *The Great War and Modern Memory* (Oxford: Oxford University Press, 2000 [1975]): 9.

20 Claire Tylee, *The Great War and Women's Consciousness: Images of Militarism and Womanhood in Women's Writings, 1914–64* (Houndmills and London: Macmillan, 1990): 19–46.

21 Michael Paris, *Warrior Nation: Images of War in British Popular Culture, 1850–2000* (London: Reaktion Books, 2000), *passim*. On wartime propaganda, see: Peter Buitenhuis, *The Great War of Words: Literature as Propaganda, 1914–18 and After* (London: B. T. Batsford, 1989 [1987]).

22 Many of Kate Luard's letters are available at the Essex Record Office, Colchester, UK, Luard family papers, files 55/13/1–4, D/Dlu 58. I am indebted to Tim Luard for providing me with transcripts of excerpts from many of these letters. See also: Christine Hallett and Tim Luard, introduction to Luard, *Unknown Warriors* (2014 edn): 9–20.

23 Anon., *Diary of a Nursing Sister*: 3.

24 Anon., *Diary of a Nursing Sister*: 40–1. For a brief account of Kate Luard's early experiences of the First World War, see: Christine E. Hallett, *Veiled Warriors: Allied Nurses of the First World War* (Oxford: Oxford University Press, 2014): Chapter 1.

25 Anon., *Diary of a Nursing Sister*: 52–3. On nursing work on hospital trains, see: Hallett, *Veiled Warriors*: Chapter 1.

26 Anon., *Diary of a Nursing Sister*: 88–90.

27 Anon., *Diary of a Nursing Sister*: 206.

28 Anon., *Diary of a Nursing Sister*: 212.

29 Vera Brittain, *Testament of Youth: An Autobiographical Study of the Years 1900–1925* (London: Virago Press, 2004 [1933]); Mary Borden, *The Forbidden Zone* (London: William Heinemann, 1929).

30 Anon., *Diary of a Nursing Sister*: 289.

31 Christine Hallett, *Containing Trauma: Nursing Work in the First World War* (Manchester: Manchester University Press, 2009): 155–93.

32 Kate Luard, *Unknown Warriors: Extracts from the Letters of K. E. Luard, R.R.C., Nursing Sister in France* (London: Chatto and Windus, 1930).

33 Luard, *Unknown Warriors* (1930): 73.

34 On memorials and mourning, see: Jay Winter, *Sites of Memory, Sites of Mourning: The Great War in European Cultural History* (Cambridge: Cambridge University Press, 1995): 78–116.

35 Luard, *Unknown Warriors* (1930): 73–4.

36 Luard, *Unknown Warriors* (1930): 74–5.

37 Luard, *Unknown Warriors* (1930): 77–8.

38 Luard, *Unknown Warriors* (1930): 80–1.

39 Luard, *Unknown Warriors* (1930): 78–81.

40 Kate Luard War Office file, WO 399/5203, supplement to the *London Gazette* (1 January 1916): 69.

41 Kate Luard War Office file, WO 399/5023.

42 Anne Summers, *Angels and Citizens: British Women as Military Nurses, 1854–1914* (London: Routledge and Kegan Paul, 1988).

43 Kate Luard War Office file, WO 399/5023, confidential report on work at No. 16 General Hospital (16 October 1915).

44 Kate Luard War Office file, WO 399/5023, confidential report from matron of No. 47 General Hospital (22 November 1918).

45 Kate Luard War Office file, WO 399/5023, confidential report from S. B. Evans, Lieut. Col. O.C., No. 41 CCS.

46 Kate Luard War Office file, WO 399/5023, letter of resignation; letter and memorandum signed by Maud McCarthy, matron.

47 Kate Luard War Office file, WO 399/5023, testimonials by Maud McCarthy (2 and 3 April 1919).

48 Anon., 'Miss K. E. Luard, R.R.C.', obituary, clipping from the Bradfield College Alumni Magazine (undated); from the private collection of Caroline Stevens.

49 Anon., 'Miss K. E. Luard, R.R.C.'.

50 The note beside the photograph and quotation is: 'Sister Kate Luard, Army Nursing Sister Reserve, No. 32 CCS (Brandhock) 7 August, 1917'. The quotation is from: Luard, *Unknown Warriors* (1930): 210. I am greatly indebted to Caroline Stevens for bringing my attention to this and other sources.

51 The 'Edith Cavell Committee' was composed of a number of influential Bostonians: William Roscoe Thayer, Philip Cabot, Rosalind Huidekoper Greene, Henry Copley Greene, and William Ernest Hocking. It announced its intention to offer the services of an American trained nurse to the BEF at a memorial service held in Steinert Hall, Boston on 11 December 1915: Anon. (ed.), *The Edith Cavell Nurse from Massachusetts: A Record of One Year's Personal Service with the British Expeditionary Force in France; Boulogne–the Somme, 1916–1917. With an Account of the Imprisonment, Trial and Death of Edith Cavell* (Boston, MA: W. A. Butterfield, 1917): i–vi.

52 Anon., *The Edith Cavell Nurse*. Edith Cavell had been executed for 'returning soldiers to the enemy'. See: Jonathan Evans, *Edith Cavell* (London: London Hospital Museum, 2008); Diana Souhami, *Edith Cavell* (London: Quercus, 2010).

53 There are four different versions of Fitzgerald's memoir/diary at the Maryland Historical Society Archives, Baltimore, Maryland. The two that were most closely consulted for this work were: Alice Fitzgerald, 'Memoirs', MS 987, Box 2; and Alice Fitzgerald, unpublished memoirs incorporating war diary, *c.* 1936, Alice Fitzgerald Papers, Md HR M2633, Md HR M2634, unpaginated. I am deeply indebted to Colleen Bowers and Dean Foreman for providing me with a complete scanned copy of this version.

54 Fitzgerald, 'Memoirs': 1–21.

55 Fitzgerald, 'Memoirs'.

56 Anon., *The Edith Cavell Nurse*.

57 Fitzgerald, 'Memoirs': 22.

58 Fitzgerald, 'Memoirs': 22.

59 Anon., *The Edith Cavell Nurse*: iv; these words are also quoted verbatim in the *BJN*'s report of Fitzgerald's appointment: Anon., 'An Edith Cavell Memorial Nurse', *BJN* (4 March 4 1916): 214.

60 It has been said that Alice Fitzgerald was 'noted for her diplomacy': Alice Howell Friedman, 'Fitzgerald, Alice Louise Florence', in Martin Kaufman (ed.), *Dictionary of American Nursing Biography* (New York: Greenwood Press, 1988): 122.

61 M. Adelaide Nutting and Lavinia L. Dock, *A History of Nursing: The Evolution of Nursing Systems from the Earliest Times to the Foundation of the First English and American Training Schools for Nurses*, 4 vols (New York and London: G. P. Putnam's Sons, 1907–12). See also: Minnie Goodnow, *Outlines of Nursing History* (W. B. Saunders: Philadelphia, 1923).

62 Anon., *The Edith Cavell Nurse*: v–vi; Friedman, 'Fitzgerald, Alice Louise Florence': 121; Anon., 'An Edith Cavell Memorial Nurse'.

63 Friedman, 'Fitzgerald, Alice Louise Florence': 121.

64 Anon., *The Edith Cavell Nurse*: 14.

65 Anon., *The Edith Cavell Nurse*: 26.

66 Fitzgerald, 'Memoirs': 35.

67 These details are taken from the unpublished memoir and diary: Fitzgerald, 'Memoirs'.

68 Anon., *The Edith Cavell Nurse*: 5.

69 Fitzgerald, 'Memoirs': 38–9.

70 Anon., *The Edith Cavell Nurse*: 15.

71 Anon., *The Edith Cavell Nurse*: 30.

72 Fitzgerald, 'Memoirs', Chapter 4, 'Along the Somme Front': 64–108.

73 Anon., *The Edith Cavell Nurse*: 24–5.

74 Anon., *The Edith Cavell Nurse*: 31–2.

75 Fitzgerald, 'Memoirs': 71. On the use of tanks on the Somme, see: Fussell, *The Great War and Modern Memory*: 16.

76 Fitzgerald, 'Memoirs': 71–2. On this episode, see also: Hallett, *Veiled Warriors*: 181.

77 Fitzgerald, 'Memoirs': 89–90.
78 Fitzgerald, 'Memoirs': 91.
79 Fitzgerald, 'Memoirs': 75. See also: Hallett, *Veiled Warriors*: 181–2.
80 Fitzgerald, 'Memoirs': 98–9.
81 Fitzgerald, 'Memoirs': 101.
82 Anon., *The Edith Cavell Nurse*: 31–2.
83 Fitzgerald, 'Memoirs': 110–11.
84 Fitzgerald, unpublished memoirs.
85 Fitzgerald 'Memoirs': 181.
86 Maggs, *The Origins of General Nursing*; Simnett, 'The Pursuit of Respectability'; Sue Hawkins, *Nursing and Women's Labour in the Nineteenth Century: The Quest for Independence* (London: Routledge, 2010).

5

American nurses in Europe

Introduction: American nurses and the war in Europe

Some nurse writers focused determinedly on the positive elements of military nursing, emphasising their own roles as effective humanitarian workers providing a highly professional service. Among these were Julia Stimson, a senior US nurse, and Helen Dore Boylston, a sister with the Harvard Unit. Yet the decision of such nurses to engage in the war ran counter to a powerful strain of pacifism in the writings of others. In August 1915, when Britain had been at war for a year, a *BJN* editorial commented on the pacifist sentiments of prominent American nurse Lavinia Dock. The article was probably authored by the journal's editor, Ethel Gordon Fenwick, a close friend of Dock's. The two women had been instrumental in the foundation of the International Council of Nurses sixteen years earlier.[1] Fenwick was firmly committed to the allied war effort; Dock, who was head of the *American Journal of Nursing*'s 'Foreign Department', was unequivocally opposed to it. Nevertheless, Fenwick decided to publish 'the beautiful human ideals of this noble and lovable little woman':[2]

> We have been asked why we do not record events happening in connection with the European War. So it may be time for us to remark that the Foreign Department, at any rate, intends to boycott this particular war. The only mention it will draw from us will be denunciation of 'war' as a specimen of man's stupidity. This war will get no advertising, no 'write ups', from the secretary of the International Council. It is a colossal piece of atavism – of return to the age of the tiger and the ape.[3]

Lavinia Dock was one of a radical breed of US nurse that was emerging at the beginning of the twentieth century. A Marxist, pacifist, and feminist, she coauthored, with Adelaide Nutting, an extensive history of nursing: a deliberately political text, stressing the significance of the nursing profession throughout the world.[4] Born into a wealthy family, Dock had trained at Bellevue Hospital, New York, graduating in 1886.[5] She had spent time working as a visiting nurse at the Henry Street Settlement on New York's impoverished 'Lower East Side', where she had, no doubt, come under the influence of the progressive Lillian Wald.[6] She was a member of the New York Women's Trade Union League, and had been instrumental in setting up the American Nurses Association.[7]

Dock's openly anti-war writing has an important place among the works of female pacifists such as Catherine Marshall in Britain, and Charlotte Perkins Gilman in the USA, who deliberately linked pacifism to feminism by suggesting that war would be less likely in a world where women wielded political power.[8] Open pacifism was, however, rare among nurses: most nurse writers contented themselves with exposing the horror of war in the hope that readers would draw their own conclusions.[9]

The American Army Nurse Corps had been founded in 1901 – a year before the formation of the British QAIMNS. It was, therefore, arguably well established by the time the USA entered the First World War in April 1917. And yet, its difficulties were similar to those encountered by the British service: subordination to a powerful military medical corps, the disadvantages associated with an entirely female workforce, and the prevailing social prejudices that linked female paid work with low social status. At the end of a pioneering era, the cultural values of US citizens were less elitist and its class system less entrenched than that in Britain.[10] And yet chauvinism was rife, and some female senior nurses appear to have been subject to bullying and harassment by male medical colleagues.[11] Paradoxically, the problem may even have been exacerbated by the relatively relaxed attitude to the class system in the USA. In Britain, their status as members of a gentry class may have offered nurses some protection. Kimberly Jensen, in her compelling paper 'A Base Hospital Is Not a Coney Island Dance Hall', presents a handful of clear examples of serious bullying on the part of medical officers, though it is unclear whether these can be viewed as typical.[12]

Julia Stimson's 'splendid women'

American nurse Julia Stimson appears to have had no difficulties in her relationships with medical officers. Her charismatic personality and apparently resolute refusal to see anything but good in any of her colleagues seems to have inoculated her against the problems encountered by some other senior nurses. Stimson was born in 1881, in Worcester, Massachusetts, into a wealthy family that clearly attached some importance to the education of women. She attended Brearley School in New York City and then the prestigious Vassar College in Poughkeepsie, New York. Following graduate studies in biology at Columbia University,

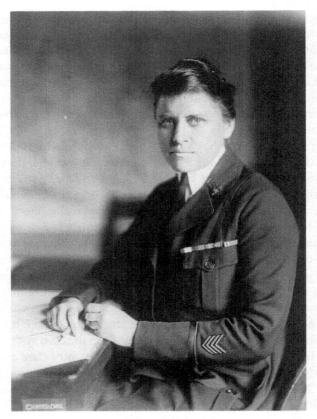

Figure 7 Portrait of Julia Stimson

New York City, from 1901 to 1903, and nurse training at the New York Hospital School of Nursing, from which she graduated in 1908, she pursued a successful career, as superintendent of nurses, first at Harlem Hospital from 1908 to 1911, and then at Barnes Hospital, Washington University, St Louis, Missouri from 1911 to 1917.[13]

Between her two periods of service as a chief nurse, Stimson took on the role of Director of Hospital Social Service at Washington University, St Louis.[14] It appears that a combination of her experience as a nurse and her awareness of the potential for philanthropy amongst the more privileged in society induced her to take a strong interest in social work. Such emphasis does seem to have been much stronger amongst American nurses at the turn of the century than amongst their British counterparts, finding its fullest expression in the work of the Henry Street Settlement from the 1890s onwards.[15] And yet, Stimson cannot be viewed as a radical. Her concern for the poor existed within the confines of a conservative and traditional view of society. In many ways, her outlook was very similar to that of Kate Luard: the world was essentially as it should be, and it was not the role of the nurse to change it, but merely to alleviate the suffering that it must necessarily contain.

Julia Stimson's real genius was as a leader. She is said to have shown 'sheer generalship' during the First World War,[16] and she appears to have achieved a remarkable level of harmony and success in her dealings with nurses and other professional colleagues. Her letters home were published in 1927 under the title *Finding Themselves*.[17] They contain clues to Stimson's personality and leadership style. The respect and affection she felt for her junior colleagues was infused with both a maternal warmth and an air of authority.

Stimson was chief nurse of one of the earliest US units to arrive in France: Base Hospital No. 21, supplied by Washington University, St Louis.[18] It took over an established British base hospital – No. 12 General Hospital, located on Rouen Race Course.[19] The hospital was large, with up to 2,000 patients. When first invited to head its nursing services, Stimson effused in a letter home about the opportunity she had been offered.[20] She expressed her 'tremendous satisfaction' at 'having a chance to ... be in the front ranks in this most dramatic event that ever was staged, and to be in the first group of women ever called out for duty with the United States Army, and in the first part of the army ever sent off in an expeditionary affair of this sort'.[21] Stimson's language, her reference to the war as a 'dramatic event' that was being 'staged', and her emphasis on being 'the first' speaks of her focus on both attainment and recognition. Sheila Rowbotham has observed that 'when they encountered opposition to their engagement in the public arena, middle class and working class women invoked motherly care, moral cleansing and class loyalty to justify stepping beyond the prescribed "womanly" sphere'.[22] Julia Stimson is a classic example of a woman who presented herself in a traditional female 'nurturing' role, while exercising enormous authority within a military setting.

Stimson's letters contain repeated expressions of concern for her staff – a concern that is mingled with admiration. On 17 June 1917, she remarks: 'my women are splendid. A few, of course, have periods of rearing, but they all have steadied down most beautifully'.[23] Stimson's tendency to write of her 'splendid women' as though they were horses who had to be broken in carries interesting undertones of the pioneering spirit of a unit from the Mid-West of the USA. Her equestrian metaphor illustrates how carefully Stimson 'handled' her nursing staff: as one might handle creatures with little sense of autonomy but much emotional volatility. She adds that she is 'proud of the spirit of cooperation' amongst her staff, and that she fosters this by posting poems on bulletin boards 'about the meaning of the war and the ideals we are fighting for'. She concludes: 'I certainly have some wonderfully splendid women with me. Some of them have queer exteriors and some queer ways, but they are fine with me.'[24] The tendency to post material on bulletin boards that a modern readership might identify as propagandist offers further evidence of Stimson's traditionalist perspective. The fact that she did not question the motives of the allies undoubtedly contributed to her strong and authoritative persona.

Stimson's ability to command the respect and affection of her staff and to sustain morale was clearly one of her strengths. But her involvement with them went much further than a desire to control their behaviour. One of her letters recounts how:

> Ruth C— has just been in to see me a moment. She is on night duty and is working very hard. She says there never in the world were such wonderful patients, that no matter how much they are suffering they are 'quite all right thank you, Sister', and they won't ask for things, and when she asks them if they are in pain, they say, 'Not too much, Sister'. The first night she says she went all to pieces, but nobody saw her; now she too is getting steadier.[25]

In the same letter, she comments that her nurses 'are beginning to show the effect of the emotional strain', adding, 'I have had about a dozen of them weeping'. She misses her own friends: 'naturally I cannot do any weeping here, since I have to be wept on; but there are times when it would be such a comfort to be braced myself'.[26] The desire to 'be braced' is characteristic of many of those who nursed the wounded during the First World War. Being a part of the army medical services (regardless of which army one was attached to) meant a lack of freedom to determine one's own movements or actions, whilst 'active service' meant an intensity of work that could be exhausting. Yet, many expressed their determination to 'stay at their posts', because the men they nursed had no choice but to do so.[27] Eventually, for some, the stress became almost unbearable:

> There was nothing really wrong on Sunday, but that day we had so many sick men to look after, and things got a bit complicated and several nurses got hysterical and I felt things were just too much. Any one would have thought so if they had seen our poor gassed men who are so terribly burnt. One of my most stolid nurses came to me that day and said 'I just don't know how I am going to stand it, taking care of so and so.' I said 'Why not?' and she replied, 'When he was brought in to us he was so badly burned we could hardly see any part of him that we could touch except the back of his neck; but that isn't the worst part, instead of cursing or moaning he was singing, and I just can't stand that.'[28]

The theme of the courage and endurance of the patients recurs regularly in Stimson's – as in other nurses' – testimony. It seems to have evoked a strong desire in nurses to emulate their patients' stoicism. One result of this was the eventual 'breakdown' of some members of staff. On 6 April 1918, Stimson wrote home to her parents that she had three nurses in hospital themselves: 'one with diphtheria, one with a kind of trench fever due to exhaustion, and the third, my dear, brave soul who came down from the evacuated CCS. She has just "exhaustion" for a diagnosis.'[29] She adds how remarkable it is that more nurses are not ill. One of her most poignant narratives is of a nurse she observes caring for a dying patient:

> It was getting dark as I went down between the A and B lines of tents. Ducking under the entrance of A.3 tent, I stopped just a moment inside the door, to get used to the darkness in the tent. The fourteen beds in the tent were all full and I thought at first that no nurse was there. Then I saw

her. She was kneeling beside the low cot of a lad whose whole head was bandaged. The tight starch bandage covered his ears and his eyes, and came down under his chin. A glance at his face showed that he was not far from the end. 'Robert, lad, what are you trying to say?' she was asking, bending over him with her arm across his shoulder and her face close to his lips. 'Say it again, boy, so that I can hear you. Did you want me to do something for you?' Slowly pulling his arms out he reached up and drew her head down to his and kissed her on the cheek. 'I think', he said, 'you must be like my sister'. Just then she saw me. 'Oh, excuse me Matron', she said as she rose, 'I didn't hear you come in.' We walked through to the connecting tent while the other thirteen men stirred and pretended to wake up.[30]

In 1918, Stimson's abilities as a leader were rewarded by her appointment as chief nurse of the American Red Cross in France. Later that year, she was transferred to the directorship of the Nursing Services for the American Expeditionary Force.[31] Her ability as a diplomat was a significant element of her impressive battery of skills. After the war, she was appointed Dean of the Army School of Nursing, a position she held until the school's closure in 1931, when she continued as superintendent of the Army Nurse Corps. In 1920, US Congress awarded army nurses relative rank, and Stimson was given the title of major. Six weeks before her death, in 1948, she was promoted to the rank of colonel (retired).[32] For Julia Stimson, there were no barriers to success or advancement. Her remarkable sense of duty and her capacity for working within the systems devised by others – and for making those systems work, through the force of her charisma and personality – ensured that she enjoyed a level of success and a recognition not afforded to many nurses in the first half of the twentieth century.

Pioneer nurse: the adventures of Helen Dore Boylston

Many US nurses appear to have relished the excitement of journeys 'into the unknown' – none more so than Helen Dore Boylston, a young nurse with the Harvard Unit, who spent the last two years of the war on the Western Front and the remainder of her life writing about the adventure of nursing.

Boylston was born in Portsmouth, New Hampshire, in 1895, when the United States of America was at the height of its pioneering

130

powers. Looking both eastwards to the sophistication and style of *fin-de-siècle* Europe and westwards towards a half-tamed wilderness, Eastern-Seaboard America was a place of unlimited opportunity, and Boylston was its creature, participating fully in its possibilities and experiencing its contradictions with the keenness of a popular writer. Her book *'Sister': The War Diary of a Nurse* was developed from a journal she kept during her time on the Western Front; but it found its final form whilst she was living a bohemian life in 1920s Albania with her close friend, confidante, and fellow-author, Rose Wilder Lane.[33]

Boylston's restless spirit, her constant quest for new experience, and her thirst for travel and adventure found expression in her recounting of her wartime experiences. It may seem surprising that nurses on the Western Front could find time and opportunity – given their difficult living conditions and long working hours – to keep full and detailed diaries. Yet, archives around the world are filled with their journals, accounts that have clearly been written contemporaneously with the events they describe – on mud-streaked paper, in tiny notebooks, often beginning with fine ink, and ending in blunt pencil.[34] Books such as *'Sister'* were the product of such meticulous diary-writing. Yet Boylston's memoir, like many others, is also, in some ways, remote from the incidents it describes. Its very clarity and simplicity belie the complexity of war nursing. It has clearly been edited and modelled to tell a particular story.

Helen Dore Boylston's father was a successful physician. It has been suggested that she herself considered training as a doctor, but chose nursing instead because the training was shorter.[35] This story may be apocryphal, but it fits with the character of a restless spirit, who clearly had no desire to be trapped in one place. She trained at one of the most prestigious North American Hospitals – the Massachusetts General Hospital, Boston – and, like Alice Fitzgerald and Julia Stimson, benefited from her upper-middle-class background, moving easily through the social milieu of this powerful institution.

Boylston was clearly at ease with herself, and this enabled her to form easy relationships with others. In northern France, she appears to have enjoyed friendships with both fellow nurses and medical officers. There is no trace in her story of elitism or snobbery. In her world, nurses, medical officers, and orderlies work in harmony, enjoy dark banter during German raids, and go off together on picnics and excursions. It may be that this world is a partly fictional one. As we have seen, the researches of Kimberley Jensen have suggested that the American Army Nurse Corps experienced more than its share of chauvinism – particularly at senior levels – and that, at times, this bordered on bullying and harassment.[36] Yet, Boylston's experiences concur with those of Julia Stimson, whose personal charm and traditional outlook on women's roles assured her a smooth social passage through the troubled waters of the American military hospital. For Boylston, it was not traditionalism, but a largely unconscious radicalism and feminism that enabled her to experience her time on the Western Front as one of camaraderie. She appears to have found chauvinism and snobbery a source of humour – something either to ridicule or to ignore.

'Sister' reads as a succession of highly entertaining vignettes of Boylston's time in northern France. The tone is light – remarkably so when one considers the nature of the subject-matter. Decades after the war, Boylston was to carve out a successful career as a writer of books for teenage girls; it may be that in the 1920s, when crafting 'Sister', she was already developing her popular style of novel writing. The narrative speaks through a strong, resonant voice, with a tone of muted humour. Boylston appears to have been, above all else, a powerful and completely natural story-teller.

The Harvard Unit – consisting of doctors, trained nurses, and male orderlies – was said by Alice Fitzgerald to have arrived in France at the end of May 1917.[37] After spending some time in Camiers, 'with leaky huts and no drainage',[38] it took over the site of the No. 13 General Hospital in Boulogne – where Fitzgerald had been serving with the BEF. The British relinquished their hospital with great reluctance, and Fitzgerald commented in her diary that 'there is much hard feeling over the whole affair', with British staff denouncing the behaviour of 'those dreadful Americans from the Harvard Unit'.[39] Boylston appears to have been largely unaware of these tensions. Her account focuses on her own individual adventures – such as a terrible throat infection, which is cured when one of her colleagues lances the abscess with an iodine-soaked probe;[40] or a battle with rats in her ward, which she wins with the assistance of the hospital's terrier, Toodles.[41] Romance also finds a place in her memoir – but it takes a light and humorous form. Friendship seems more important, with Boylston and her friends finding great pleasure in each other's company on long walks.[42]

Boylston's text offers simple, vivid descriptions of a world in which she takes an eager, yet relaxed, interest. One passage, written while waiting for night duty to begin, offers a nostalgic reflection on how life in a French base hospital reminds Boylston of camping in Maine:

> The smoky smell in the air is making me a little homesick for the old days when I went fishing down in the Maine woods with Dad. I remember the smell of the hot pine-needles and dry leaves and burnt underbrush; the great broad lake, blue and motionless in the summer heat; the dry buzz of insects; and the nights, the beautiful, lonely nights when the lake was full of stars and the woods lay heavy with blackness along the shores, and there was no sound except the far-off call of a loon, or the sad, questioning 'Quosh?' of a blue heron sweeping through the night ... How far away and long ago it seems! I wonder sometimes if it really happened. I wouldn't go back. I wouldn't give up these days in France, but I can't help remembering when there is a smell of wood-smoke in the air.[43]

Boylston's skill lies in the simplicity of her sentences. The pathetic fallacy achieved by juxtaposing the camp fires of a military base hospital with the smoky smell of a peaceful lakeshore in Maine evokes a sense of nostalgia and creates a mood of peaceful longing for something the reader can sense but not fully understand. This passage is followed immediately by a humorous one, in which nurses, British VADs, and medical officers take a walk 'carrying steamer-rugs and poetry', and in which 'an ardent VAD [begins] a frenzied pursuit of one of our shyest medical officers'.[44]

In May 1918, soon after the commencement of the German counter-offensive on the Western Front, Boylston's unit became the target of a series of relentless bombing raids. It is not known what she actually wrote in her diary during this time, but, years later, sitting at her table in the Albanian residence she was sharing with Rose Wilder Lane, she chose to model these events into a remarkable adventure. Some of the episodes in her memoir could almost have been lifted straight out of a 'girl's own adventure' story. One example recounts an episode when the hospital is bombed from the air by German Gothas. The episode begins with Boylston working with a medical officer, caring for a dying patient. They hear the guns at Boulogne, and then the approach of the German planes:

> 'Good God!' Eddie said. 'We're in for it!'
>
> At that instant there came a flash from the beach, a long whistling sigh, a terrific jar, and then a faint *b-o-o-ng* directly overhead. Archie had spoken! A moment later every gun for miles around had turned loose and was firing frantically, the shells whining in a dozen different keys. And all the time, *hiss-ss-ss*, a tremendous shock, and a blinding red glare. The planes circled closer and closer, until even the machine-guns opened fire on them, with their ridiculous *put-put-put*. It was horrible, and yet it had a kind of dreadful beauty – the searchlights swinging and crossing; the yellow blaze of flares and star-shells; the lightning flash of the guns; and sometimes a great gold bug swooping out of the sky – Fritz, caught in the searchlights. Or again, a hideous black bug moving against the moon.
>
> The boys, terrified, were beginning to shout for 'sister', and I ran across to B5, where they were the most helpless. Eddie followed me, and we walked up and down between the beds, trying to quiet the boys by appearing calm ourselves. They were frantic with terror, and I can't say that I was much better.[45]

Boylston describes how, later, while moving between wards, she is almost caught in the blast of an exploding shell. She writes of 'living ten years' as she waits for the bomb to land, and then of seeing a 'blood-red flare' even with her hands over her closed eyes, and of feeling earth and stones 'pattering down'. She adds: 'When I crawled to my feet I found that I was shaking all over, which surprised me, for I was still not conscious of any particular emotion.[46]

The apparent simplicity of Boylston's style belies her skill in creating a text that draws in the reader, sustaining a feeling of suspense while presenting a succession of highly visual images. The text has an auditory quality too: reading a narrative that contains the '*b-o-o-ng*' of heavy artillery, the '*hiss-ss-ss*' of shrapnel, and the '*put-put-put*' of machine guns conveys a feeling of having returned to childhood – of listening to a story read aloud. It is not difficult to understand why Boylston later became a successful children's novelist. Far from recreating a Western-Front base hospital, these images construct something entirely original. In the style of G. A. Henty, they enable the reader to experience vicariously the excitement of war without being tarnished by its grimmer realities.[47]

Many nurses belonging to US hospital units during the First World War wrote diaries, but very few ever intended their works to be published. Canadian-born Ella Mae Bongard travelled to France as a fully trained member of a medical unit sent out by the Presbyterian Hospital of New York, and was posted to Etretat on the French coast. Her diary does not appear to have been written with publication in mind, and was, in fact, only published many years after her death, by her son, Eric Scott. Her diary entries offer an interesting contrast to Boylston's deliberately engaging story-telling:

> January 22, & 23, 1918. I feel a little like Lady Macbeth these days – 'Tomorrow & Tomorrow & Tomorrow creeps in this petty pace from day to day' etc. But of course I know it's just night duty. The other night I was sent up to officers to special a very sick man. He was a young aviator of 19 & he had one leg off, the other one fractured, a fractured skull and was then developing tetanus. It hardly seems fair for one person to have to go through so much. That was about a week ago and now I hear that he is a little better and they have some hopes of his recovery. He may want to live but I don't believe I should under the circumstances.[48]

Bongard's writing conveys a quiet calmness, its laconic phrases contrasting with Boylston's adventure-writing style.

Helen Dore Boylston's 'Sister' ends with the armistice, and Boylston's reaction to peace is characteristic:

> November 11.
> In ten minutes the war will be over. Hostilities are to cease at eleven o'clock, and it is ten minutes to eleven now …
> There go the bells! And the drums! And the sirens! And the bagpipes! And cheering that swells louder and louder! The war is over – and I never felt so sick in my life. Everything is over.
> But it shan't be! I *won't* stop living.[49]

Boylston's outburst – so different in both perspective and style to many other nurses' reminiscences of the armistice – offers a clear insight into her thirst for variety and adventure. And yet she was not unique. Many of those who had experienced both the excitement and the horror of wartime nursing were unable – often for reasons they could not express – to return to civilian nursing after the armistice. Many left nursing altogether. Others moved into relief work.[50] Boylston herself spent several years after the war working for the Red Cross in Albania, Poland, Russia, Italy, and Germany. Yet, ultimately Red Cross relief work was no more satisfying than civilian nursing, and she returned to the Massachusetts General Hospital.[51]

Boylston met fellow Red Cross worker Rose Wilder Lane on a train from Paris to Warsaw in 1920, and the two became close friends. Both craved adventure and longed for a more independent way of life. By the mid-1920s they had formed a plan to travel overland in a Model T Ford from Paris to Albania, to establish a home in a land free from the constraints of western power-politics and bureaucracy.[52] Boylston had already spent time in Albania working for the Red Cross and had convinced Lane that Albanian culture was pure and unsullied – free from both the corrupt political and imperialist forces that had almost destroyed Europe and the 'crassly commercial' atmosphere of the USA.[53]

Lane was the rebellious and talented daughter of Laura Ingalls Wilder, who would later become famous as author of a series of books including *The Little House on the Prairie*.[54] Boylston, although eight years her junior, was clearly the more adventurous of the two; she was the expedition's driver and car-mechanic. The addition of the women's French maid, Yvonne, meant that an unlikely trio of friends made their way through France and Italy during the summer of 1926.

For biographer William Holtz, Boylston and Lane personified American confidence and materialism. Their relationship with their car, which they named 'Zenobia' and wrote of as though it were a human being, was a classic example of the 'American love affair with the automobile'.[55] As they travelled through Europe, the two women composed a series of long, jointly written letters home, sending copies to their families, and to their stockbroker and close friend, George Palmer. Put together, these letters provide an account of their deliberately intrepid journey. Through Holtz's edited text, a modern reader can learn of their adventures in France, of the dangers they faced in the Italian Apennines, of the dismay they felt when almost all of their possessions were stolen in Naples, and of the idiosyncrasies of peasants in various lands, all of whom are presented as humorous stereotypes.[56] For Holtz, the women's pursuit of adventure was deeply influenced by 'their commitment to a vision of America as a special case in history, a chosen land in which a chosen people would forge a great nation by simply pursuing their individual destinies'.[57]

Throughout the story, Boylston is referred to as 'Troub', the nickname she had been given by her colleagues in the Harvard Unit.[58] The highlight of the women's journey is reached towards its end, when 'Troub' drives Zenobia from a small sailing-boat onto the harbour of Durazzo, across two narrow planks that bend and crack under the automobile's wheels:

> When I saw her she stood there swaying. Two planks, eight inches wide, had been inserted under her front wheels, and led upward at an acute angle to the edge of the wharf. Under them the lapping water licked its lips. Troub was at the wheel, enclosed in the glass box of that sedan. On the wharf a wild-eyed Yvonne clutched all our purses and stared, frantic. Some twenty or thirty Albanians swarmed over Zenobia and the sail boat, tipping the boat, the car and the planks first to one side and then far to the other. I expected the whole thing to capsize momentarily.[59]

The two women remained in Albania for less than two years. Returning to America, and to the disastrous stock-market crash of 1929, each found herself in need of regular employment. Boylston returned, once more, to nursing, pursuing a successful career at the Massachusetts General Hospital and in Connecticut.[60]

Eventually, in the 1930s, Boylston found fame writing books for teenage girls: firstly relating the adventures of 'Sue Barton', an American nurse,[61] and then of romantic 'Carol Page', a successful actress.[62] Perhaps 'Troub' herself was as much an actress as a nurse, presenting herself as 'the all-American [girl] of magazine fiction'.[63] This act was convincing because she herself believed so fully in it. Yet, Deborah Philips asserts that Boylston's *Sue Barton* books, for all their 'pioneer' spirit, offer a realistic, rather than romanticised, vision of nursing,[64] providing an important impetus to the growing conviction amongst young girls that their careers mattered. For Sue, her love of nursing takes precedence over her love of handsome doctor Bill Barry. Although their romance simmers through the first three books in the series, it is not until the fourth, *Sue Barton, Rural Nurse*, that Sue consents to marry Bill.[65] Helen Dore Boylston's own determination to make her mark in the world was probably influenced by her upbringing in a wealthy but active professional household. Her father had taken her on camping trips in the Maine countryside – an activity normally reserved for boys – and had encouraged her to 'show the world what you can do before you settle down'.[66] Boylston appears to have taken his advice so seriously that she never really did 'settle down'.

137

Conclusion: far-off lands and strange adventures

The published memoirs of First World War nurses sometimes read like travelogues. For Julia Stimson, service with the ANC meant a loss of control over her own life – a prospect that she found exciting. One of her earliest letters comments on the thrill of not knowing where in the world she is to be posted. Upon finding herself in France, she appears to have revelled in the challenge of supervising a nursing staff in a new and strange environment. For Helen Dore Boylston, the travelling never seems to have stopped – or, at any rate, it lasted for as long as her funds would allow. It was only the stock-market crash of 1929 and the need to stay in one place and earn a living that turned her adventurous spirit inwards to the writing of children's fiction. Many early-twentieth-century women appear to have experienced a compulsion to travel,[67] a compulsion that was perhaps most clearly expressed in Rose Wilder Lane's description of an Albanian sunset:

> The mountains were sliced off along their tops, neatly, in a straight line, by a dark blue mist that covered the eastern sky. Beneath this line, between the nearer mountain peaks, the far valleys and farther mountain peaks were revealed in sunshine. They were vaguely beautiful – something as lovely as our waking dreams of lands we shall never see. We continue to cling to the belief that when we see them they will be beautiful, but an implacable circle of reality moves with us wherever we go.[68]

The longing to move beyond their 'circle of reality' drove many women to offer their services as nurses in the First World War. For others, it was patriotism that moved them. Their travels – though experienced as exciting, and described in terms of wonderment – were incidental to their desire to serve in the Great War: the greatest event in living memory and the conflict to which so many brothers, friends, and lovers had committed themselves. For many, their experiences brought satisfaction in service. For others, the war left them with an unfulfilled longing – to see the 'farther mountain peaks'.

Notes

1 Fenwick was first president and Dock first secretary to the International Council of Nurses: Barbara Brush, Joan Lynaugh, Geertje Boschma, Anne Marie Rafferty, Meryn Stuart, and Nancy J. Tomes, *Nurses of All Nations: A History*

of the International Council of Nurses, 1899–1999 (Philadelphia: Lippincott, Williams, and Wilkins, 1999).

2 Anon., Column, *BJN* (7 August 1915): 118–19 (119).

3 Lavinia Dock, Column published in the *American Journal of Nursing*, quoted verbatim in *BJN* (7 August 1915): 118–19.

4 M. Adelaide Nutting and Lavinia L. Dock, *A History of Nursing: The Evolution of Nursing Systems from the Earliest Times to the Foundation of the First English and American Training Schools for Nurses*, 4 vols (New York and London: G. P. Putnam's Sons, 1907–12).

5 Deborah Philips, 'Healthy Heroines: Sue Barton, Lillian Wald, Lavinia Lloyd Dock and the Henry Street Settlement', *Journal of American Studies*, 33.1 (1999): 65–82.

6 Although Dock was probably the more radical of the two: Philips, 'Healthy Heroines'.

7 Philips, 'Healthy Heroines'.

8 Catherine Marshall, *Militarism versus Feminism* (London: Virago, 1987 [1915]); Charlotte Perkins Gilman, *Herland* (New York: Pantheon, 1979 [1915]). On the work of Charlotte Perkins Gilman, see: Claire Tylee, *The Great War and Women's Consciousness: Images of Militarism and Womanhood in Women's Writings, 1914–64* (Houndmills and London: Macmillan, 1990): 41. Tylee also comments on the writings of Olive Schreiner, who states that 'the day that women shared in government with men would be the day that heralded the death of war' (41).

9 This was a particular trait in the writings of British and Dominion nurses. See: Kate Finzi, *Eighteen Months in the War Zone: The Record of One Woman's Work on the Western Front* (London: Cassell, 1916); Irene Rathbone, *We That Were Young: A Novel* (New York: The Feminist Press, 1989 [1932]); May Tilton, *The Grey Battalion* (Sydney: Angus and Robertson, 1933).

10 Margaret Deland, *Small Things* (New York: D. Appleton, 1919): 8.

11 Kimberly Jensen, *Mobilizing Minerva: American Women in the First World War* (Urbana and Chicago: University of Illinois Press, 2008), Chapter 7, 'A Base Hospital Is Not a Coney Island Dance Hall: Nurses, Citizenship, Hostile Work Environment and Military Rank': 116–41.

12 Jensen, *Mobilizing Minerva*: 116–41. See also: Kimberly Jensen, 'A Base Hospital Is Not a Coney Island Dance Hall: American Women Nurses, Hostile Work Environment, and Military Rank in the First World War', *Frontiers*, 26.2 (2005): 206–35.

13 Alice Howell Friedman, 'Stimson, Julia Catherine', in Martin Kaufman (ed.), *Dictionary of American Nursing Biography* (New York: Greenwood Press, 1988): 350.

14 Friedman, 'Stimson, Julia Catherine': 350.

15 Karen Buhler-Wilkerson, *No Place like Home: A History of Nursing and Home Care in the United States* (Baltimore: Johns Hopkins University Press, 2001).

16 Friedman, 'Stimson, Julia Catherine': 350–1.

17 Julia Stimson, *Finding Themselves: The Letters of an American Army Chief Nurse at a British Hospital in France* (New York: Macmillan, 1927).

18 Mary T. Sarnecky, *A History of the US Army Nurse Corps* (Philadelphia: University of Pennsylvania Press, 1999): 83.

19 Stimson, *Finding Themselves*: frontispiece; Jensen, *Mobilizing Minerva*: 136.

20 Stimson, *Finding Themselves*: 3–4.

21 Stimson, *Finding Themselves*: 3–4.

22 Sheila Rowbotham, *Dreamers of a New Day: Women who Invented the Twentieth Century* (London: Verso, 2010): 2.

23 Stimson, *Finding Themselves*: 63.

24 Stimson, *Finding Themselves*: 63.

25 Stimson, *Finding Themselves*: 43–4.

26 Stimson, *Finding Themselves*: 92.

27 Christine Hallett, *Containing Trauma: Nursing Work in the First World War* (Manchester: Manchester University Press, 2009): 194–218.

28 Stimson, *Finding Themselves*: 93.

29 Stimson, *Finding Themselves*: 220.

30 Stimson, *Finding Themselves*: 223.

31 Friedman, 'Stimson, Julia Catherine': 350–1.

32 Sarnecky, *A History of the Army Nurse Corps*: 100–1. See also: Friedman, 'Stimson, Julia Catherine': 351.

33 Helen Dore Boylston, *'Sister': The War Diary of a Nurse* (New York: Ives Washburn, 1927). The diary was, initially, serialised as "Coming of Age", in the popular journal *Atlantic Monthly*, from September to November 1925: William Holtz (ed.), *Travels with Zenobia: Paris to Albania by Model T Ford* (Columbia and London: University of Missouri Press, 1983): 6–7, 9.

34 Santanu Das, *Touch and Intimacy in First World War Literature* (Cambridge: Cambridge University Press, 2005): 175–203; Hallett, *Containing Trauma*: 10–15.

35 Holtz, *Travels with Zenobia*: 6.

36 Jensen, 'A Base Hospital Is Not a Coney Island Dance Hall'.

37 Although there is evidence that a unit from Harvard University was in France much earlier than this. Alice Fitzgerald, unpublished memoirs incorporating war diary, *c.* 1936, Alice Fitzgerald Papers, Md HR M2633, Md HR M 2634, Maryland Historical Society Archives, Baltimore, Maryland, USA.

38 Fitzgerald, unpublished memoirs.

39 Fitzgerald, unpublished memoirs.

40 Boylston, *'Sister'*: 88–9.

41 Boylston, *'Sister'*: 93–4.

42 Boylston, *'Sister'*: 86–7.

43 Boylston, *'Sister'*: 90–2.

44 There is evidence that contingents of British VADs were left in general hospitals following their evacuation by their British units, until fully trained American 'reinforcements' could be brought from the USA: Boylston, 'Sister': 92.

45 Boylston, 'Sister': 97–103.

46 Boylston, 'Sister': 102.

47 G. A. Henty, *The Collected Works of G. A. Henty*, 7 vols (Alvin, TX: Halcyon Classics, 2011). On G. A. Henty, see: Mawuena Kossi Logan, *Narrating Africa: George Henty and the Fiction of Empire* (London: Taylor and Francis, 2007).

48 Eric Scott (ed.), *Nobody Ever Wins a War: The World War I Diaries of Ella Mae Bongard, R.N.* (Ottawa: Janeric Enterprises, 1997): 29.

49 Boylston, 'Sister': 173–4.

50 Christine E. Hallett, *Veiled Warriors: Allied Nurses of the First World War* (Oxford: Oxford University Press, 2014): Conclusion.

51 Philips, 'Healthy Heroines': 65–82; Holtz, *Travels with Zenobia*: 6–7.

52 Their letters are edited by William Holtz, who also offers numerous insights into their backgrounds and motivations: Holtz, *Travels with Zenobia*: passim.

53 Holtz, *Travels with Zenobia*: 6–7, 10.

54 *Little House on the Prairie* was one of a highly successful series of children's novels recounting Wilder's childhood as part of a pioneering American family. On the careers of both Laura Ingalls Wilder and Rose Wilder Lane, see: Holtz, *Travels with Zenobia*: 2–5.

55 Holtz, *Travels with Zenobia*: 12.

56 Holtz, *Travels with Zenobia*: passim.

57 Holtz, *Travels with Zenobia*: 20.

58 It is probable that she first acquired this nickname in childhood. See: Holtz, *Travels with Zenobia*: 5.

59 Holtz, *Travels with Zenobia*: 88–9.

60 Philips, 'Healthy Heroines': 67.

61 Boylston wrote thirteen highly successful children's books. The 'Sue Barton' series consists of: *Sue Barton, Student Nurse* (1936); *Sue Barton, Senior Nurse* (1937); *Sue Barton, Visiting Nurse* (1938); *Sue Barton, Rural Nurse* (1939); *Sue Barton, Superintendent of Nurses* (1940); *Sue Barton, Neighbourhood Nurse* (1949); *Sue Barton, Staff Nurse* (1952). All went into several editions and reprints.

62 The 'Carol' books are: *Carol Goes Backstage* (1941); *Carol Plays Summer Stock* (1942); *Carol on Broadway* (1944); *Carol on Tour* (1946); *Carol Goes on the Stage* (1947). Boylston is believed to have obtained material for these novels from an actress friend, Eva Le Galliene. She also wrote a biography of famous Civil War volunteer nurse Clara Barton: Helen Dore Boylston, *Clara Barton: Founder of the American Red Cross* (New York: Random House,

1955). On Helen Dore Boylston as a children's author, see also: Sally Mitchell, 'Helen Dore Boylston', in Lina Mainiero (ed.), *American Women Writers* (New York: Frederick Ungar, 1979): 209–11; Brian Doyle (ed.), *The Who's Who of Children's Literature* (New York: Schocken Books, 1968): 35.

63 Holtz, *Travels with Zenobia*: 22.

64 Philips, 'Healthy Heroines': 78.

65 Helen Dore Boylston, *Sue Barton, Rural Nurse* (New York: Image Cascade, 2008 [1939]).

66 Philips, 'Healthy Heroines': 81.

67 On travel literature, see: Alan Ogden, 'Romanian Culture in the Twentieth Century: The View of English Travel Writers before the Second World War', *Romanian Civilization*, 19.3 (2000): 44–54; Alba Amoia and Bettina Knapp, *Women Travel Writers: From 1750 to the Present* (New York: Continuum, 2005); Richard De Ritter, 'Reading "Voyages and Travels": Jane West, Patriotism and the Reformation of Female Sensibility', *Romanticism*, 17 (2011): 240–50; Juanita Cabello, 'On the Touristic Stage of 1920s and '30s Mexico: Katherine Anne Porter and a Modernist Tradition of Women Travel Writers', *Women's Studies*, 41.4 (2012): 413–35.

68 Holtz, *Travels with Zenobia*: 99.

6

The war nurse as free agent

Introduction: the rewards of professional nursing

In the second decade of the twentieth century, the nursing professions in both Britain and the USA had attained a level of recognition
that permitted their members considerable personal and professional
autonomy. During training their lives were circumscribed by the
patriarchal hierarchies of early-twentieth-century hospital life; but,
once they had attained the level of 'senior probationer', nurses exercised high levels of responsibility – often running wards and supervising junior staff. Their work was vital to the recovery of their patients.
Although physicians and surgeons rarely expressed open admiration
for nursing work, it was implicitly understood that medical and surgical interventions could not be successful without the presence of a
cadre of disciplined and knowledgeable bedside carers.[1]

Nurse training schools – particularly those in the prestigious hospitals of cities such as London, Philadelphia, and Baltimore – were
highly disciplined environments in which survival and ultimate success depended on the ability to display obedience and compliance.
Yet, once qualified, a nurse could use her certificate as a permit to
enter worlds that were, mostly, denied to other women. Indeed, in the
context of the First World War, it was only the wealthiest and most
socially elevated (British) women who could carve out opportunities
similar to those of professional nurses. Elsie Knocker and Violetta
Thurstan stand as examples of women who used their nursing qualifications as a means of entering the male 'zone of the armies' – a space

within about ten kilometres of the front lines from which women were normally barred.

Heroine of Pervyse: the adventures of Elsie Knocker

There was, following the formation of the trench system on the Western Front, an absolute embargo on permitting women to work close to the front-line trenches. Hence, the largely freelance efforts of two determined women, Elsie Knocker and Mairi Chisholm, who set up their own independent dressing station in the Belgian village of Pervyse, were extraordinary. Knocker and Chisholm's 'Cellar-House' was so close to the front line that they were able to take soup and coffee into the trenches for the soldiers and carry the wounded on stretchers back to their cellar, treating them for shock, dressing their wounds, and giving them the opportunity to rest before being taken by ambulance back 'down the line' to a field hospital in Furnes.[2]

Elsie Knocker was a persuasive communicator. She convinced the Belgian military authorities to allow her and Chisholm to establish the only forward field dressing station run by women in the so-called 'zone of the armies'.[3] Her powerful communication skills also enabled her to publicise the work of the 'Cellar-House of Pervyse' to large audiences in Britain.[4] Well before the end of the war, she had been awarded the highest military honours available to women, by both the British and Belgian Governments. She was publicly lauded as one of the 'Heroines of Pervyse' and street artists chalked her portrait onto the pavements of London.[5] Yet, her early life had been difficult. Having lost both parents to infectious diseases while still a small child, she had been adopted by an older couple who, she believed, had really wished for a son. Her relationship with this kind but detached couple was often tense and difficult, resulting in both tomboyish behaviour, and a refusal to recognise the boundaries set by others. It is clear that her childhood experiences also infused her with a powerful sense of self-sufficiency and a belief that she was the master of her own destiny.

Knocker's early life was one of impoverished gentility. Her adoptive father was a housemaster of a public school and, although she had been left a small legacy by her natural father, this was not enough to support a genteel lifestyle. She attended finishing school at Lausanne and then began training as a children's nurse in Sevenoaks.[6] In 1906 she married, and travelled with her husband – an unhappy and abusive man – to Singapore, where she realised she was pregnant. Having returned to England, where her son Kenneth was born on 1 February 1907, Knocker took the unusual and courageous step of petitioning for divorce in 1911. In the first decades of the twentieth century it was almost unheard of for a wife to sue for divorce, and she was obliged to pay all the costs of the proceedings.[7] Realising that she must now support both herself and her son, Knocker returned to hospital work, this time training as a midwife at Queen Charlotte's Hospital, Marylebone, London. Just as she completed her training, an uncle died, leaving an inheritance that enabled her to establish a home with her brother and son in Fordingbridge. It was here that Knocker bought a Chater-Lea motorcycle, enabling her to develop the driving and mechanical skills that, along with her nursing skills, would be her entrée into war work in 1914.[8]

Elsie Knocker and Mairi Chisholm began their war service as ambulance drivers with Hector Munro's Flying Ambulance Corps, ferrying the wounded over rough terrain to hospital. They noticed that wounded men were spending very little time in forward field dressing stations. The normal practice was to dress their wounds and administer morphine, before transferring them to distant field hospitals. A trained nurse, Knocker realised that removing dangerously wounded and physiologically fragile men from the front lines, putting them straight into ambulances, and then bumping them over shell-torn Belgian pavé roads was killing more casualties than it was saving. What was needed was the opportunity to stabilise the wounded, treat them for shock, and warm and reassure them, before moving them down the line.[9] This meant keeping a shocked casualty for several hours in a forward field dressing station. Knocker managed to persuade the Belgian military authorities to permit her to establish her 'Cellar-House' in the tiny and almost totally ruined village of Pervyse, directly behind the Belgian front-line trenches. Casualties came with problems ranging from minor injuries, such as barbed-wire grazes, to serious shrapnel- and bullet-wounds.[10] During most of their three-and-a-half years in the Cellar-House, their section

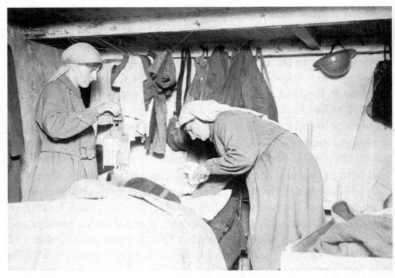

Figure 8 Elsie Knocker and Mairi Chisholm attend to a patient in
their Cellar-House in Pervyse

of the line was quiet, and the two women treated numerous cases of
minor illness or injury. At times, though, they participated in the
evacuation of serious casualties during the 'rushes' created by failed
assaults on the front line. Knocker also became adept at tooth extrac-
tion after the British Red Cross Society sent her a complete set of den-
tal instruments. Her fame as a dentist – by her own account – 'spread
far and wide'.[11] In 1916, Arthur Gleason, who had worked for five
months as a volunteer for Hector Munro's Flying Ambulance Corps,
commented that the women had been warned that their sector of the
line would, eventually, come under severe attack and might be 'wiped
out'. He also observed that their response was simply to 'go on with
their cool, expert work', adding: 'The only way to stop them is to stop
the war.'[12]

During her visits to England to campaign for funds, Knocker gave
lectures, describing her philosophy of shock treatment and narrating stories of Belgian soldiers who had recovered in her Cellar-House
after having been given up for dead by their military and medical
colleagues.[13] In her own personal diary, she expanded on some of

these success stories. On 26 January 1915, for example, she noted the following:

> One man had a burst main artery and also smashed his hand to smithereens. They took him over to the other poste where he certainly would have died – they put him on straw with his feet hanging down and his head up – whereas with such haemorrhage it naturally ought to have been the other way round – I took him in hand however and gave him a saline injection and got his feet raised and his head down and … I was able to get him removed to my poste and to attend to him there … I got him over to my blessé bed – with nice warm blankets and hot water bottles – another saline injection – water to drink – and a morphia injection. I then closed the shutters, made up the fire and left him in peace … I refused to have him moved for at least an hour … When a man is suffering from shock and he is taken over these roads and at once put under a serious operation he cannot withstand the shock … I kept him until 3.30 and he was able to get nice and warm and rested and he was able to say 'merci' when he went off and he looked so much better – I was glad to see it – and hope he will recover.[14]

It was only with great difficulty that Knocker obtained the permission of the Belgian authorities to set up her dressing station right on the front lines.[15] The British never gave any woman such permission, and the allied forces made a decision en masse, early in 1915, to forbid all such initiatives.[16] However, by this time the two so-called 'Heroines of Pervyse' had made such names for themselves in both Belgium and Britain that they were permitted to remain on the front lines. The British even came to value their presence and, early in 1915, supplied them with binoculars and asked them to 'spot' the movement of British planes.[17] On occasions they would move deep into no man's land with stretchers to rescue aviators who had crash-landed.[18] Even after the British army took over their sector in 1917, they remained in place until actually shelled out of their cellar by German gas shells, and invalided home. They were decorated for their heroism, being made Chevaliers of the Order of St Leopold (a Belgian decoration) and awarded the Order of St John of Jerusalem and the British Military Medal.[19] Romance also featured in Knocker's story. During her time in the 'Cellar-House of Pervyse', she met and married the Baron Harold de T'Serclaes de Rattendael, a Belgian pilot with 'an air of recklessness and gaiety'.[20]

The Baroness de T'Serclaes's memoir, *Flanders and Other Fields*, reads partly as adventure story, partly as reflection on war, and partly as a meditation on her own life – an affirmation of the meaning and significance of her nursing knowledge and work. Her conviction that offering wounded and shocked men rest, quiet, and fluids before moving them to a hospital was, in some ways, well founded. In others, it may have been flawed. Injuries sustained in the muddy fields of Flanders were liable to contamination with anaerobic bacteria, causing infections such as gas gangrene that, if not treated quickly, could prove fatal.[21] Although delaying the movement of a wounded man could enable his body to recover from shock, it might also allow a dangerous infection to take hold and spread. During the winter of 1914–15, it became clear to the allied military medical services that surgery to remove infected matter from wounds had to be performed as quickly as possible following an injury. Yet, it was also clear that it was fruitless to attempt to operate upon severely shocked patients until the shock itself had been alleviated. T'Serclaes was certain that her actions in keeping patients quiet in her Cellar-House, and delaying their journey to the base, saved lives. Indeed, she came to believe that she herself had the power to 'bring back' men from the brink of death:

> The stress of the life we were living had begun to reveal something in me which I had never suspected and which could not, surely have been the produce of the few absurd years on earth of which I was aware. I possessed a kind of power which seemed to be able to drag men back literally from the jaws of death. I was a fully trained nurse in the technical sense, but this was something more than technical efficiency. It was the breathing back of the Life Force, a kind of spiritual resuscitation.[22]

T'Serclaes was not the only nurse writer to express a sense of her power in such spiritual terms. Mary Borden, in *The Forbidden Zone*, wrote of dragging men back from the brink of death,[23] while Irene Rathbone recounted an incident in a British base hospital in which the nurse was forbidden to stay beyond her hours of duty with a dying patient, even though she believed she had the power to keep him alive.[24]

One of the most dramatic episodes in *Flanders and Other Fields* was T'Serclaes and Chisolm's final exit from their Cellar-House in the middle of a gas-attack. Both were badly poisoned, and had to be taken by ambulance to a field hospital, where T'Serclaes discovered what it was like to be a military casualty:

> I was coughing and gasping for breath, together with dozens of soldiers all around me, until I thought my lungs must burst or be torn from my body

… A nurse came and stripped off all my clothes, explaining that they were impregnated with gas and must be destroyed. At that I felt utterly miserable and helpless. A soldier somewhere to my right tried to comfort me by saying, 'Cheer up, gal, you've just got to the fifth stage. When you get to the eighth you'll be alright.' I asked him to explain, and this was the sequence. (1) The first shock. (2) The realization of what has happened and the panic. (3) The rescue – if you're lucky. (4) The dash to the casualty clearing station. (5) The nasty demoralization of being just a lump of flesh that can be stripped, injected, lugged around, and expected to have no emotions. The sixth stage was when you were lifted up and carted away, either to the mortuary or to a ward bed; the seventh was when you came to and realized that you were getting better; the eighth was when you could appreciate the warmth of your nice neat bed and fall luxuriously asleep.[25]

T'Serclaes and Chisholm never returned to Pervyse. Between the wars, T'Serclaes undertook a range of poorly paid jobs, working variously as a housekeeper, a hotelier, and a nurse.[26] During the General Strike of 1926, she discovered a new opportunity for adventure when she set up a first aid post in a disused butcher's shop in Poplar High Street, one of the most volatile areas of east London. She became 'the most spectacularly unusual district nurse the borough had ever known'.[27] During the Second World War, she served in the Women's Royal Air Force.[28]

In *Flanders and Other Fields* T'Serclaes maps change over time in her own perceptions of warfare. Written five decades after the First World War, with the benefits of both hindsight and a recognition of a massive shift in public opinion since 1918, it contains numerous expressions of pacifist sentiment. T'Serclaes's account of the First World War opens with a rehearsal of the numerous tales of German atrocities, current during the first months of the war. It then shifts to recount stories of occasional camaraderie between front-line troops on opposing sides, such as when, at Christmas or Easter, the German troops would hold up placards joking 'Let's All Go Home!'.[29] It addresses the view, which was current in the 1960s, that the troops of the First World War were betrayed by their political and military leaders. T'Serclaes's 'war lords sitting round a warm fire, sipping brandy and "organizing" such a cruel mess'[30] were the 'donkeys' referred to by some mid-century historians.[31]

Ultimately, T'Serclaes expresses largely pacifist sentiments, writing of her hope that the world will not see another such war. Her perceptions of the First World War may well have been coloured by her later experiences of the Second World War – the war in which her son, a bomber pilot, was killed on active service. She ends her book with her sense of the pity and anger she felt when she watched the suffering of infantrymen 'weighted down with all their kit, but especially … with the intolerable burden of the stupidities of statesmen'. And yet, she also honestly reflects that: 'Only in time of war have I found any real sense of purpose and happiness. Only then have I moved with honour among the sort of people whom I regard as my sort of people.'[32] The Baroness de T'Serclaes's feelings about war were ambivalent. Horrific, and yet empowering, war had both granted her the opportunity to be the person she most wanted to be, and killed the person she most loved.

Violetta Thurstan: intrepid, travelling nurse

In a novel written towards the end of her life, Violetta Thurstan likened her heroine – who bore a remarkable similarity to herself – to a storm petrel, a tiny bird known to skim the surface of the world's most powerful oceans, swooping repeatedly into the waves to feed on sea creatures swept to the surface.[33] For anyone reading her memoirs, the storm petrel does indeed seem to be a fitting metaphor for Thurstan – a small and apparently fragile woman, standing at a height of just under five feet, who craved the excitement and challenge of wartime nursing, and whose spirit was fed by her encounters with the storm of the most destructive war that had ever been fought.

Like Kate Luard or Julia Stimson, Thurstan chose not to judge the military or political leaders of her time. She saw war almost as a force of nature – something that would sweep over and destroy her compatriots if they did not mobilise themselves to meet it. She also saw it as something with which all must engage. Her own form of engagement was like the intermittent swooping of a tiny bird into the teeth of a gale – first in Belgium, then Russia, France, and Macedonia. Each time, danger, in the form of capture, disease, or injury, forced a withdrawal and a period of recovery, before a further re-engagement.

Trained at the turn of the century at The London Hospital – one of the most rigorous and constraining nurse training schools of her time – she broke free of the limitations imposed by the hospital system to become one of a new, emerging breed of nurse: the professional woman who practised when and where she wished. Violetta

Thurstan's nurse training was a ticket to freedom and she used it to claim many forms of freedom: she practised nursing in at least five different countries, she interpreted the medical science behind the most advanced British nursing procedures of her day,[34] and she wrote her own memoir – and then rewrote it in a different form.[35] This was, indeed, the greatest of her freedoms: the freedom to tell and retell her own story – to create and recreate her life – in letters; journal articles; autobiographical works; and, finally, towards the end of her life, a series of highly imaginative novels.[36]

Thurstan's life and writings were steeped in the nursing issues of her time. The London Hospital was known for both the rigidity of its discipline and the thoroughness of its training.[37] Thurstan transferred from the hospital's preliminary training school on 29 December 1900,[38] and spent the next two years acquiring a 'Certificate of Training' in which her work was said to be 'satisfactory', her conduct 'very good', and her sick-room cookery 'excellent'.[39] Her training clearly gave her confidence in her own abilities. Her technical writings are redolent of a sense of certainty in her knowledge and practice skills. Yet, after leaving The London, Thurstan turned against the views and values of its matron, Eva Luckes, by becoming one of the most vociferous of those nurses who campaigned openly for a state register.[40] She aligned herself with those nurse leaders of her day who were committed to making nursing an autonomous and independent profession: women such as Ethel Gordon Fenwick and Isla Stewart.[41]

Violetta Thurstan was born on 4 February 1879 in Hastings, Sussex, and named 'Anna Violet'.[42] Her father, Dr Edward Paget Thurstan, travelled extensively, and appears, to have spent a large amount of his time apart from his children.[43] It is not clear when 'Violetta' changed her name.[44] She and her three brothers clearly had a fractured childhood, moving frequently, and spending time in Cornwall, Devon, and the Canary Islands.[45] Like the sons of the Luard family, the Thurstan boys attended private schools, and two of the three joined the armed services. Violetta obtained part of her schooling at the Ladies College in Guernsey, and appears also to have attended a school in Germany. In adulthood, she had a remarkable mastery of a number of European languages, including French, German, and Spanish.[46]

In the last few years of the nineteenth century, it was still possible to 'become' a nurse simply by joining the staff of one of the lower-status hospitals, such as a fever hospital or a hospital for children. Any young British woman with ambition soon realised, however, that it was impossible to advance a nursing career without a training from one of the prestigious voluntary hospitals – preferably in London. After obtaining experience at a 'Home for the Incurables' in London, the East London Hospital for Children in Shadwell, and the Fever Hospital in Guernsey,[47] Thurstan entered The London Hospital as 'probationer Anna Violet Thurstan' in 1900.[48] Here, she appears to have been largely successful, winning the praise and affection of the ward sisters with whom she practised.[49] In spite of this, Matron Eva Luckes appears to have taken something of a dislike to probationer Thurstan, referring to her in the London's 'Register of Probationers' as 'a well-meaning gentle ['feeble' crossed out] little woman with very little strength of character and very nervous and diffident as to her own powers'.[50] A later report condemned 'Anna V. Thurstan' as 'young on her appointment and ... young and childish in her ways. This being so she was spoilt in many ways and did not develop as she ought to have done. She remained unpunctual and untidy to the end and was fond of being made a great deal of'.[51] Like many reports written by a superior about a junior employee (which nurse probationers effectively were), this report probably gives a greater insight into the personality and prejudices of its writer than those of its subject.

Thurstan ended her career at the London as Assistant Sister at Tredegar House, caring for the hospital's population of nurse probationers. There were rumours that she disliked the work, and was planning to leave and start her own business: a children's convalescent home.[52] This may have further alienated Eva Luckes, whose final report on Thurstan comments that 'she had great ideas of her own capabilities but she was very unpractical'.[53] Eventually, Luckes decided to recommend Thurstan for the position of matron at a small convalescent home for children in Hythe. One of her reasons for transferring Thurstan to such an 'easy' position was her concern that her former probationer's health was 'not robust'. This is borne out by the fact that Thurstan's probation record refers to a number of instances when her health 'broke down'.[54] Yet Violetta Thurstan's career went on to span two world wars, a range of gruelling experiences on several war fronts, and frequent injury and illness; and she lived to the age of ninety-nine.

Upon leaving the London Hospital, Thurstan pursued further education, enrolling on a correspondence course at St Andrews University, studying French, geography, fine art, physiology, and English, and acquiring the qualification of 'Lady Literate in Arts' in 1914.[55] In 1913 she had joined the Westminster 146 VAD, run by the British Red Cross.[56] By 1914, Thurstan, like many young people of her time, was poised for war.

Thurstan was clearly a restless spirit. Prior to her move to London, it was reported that she had undertaken temporary work in a surgical hospital in Spain; been Home Sister at the Royal Infirmary, Bristol; held the position of Matron of the Children's Invalid Home, Duxhurst; and, for two-and-a-half years, held a position as Lady Superintendent of the West Riding Nursing Association.[57] These later roles entitled her to membership of the Matrons' Council, to which she was duly elected in February 1913.[58] In that same year, she accepted the position of matron of the new Civil Hospital in La Spezia, Italy, though the building of the hospital was delayed and it is not clear whether she ever took up the position.[59] As a committed and influential member of the movement for the professionalisation of nursing, Thurstan spent much of her time touring the country giving lectures on subjects such as 'The History of Nursing' or 'Some Aspects of Women's Work in the Past'.[60] In 1913, she was just beginning a long association with the *BJN*. During and after the war years, her letters and accounts appeared frequently, along with articles about her exploits and verbatim accounts of interviews with this 'intrepid' nurse.[61]

In September 1914, the Order of St John of Jerusalem invited Thurstan to lead a party of nurses to Brussels to work for the Belgian Red Cross. Her party was selected by the National Union of Trained Nurses (NUTN), a nascent nurses' organisation with which she had just begun what was to be a long and fruitful collaboration.[62] Hundreds of British nurses and volunteers travelled to Belgium in the first weeks of the war. Thurstan was one of those who refused to retreat. Her entire party remained in Brussels, where she soon found herself a prisoner, treating thousands of German soldiers for trench foot.[63] Finding this experience unpleasant, she responded to a request from the Burgomaster of Charleroi to run a small hospital caring for the wounded of several nations.

Thurstan's experience in Charleroi was recounted in her memoir, *Field Hospital and Flying Column*, as one of both hardship and mental stress.[64] Thurstan, with two colleagues, cared for large numbers of wounded soldiers with almost no help. Her narrative is punctuated by episodes in which she defies arrogant German officers who issue unreasonable commands; is almost captured as a spy; and uses her language skills and quick thinking to elude danger.[65] It is not clear what Thurstan's purpose was in writing this book, which, like the work of several other nurse writers, reads very much like a collection of 'girls' own adventure' stories. It may be that she merely wanted to set down an account of her extraordinary experiences. The pace and tone of the book, along with its plain, direct language, suggest that she wanted others to know the adventure of her life – an adventure of which she was the heroine. Thurstan's writing offers, perhaps, one of the clearest examples of the sense of thrill and adventure that infused the 'war fever' of the first months of the First World War and that has been characterised by later writers as the 'innocence' that made it so easy to recruit soldiers to fight on the front lines.[66] It was, perhaps, the same spirit that drove nurses and volunteers to offer their services to the wounded in such large numbers.

In addition to *Field Hospital and Flying Column*, which was published in the spring of 1915, Thurstan also wrote a series of articles and letters for the *BJN*, permitting the journal's readership to follow her adventures. In recounting her experiences in Charleroi, she wrote: 'The day we came there were seventy very badly wounded – French and German – sent here, and there were only our three selves with some Red Cross people from the town who had attended six lectures, and who nearly drove us quite mad.'[67]

In October, Thurstan, along with a large number of other British nurses, was removed from Belgium on a locked train, and deported to neutral Denmark.[68] The Danes appear to have treated the British nurses as celebrities[69] and, while attending a dinner as a special guest, Thurstan met Prince Gustav, nephew of the Dowager Russian Empress, Marie Federovna, who was Head of the Red Cross in Russia.[70] A careful piece of dinnertime diplomacy appears to have won Thurstan and three companions an invitation to join the Russian Red Cross and transfer their services to the Eastern Front.[71] Following what she describes as an exciting journey through Sweden and Finland via the

Arctic Circle in winter, Thurstan reached her first posting in Warsaw (at that time part of the Russian Empire), where she was placed in a Red Cross Hospital run by Russian Sisters of Mercy.[72]

For Thurstan, offering British nursing expertise in regions where nurse training was considered to be underdeveloped was an adventure in itself. She found her Russian colleagues 'amiable' and the Sister Superior a kind and effective leader, who had worked with English nurses during the Russo-Japanese War.[73] Still, wartime conditions meant that staff were short, conditions poor, and the work hard. Two of her group returned to England within weeks, leaving only Thurstan

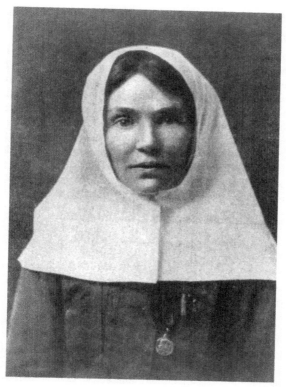

Figure 9 Portrait of Violetta Thurstan in her Russian Red Cross uniform

and experienced St John's Ambulance volunteer nurse Elizabeth Greg to continue the work.[74]

In *Field Hospital and Flying Column*, Thurstan comments on the differences between nursing in Russia and nursing in England. At first, she was amazed at the poor staffing: twenty sisters to a thousand patients. Then she began to realise that much of the real nursing was undertaken by orderlies known as 'sanitars', with sisters supervising, performing technical procedures, and undertaking lighter work. Nevertheless, wartime conditions were harsh, with each nurse working long hours every day, and then – three times per week – remaining on duty all night. She found that 'English views on ventilation are not at all accepted in Russia', where 'the Sisters were genuinely frightened for the safety of the patients when I opened the windows of a hot, stuffy ward one night'.[75] She added that:

> the art of nursing as practised in England does not exist in Russia – even the trained Sisters do things every hour that would horrify us in England. One example of this is their custom of giving strong narcotic or stimulating drugs indiscriminately, such as morphine, codeine, camphor, or ether without doctor's orders. When untrained Sisters and inexperienced dressers do this (which constantly happens) the results are sometimes very deplorable. I have myself seen a dresser give a strong hypodermic stimulant to a man with a very serious haemorrhage. The bleeding vessel was deep down and very difficult to find, and the haemorrhage became so severe after the stimulant that for a long time his life was despaired of from extreme exhaustion due to loss of blood.[76]

Thurstan's observations provide insight into her own priorities as a British nurse. She clearly valued the surgical dressing technique of the Russians, and their attention to asepsis, but deplored what she saw as their failure to offer fundamental nursing care. Years after her experience in Russia, she reflected on these differences in an article for the *BJN*:

> Russian sisters are extremely well trained in the matter of asepsis, and are far beyond ourselves in many ways in this respect … Most of their training time is given up to surgical work; indeed at some of the training schools in Petrograd no medical cases are taken at all. The result is, of course, that the bandaging and dressing is exquisitely done and an example to most English nurses, while the art of nursing, as we have it in England, is – apart from the wound – entirely unknown. That is to say, if a man is admitted with a severe wound in the chest, the wound is most carefully and adequately treated and

beautifully bandaged, while the pneumonia that accompanies it is hardly nursed at all. There is little or no sponging down of feverish patients, no 'art of bedmaking' – the 'sedeilka', or ward maid, generally makes the bed – and very little idea of bringing dainty little dishes to tempt the patient's appetite; if they do not like, or do not want, what is provided, they simply leave it.[77]

While still in Warsaw, Thurstan and Greg were transferred by the Red Cross to what was to prove their most adventurous posting: a flying column, or *letuchka* – a highly mobile unit that would follow the advances and retreats of the Russian army, remaining as close as possible to the front lines in order to receive the wounded from the battlefield without delay.[78] Violetta Thurstan's adventures with the Russian flying column brought her closer to the front lines than almost any woman of her time. She recounted her experiences as a series of intrepid exploits.[79] During these adventures, she wrote a rather breathless article to the honorary secretary of the National Union for Trained Nurses, which was published in the *BJN*:

Warsaw, December 9th, 1914.
   I have had the most exciting time I have ever had in my life. I must tell you about it … Shells were coming at the rate of ten a minute. There were aeroplanes just over us dropping bombs every minute. We got out without anyone being hurt. I never enjoyed anything so much in my life … I can't describe what it was like, but it was splendid.[80]

Thurstan's English companion in Russia, Elizabeth Greg, offers a very different perspective. An 'Honorary Serving Sister of the Order of St John of Jerusalem', Greg had served in Bulgaria from 1912 to 1913 during the Balkan War, as a VAD probationer with Mabel St Clair Stobart's Women's Sick and Wounded Convoy Corps. She appears to have had a considerable amount of wartime nursing experience, but little formal training. In a letter home to a friend she writes of 'Miss T' being 'in great state of excitement being so near things', adding, 'I should not be surprised if she broke down from overstress – solid, stout people who can sleep and eat everything should really come on these jobs.'[81]

In January 1915, Thurstan did, indeed, break down. The semi-trained Elizabeth Greg believed that she was 'altogether too delicate and highly strung and also over-trained for the work she was doing'.[82] In fact there appears to have been much more to Thurstan's 'breakdown' than her apparent delicacy. Evidence (although much of it from one source: the *BJN*) suggests that she had experienced a run of bad luck, having first been wounded by shrapnel while dressing a patient in a forward field hospital, then shocked by the close impact of a shell, and, finally, having contracted pleurisy.[83] She returned to England in April 1915. Greg wrote to her aunt that Thurstan 'was quite broken down – poor thing – She should never have been a nurse – at least being one was too much for anyone so frail – in a quiet civil hospital a matron or a head sister – where there were no shots and shells she might have kept well, but she was too highly strung for the kind of life we have been having.'[84] Greg's judgement of Thurstan is reminiscent of the London Hospital's reports of their 'frail' probationer. Yet, Thurstan went on to serve in Belgium, France, and Macedonia, and to be awarded a Military Medal for courage.

Towards the end of *Field Hospital and Flying Column*, Thurstan comments that 'War would be the most glorious game in the world if it were not for the killing and wounding. In it one tastes the joy of comradeship to the full, the taking and giving, and helping and being helped in a way that would be impossible to conceive in the ordinary world.'[85] Her perception of war as another world is characteristic of her tendency to romanticise her experience. Many decades after the war, she wrote another, somewhat revised, memoir of her experiences, which was published in 1978 just before her death. In this later account, which she titled *The Hounds of War Unleashed*, Thurstan tells of a love affair with Nicholas, an ambulance driver belonging to the flying column, who dies tragically in the early spring of 1915.[86]

Had Violetta Thurstan left only one memoir of her experiences in Belgium and Russia, the directness of her writing and the certainty of her expression might have convinced most readers that her account was a full and accurate narrative of events. The existence of another account, which deviates from the first, creates uncertainty about both. It is tempting to suppose that *The Hounds of War Unleashed*, published when Thurstan was in her late nineties, is the less accurate of the two – that it may, in fact, contain fictional elements. Yet, it is also possible that it was the final confessional of a woman now facing death, writing in a more permissive era, when an element of romance might make a memoir more interesting to its readers. Thurstan's own romantic vision of life undoubtedly influenced the style of both memoirs.

After spending several months in England, convalescing, working as elected Organising and General (Central) Secretary to the NUTN,[87] and touring the country to give lectures on her wartime experiences,[88] Thurstan once more embarked for Russia, this time as the NUTN's representative, to offer its support to the Russian Government in alleviating the plight of millions of refugees.[89] Her remit was to examine the possibility of staffing a maternity unit in one of the major Russian cities,[90] yet she travelled widely, examining the refugee problem in detail. The result was a book, *The People who Run*, which explores the realities of life for 'those five and a half million dazed and terrified people who fled away from their homes in the summer and autumn of 1915, before the great German advance into Russia'.[91]

Thurstan was obviously deeply moved by the plight of the Russian refugees, bringing her romantic perception of the Russian character to her book. For the *BJN* she recounted her memories, stating that 'the bells of Russia ... are the most beautiful in the world, deep, mellow and irresistible, incessantly calling the faithful to church'.[92] Thurstan herself may have been experiencing a sense of homesickness for the Russia in which she had spent only a few months, but to which she appears to have grown attached. In writing of the refugees, she expanded on the subject of the romance of the Russian nation:

> Romance is a rare and almost a despised quality in our materialistic world. But there are those for whom it is the breath of life, and they will know where to look for it, for it does still exist in certain places in spite of 'organization', 'standardization', 'cooperation', and other estimable and modern methods which, if we are not careful, are apt to smother and kill it. And the soil in which this rare plant flourishes is almost always to be found in those countries – such as Russia, Spain, Ireland – which have a curious instinct for suffering and a supreme indifference to the necessities of life.[93]

Thurstan's highly romantic perspective is easy for a modern readership to condemn. A twenty-first-century audience comes to such writings through the prism – both distorting and clarifying – of later perspectives that condemned the First World War as an act of destruction perpetrated upon an innocent generation.[94] Only more recently have some academics begun to focus with greater appreciation on the attitudes of the war generation.[95] Reading Violetta Thurstan's passionate and apparently naive texts returns us to the certainties of that generation – certainties that existed in many minds before hindsight had begun to dissolve them. One of the consequences of Thurstan's passionate support for engagement in the war was her tendency to promote what has come later to be seen as war propaganda. In her frequent lectures, in various parts of Britain, on her experiences in Belgium and Russia, she appears to have given much attention to German atrocities such as the deliberate 'firing' of Belgian towns.[96] She is also reported to have lectured for Lord Derby's appeal to men to enlist voluntarily in order to avoid conscription.[97]

On 11 November 1916, Violetta Thurstan departed, once more, for Belgium. She had been invited by the Joint War Committee of the Red Cross and Order of St John of Jerusalem to take on the role of matron to the prestigious Hôpital de l'Océan at La Panne, on the narrow coastal strip of Belgium that was still in allied hands – an institution that prided itself on being at the leading edge of wartime surgical advance. Its director was the famous Belgian surgeon Dr Antoine Depage, who had previously worked closely with Edith Cavell, and whose hospital was staffed by Belgian, French, Canadian, and British trained nurses; British VADs; and Belgian 'Red Cross ladies'.[98] A column in the *BJN* referred to it as 'not only a hospital, but a university, with a cosmopolitan staff', which used 'microbe charts' to monitor wound recovery in its patients, and had its own social club.[99]

It was during her time as matron at L'Hôpital de l'Océan that Thurstan wrote her technical book on nursing practice: *A Text Book of War Nursing*.[100] Differing in many respects from her other books, it laid down Thurstan's knowledge of wartime nursing practice – a knowledge that was built on her rigorous training at The London Hospital and on her later extensive experience on both Western and Eastern Fronts. The book is infused with Thurstan's sense of the judgement and autonomy of the trained nurse and offers an insight into her philosophy of modern nursing: that the nurse should understand the science behind her practice, and yet should also show deference and obedience to the doctor. A remarkably avant-garde piece of writing, *A Text Book of War Nursing* has received far less attention than Thurstan's other works, and yet this obscure textbook was possibly her most important work, because of its rare contribution to the nursing knowledge of its time. Written in a prosaic style – abandoning the overt romanticism of *Field Hospital and Flying Column* and *The People who Run* – it nevertheless uses rousing language to expound the virtues of the 'fully trained nurse' who can 'go on steadily day by day though most of the excitement and novelty has worn off, teaching batch after batch of raw probationers and orderlies, expending the very best of themselves on the various people with whom they come into contact every day'.[101]

Thurstan's second serious wounding is said to have taken place while she was working at 'a very advanced post in the war zone' in September 1917.[102] Evidence for the incident is sketchy. Reports state that Thurstan was injured by a falling roof, brought down by bombing from a German plane, yet 'recovered enough to help the stretcher-bearers carrying the wounded away, over fields of sugar-beet, in pouring rain, to the next line ambulance'.[103] For this action, she was awarded the Military Medal – an extremely rare accolade for a woman.[104]

From December 1917 to June 1918, Thurstan worked under the auspices of the Scottish Women's Hospitals. Her posting was to Macedonia, where she took on the role of the matron at a hospital in Ostrovo.[105] Here, she is said to have acted heroically in restoring order to the field hospital, which had been 'practically blown to pieces' in a blizzard. Again, illness – this time a bout of malaria – forced her to return to England.[106]

Immediately after the war, Thurstan enlisted in the Women's Royal Air Force, rising to the position of Deputy Assistant Commandant in 1919.[107] Following her demobilisation, she spent time in Egypt as Director of Bedouin Industries, assisting women in refugee camps.[108] Here, she appears to have acquired the weaving skills that were to be so important to her in old age, much of which she spent creating, exhibiting, and selling woven carpets, using natural dyeing techniques and becoming renowned as an expert on a range of ancient weaving and dyeing processes.[109] She appears not to have lost her deep romanticism, recounting for the benefit of *BJN* readers a night she spent camping in the desert, under the stars, which 'on a windless night is a foretaste of Paradise'.[110]

Thurstan was in Spain during the Civil War. It has been reported that she was offered the role of supervisor to the Universities Ambulance;[111] yet, it is also believed that she assisted prisoners to escape from Almeria during the siege, at the end of which she was expelled from Spain.[112] During the Second World War, now well into her sixties (but declaring her age to be forty-seven), she joined the Women's Royal Naval Service, and worked for Naval Intelligence, boarding ships and assisting with searches for contraband.[113] In later life, she worked in a variety of postings with the United Nations Relief and Rehabilitation Association, in Egypt, Italy, Austria, and Serbia. A fervent Catholic (having converted soon after the First World War), she worked with displaced persons on a Catholic Relief Programme. Following her eventual retirement (which came rather late in life) she returned to Cornwall, where she spent her time spinning, weaving, and writing novels.

Violetta Thurstan died on 13 April 1978 in Penryn, Cornwall, at the age, most probably, of ninety-nine. Her funeral was conducted with the full rites of the Catholic Church, and she was, at her own request, buried with her eight military medals.[114]

Conclusion: intrepid nurses

The nurses of the early twentieth century have often been portrayed as a somewhat oppressed group, whose freedoms were constrained and whose opportunities for self-expression were curtailed by the masculine hierarchies of modern hospitals.[115] The careers of Elsie Knocker and Violetta Thurstan suggest that, if an independently minded woman could survive the rigours of a two- or three-year hospital training, she might then use her skills to develop a highly independent career. For nurses as for other women, the First World War appears to have opened up hitherto undreamed-of opportunities.

Women's historians have observed that war did, indeed, permit some women to escape the constraints of patriarchal societies.[116] Yet, they have also pointed out that the freedoms and opportunities gained during the war were not always retained after the armistice. Many women who had taken on the work of men during the war – notably those who had served in the munitions industry or 'land army' – were obliged to relinquish such work at the war's end.[117] The fate of nurses could be very different. Their hospital training certificates, along with their wartime experience, permitted them to present themselves as highly desirable recruits for relief agencies such as the Red Cross. Hence, they were able to retain the independent work-patterns they had carved out for themselves during wartime. The Baroness de T'Serclaes – always an adventure-seeker – worked as a district nurse in Poplar, East London, during the General Strike of 1926. Violetta Thurstan enlisted with the Women's Royal Air Force before working for a range of relief agencies, then travelling to Egypt to take up the position of 'Director of Bedouin Industries' supporting the development of the predominantly female weaving industry. Such women used their nursing qualifications to remain outside the 'cage' of patriarchal social and cultural norms that limited opportunity for most women of their times.[118]

Notes

1 On British nurse training, see: Ann Bradshaw, *The Nurse Apprentice, 1860–1977* (Aldershot: Ashgate, 2001); Christine E. Hallett, 'Nursing 1830–1920: Forging a Profession', in Anne Borsay and Billie Hunter (eds), *Nursing and Midwifery in Britain since 1700* (London: Palgrave, 2012). On American nurse training, see: Patricia D'Antonio, *American Nursing: A History of Knowledge, Authority and the Meaning of Work* (Baltimore: Johns Hopkins University Press, 2010).

2 Baroness de T'Serclaes, *Flanders and Other Fields* (London: George G. Harrap, 1964): 52–101; G. E. Mitton (ed.), *The Cellar-House of Pervyse: A Tale of Uncommon Things from the Journals and Letters of the Baroness de T'Serclaes and Mairi Chisholm* (London: A. and E. Black, 1916): *passim*; Diane Atkinson, *Elsie and Mairi Go to War: Two Extraordinary Women on the Western Front* (London: Preface Publishing, 2009): 79–189.

3 Mitton, *The Cellar-House of Pervyse: passim*.

4 T'Serclaes, *Flanders and Other Fields*: 72–82.

5 T'Serclaes, *Flanders and Other Fields*: 17.

6 Atkinson, *Elsie and Mairi Go to War*: 10–15.

7 Atkinson, *Elsie and Mairi Go to War*: 17–19.

8 T'Serclaes, *Flanders and Other Fields*: 30–5.

9 T'Serclaes, *Flanders and Other Fields*: 62–3.

10 T'Serclaes, *Flanders and Other Fields*: 66–7.

11 T'Serclaes, *Flanders and Other Fields*: 69.

12 Arthur Gleason and Helen Hayes Gleason, *Golden Lads: A Thrilling Account of How the Invading War Machine Crushed Belgium* (New York: A. L. Burt, 1916).

13 T'Serclaes, *Flanders and Other Fields*: 78–9.

14 Baroness de T'Serclaes, MS diary; 9029-2, Imperial War Museum, London.

15 T'Serclaes, *Flanders and Other Fields*: 63–4.

16 Claire Tylee: *The Great War and Women's Consciousness: Images of Militarism and Womanhood in Women's Writings, 1914–64* (Houndmills and London: Macmillan, 1990): 31.

17 T'Serclaes, *Flanders and Other Fields*: 70.

18 T'Serclaes, *Flanders and Other Fields*: 96.

19 T'Serclaes, *Flanders and Other Fields*: 76, 96; T'Serclaes, MS diary, entry for 27 January 1915.

20 T'Serclaes, *Flanders and Other Fields*: 83.

21 On gas gangrene and other anaerobic infections, see: Christine Hallett, *Containing Trauma: Nursing Work in the First World War* (Manchester: Manchester University Press, 2009): 49–59; Mark Harrison, *The Medical War: British Military Medicine in the First World War* (Oxford: Oxford University Press, 2010): 27–31.

22 T'Serclaes, *Flanders and Other Fields*.

23 Mary Borden, *The Forbidden Zone* (London: William Heinemann, 1929): 143–6.

24 Irene Rathbone, *We That Were Young: A Novel* (New York: The Feminist Press, 1989 [1932]).

25 T'Serclaes, *Flanders and Other Fields*: 99–100.

26 T'Serclaes, *Flanders and Other Fields*: 100–14. Elsie Knocker separated from her husband, the Baron de T'Serclaes, and was forced to find work to support herself and her son. On her life after the war, see: Atkinson, *Elsie and Mairi Go to War*: 201–38.

27 T'Serclaes, *Flanders and Other Fields*: 130.

28 T'Serclaes, *Flanders and Other Fields*: 144–202.

29 T'Serclaes, *Flanders and Other Fields*: 91.

30 T'Serclaes, *Flanders and Other Fields*: 49.

31 Alan Clark, *The Donkeys* (London: Pimlico, 1991 [1961]). See also: J. Laffin, *British Butchers and Bunglers of World War One* (Stroud: Sutton, 1988).

32 T'Serclaes, *Flanders and Other Fields*: 213–14.

33 Violetta Thurstan, *Stormy Petrel* (Falmouth: Violetta Thurstan, 1964).

34 Violetta Thurstan, *A Text Book of War Nursing* (London: G. P. Putnam's Sons, 1917).

35 Violetta Thurstan, *Field Hospital and Flying Column: Being the Journal of an English Nursing Sister in Belgium and Russia* (London: G. P. Putnam's Sons, 1915); Violetta Thurstan, *The Hounds of War Unleashed* (St Ives, Cornwall: United Writers Publications, 1978).

36 Thurstan, *Stormy Petrel*; Violetta Thurstan, *The Foolish Virgin* (Marazion: Wordens of Cornwall, 1966). See also the unpublished partial manuscripts held by the Hypatia Trust at the Jamieson Library, Penzance, Cornwall: *The Lucky Mary*; *The Demon*; *The Three Miss Trotts of Polperi*; *Moussa, The Snake Charmer*; *Lunch with the Sheikh*.

37 On Eva Luckes's style as matron of the London Hospital, see: Susan McGann, *The Battle of the Nurses: A Study of Eight Women who Influenced the Development of Professional Nursing, 1880–1930* (London: Scutari Press, 1992): 10–20. For a broader overview of the hospital and its training school, see: Edith R. Parker and Sheila M. Collins, *Learning to Care: A History of Nursing and Midwifery Education at the Royal London Hospital, 1740–1993* (London: Royal London Hospital Archives and Museum, 1998): *passim*.

38 Register of Probationers, no. 7, entry for Anna Violet Thurstan, Archives of the Royal London Hospital, Aldgate, London.

39 Register of Probationers, no. 8, entry for Anna Violet Thurstan, Archives of the Royal London Hospital, Aldgate, London.

40 Violetta Thurstan, 'ABC of State Registration', *BJN* (6 May 1916): 404.

41 Violetta Thurstan registered as a nurse soon after the passing of the Nurses Registration Act in December 1919. She was nurse no. 8177, registered in the name Anna Violetta Thurstan on 27 October 1922. Register for Nurses, 1923, General Part, Archive of the Nursing and Midwifery Council, London.

42 Thurstan herself gave different accounts of her date of birth, probably habitually moving it back in order to be able to obtain positions in adulthood that would normally have been reserved for younger women. Hence, some accounts give her date of birth as 1881: Liz Walton, 'Nurse Violetta Thurstan', *Channel Islands Great War Study Group Journal*, 15 (August 2007): 6–11 (6).

43 Walton, 'Nurse Violetta Thurstan': 6.

44 Her 'correct' name, 'Anna Violet', does appear on the register of the London Hospital. Register of Probationers, no. 8.

45 On Violetta Thurstan, see: Melissa Hardie-Budden, 'Thurstan, Anna Violet (1879–1978)', in *Oxford Dictionary of National Biography* (Oxford: Oxford University Press, 2008).

46 On Violetta Thurstan's early life, see: Muriel Somerfield and Ann Bellingham, *Violetta Thurstan: A Celebration* (Penzance: Jamieson Library, 1993): 1–10.

47 Register of Probationers, no. 8.

48 Register of Probationers, nos 7 and 8.

49 See, for example, a report by the sister on 'Mellish Ward' for the week ending 1 February 1902: 'She is a nice little woman and the patients like her very much'. Register of Probationers, no. 8.

50 Report on 'Mellish Ward', Register of Probationers, no. 8.

51 Report on 'Mellish Ward', Register of Probationers, no. 8.

52 Report on 'Mellish Ward', Register of Probationers, no. 8.

53 Report on 'Mellish Ward', Register of Probationers, no. 8.

54 Report on 'Mellish Ward', Register of Probationers, no. 8.

55 Somerfield and Bellingham, *Violetta Thurstan*: 9–10; Walton, 'Nurse Violetta Thurstan': 7.

56 Walton, 'Nurse Violetta Thurstan': 7.

57 Anon., 'Nurses of Note: Miss Violetta Thurstan', *BJN* (15 February 1913): 130.

58 Anon., Account of a meeting of the Matrons' Council, *BJN* (8 February 1913): 106.

59 Anon., 'Appointments', *BJN* (8 February 1913): 108–9; Anon., Column, *BJN* (12 April 1913): 288; Anon., 'The Dublin Nursing Conference and Exhibition', *BJN* (26 April 1913): 329; Anon., 'The Spezia Hospital', *BJN* (10 May 1913): 367.

60 Anon., 'Nursing Echoes', *BJN* (31 January 1914): 89; Anon., 'Coming Events', *BJN* (9 May 1914): 424; Anon., 'League News', *BJN* (27 June 1914): 584. In 1915, when Thurstan took on the role of Organising Secretary of the National Union of Trained Nurses (NUTN), she supported the work of the union in campaigning for nurse registration. She also gave at least one personal donation of funds to the Society for the State Registration of Trained Nurses: Anon., Column, *BJN* (19 June 1915): 526; Anon., Column, *BJN* (11 March 1916): 224; Violetta Thurstan, 'ABC of State Registration'; Anon., 'National Union of Trained Nurses', *BJN* (17 June 1916): 525; Anon., 'National Union of Trained Nurses', *BJN* (14 October 1916): 315; Anon., 'National Union of Trained Nurses', *BJN* (21 October 1916): 335.

61 Anon., 'Nurses of Note: Miss Violetta Thurstan'; Violetta Thurstan, 'The British Red Cross Society', *BJN* (24 January 1914): 65–6.

62 Anon., 'Active Service', *BJN* (22 August 1914): 158; Anon., Column, *BJN* (19 September 1914): 224.

63 Thurstan, *Field Hospital and Flying Column*: 20.

64 Thurstan, *Field Hospital and Flying Column*: 16–52.

65 On these experiences, see also a series of articles Thurstan wrote for the *BJN*, among them: Violetta Thurstan, 'From Brussels', *BJN* (10 October 1914): 286–7; Violetta Thurstan, 'An International Welcome', *BJN* (24 October 1914): 322.

66 Paul Fussell, *The Great War and Modern Memory* (Oxford: Oxford University Press, 2000 [1975]); Eric Leed, *No Man's Land: Combat and Identity in World War One* (New York: Cambridge University Press, 1979); Modris Ecksteins, *Rites of Spring: The Great War and the Birth of the Modern Age* (Boston, MA: Houghton Mifflin, 1989).

67 Violetta Thurstan, 'Letters from the Front', *BJN* (26 September 1914): 246–7. On her continuing adventures in Belgium, see also: Thurstan, 'From Brussels'.

68 Thurstan, 'An International Welcome', *BJN* (24 October 1914): 322.

69 The Danish nurses appear to have been acting, in part, under the auspices of the Danish Council of Nurses and the International Council of Nurses; Thurstan was a member of the latter and had already met a number of prominent Danish nurses at a meeting of the council in Cologne in 1912. See: Thurstan, 'An International Welcome'. See also: Anon., 'The National Council of Trained Nurses', *BJN* (13 March 1915): 210.

70 Thurstan, *Field Hospital and Flying Column*: 110. See also: Somerfield and Bellingham, *Violetta Thurstan*: 15.

71 'Miss Thurstan, Miss Wilkinson and Mrs Nicholson, accompanied by Miss Greg, have left Copenhagen for Petrograd': Anon., Column, *BJN* (24 October 1914): 324. See also: M. B. (probably Margaret Breay), '"With a Flying Column of the Russian Red Cross": Miss Violetta Thurstan', *BJN* (13 March 1915): 207–10. One of Thurstan's companions, Sister Martin-Nicholson, later wrote a memoir of her experiences: Sister Martin-Nicholson, *My Experiences on Three Fronts* (London: George Allen and Unwin, 1916). Elizabeth Greg subsequently condemned Martin-Nicholson as 'a real adventuress': Miss Elizabeth Agnes Greg, letters, 01/17/1, Imperial War Museum, London. An anonymous review of *My Experiences on Three Fronts* can be found in: *BJN* (30 December 1916): 527.

72 Thurstan, *Field Hospital and Flying Column*: 113.

73 Thurstan, *Field Hospital and Flying Column*: 114–15.

74 Although Thurstan refers to her English companion only as 'Sister G', corroborative evidence suggests persuasively that 'Sister G' was Elizabeth Greg, whose letters home refer to her work with 'Miss Thurstan' in Russia. See: Greg, letters.

75 Thurstan, *Field Hospital and Flying Column*: 117.

76 Thurstan, *Field Hospital and Flying Column*: 120–1.

77 Violetta Thurstan, 'Russian Red Cross Sisters', *BJN* (27 January 1917): 62. See also Christine E. Hallett, *Veiled Warriors: Allied Nurses of the First World War* (Oxford: Oxford University Press, 2014): Chapter 3.

78 Thurstan, *Field Hospital and Flying Column*: 125–7.

79 Thurstan, *Field Hospital and Flying Column*. See, for example: 144–60, 172.

80 Violetta Thurstan, 'From Warsaw', *BJN* (9 January 1915): 30.

81 Greg, letters.

82 Greg, letters.

83 Anon., Column, *BJN* (13 February 1915): 130–3 (132); Anon., Column, *BJN* (20 February 1915): 146; M. B., 'With a Flying Column of the Russian Red Cross'.

84 Greg, letters.

85 Thurstan, *Field Hospital and Flying Column*: 174.

86 Thurstan, *The Hounds of War Unleashed*.

87 The NUTN campaigned openly for nurse registration. See: Anon., 'National Union of Trained Nurses', *BJN* (3 April 1915): 279; Anon., Column, *BJN* (6 November 1915): 385; Anon., 'National Union of Trained Nurses' (31 July 1920); Anon., Column, *BJN* (19 June 1915).

88 Anon., 'Coming Events', *BJN* (17 April 1915): 330; Anon., 'Book of the Week', *BJN* (24 April 1915): 352; Anon., Column, *BJN* (1 May 1915): 371, 377; Anon., Column, *BJN* (5 June 1915): 489; Anon., Column, *BJN* (26 June 1915): 550; Anon., Column, *BJN* (27 November 1915): 445; Anon., Column, *BJN* (24 July 1915): 78; Anon., Column, *BJN* (6 October 1915): 317; Anon., Column, *BJN* (23 October 1915): 340.

89 Anon., Column, *BJN* (11 December 1915): 481.

90 Anon., Column, *BJN* (8 January 1916): 29; Anon., Column, *BJN* (5 February 1916): 115–16; Anon., Column, *BJN* (4 March 1916): 214; Anon., Column, *BJN* (11 March 1916).

91 Violetta Thurstan, *The People who Run: Being the Tragedy of the Refugees in Russia* (London: G. P. Putnam's Sons, 1916): 1. See also the reviews in *BJN*: Anon., review of Violetta Thurstan, *The People who Run*, *BJN* (8 April 1916): 327–8; Anon., 'A School for Mothers in Petrograd', *BJN* (6 May 1916): 411; Anon., 'Refugees in Russia', *BJN* (27 May 1916): 462; Anon., Review of Violetta Thurstan, *The People who Run*, *BJN* (1 July 1916): 13; Anon., 'The Horrors of Deportation', *BJN* (12 August 1916): 134; Anon., Column, *BJN* (9 December 1916): 477.

92 Anon., Column, *BJN* (18 March 1916): 243.

93 Thurstan, *The People who Run*: 11–12.

94 Tylee, *The Great War and Women's Consciousness*.

95 Alan Bishop and Mark Bostridge, *Letters from a Lost Generation: First World War Letters of Vera Brittain and Four Friends* (London: Abacus, 1999); Adrian Gregory, *The Last Great War: British Society and the First World War* (Cambridge: Cambridge University Press, 2008); Hallett, *Veiled Warriors*.

96 See, for example, a report on Violetta Thurstan's speech to the Matrons' Council on 1 May 1915: Anon., Column, *BJN* (8 May 1915): 385.

97 Anon., 'Miss Violetta Thurstan on Active Service in Spain', *BJN* (March 1937): 79.

98 Anon., 'National Union of Trained Nurses', *BJN* (28 October 1916): 355; Anon., Column, *BJN* (4 November 1916): 377; Anon., Column, *BJN* (1 November 1916): 387. See also: Hallett, *Veiled Warriors*: Chapter 1.

99 Anon., 'Nursing at La Panne', *BJN* (10 March 1917): 169. On L'Hôpital de l'Océan, see also: Anon., 'Care of the Wounded', *BJN* (14 April 1917): 25; Anon., Column, *BJN* (16 June 1917): 415; Henrietta Tayler, *A Scottish Nurse at War: Being a Record of What One Semi-Trained Nurse Has Been Privileged to See and Do during Four and a Half Years of War* (London: John Lane, 1920): 29–45.

100 Thurstan, *A Text Book of War Nursing*. See also the advance notice in *BJN*: Anon., Column, *BJN* (14 July 1917): 21; Anon., Column, *BJN* (15 September 1917): 165; Anon., review of Violetta Thurstan, *A Text Book of War Nursing*, *BJN* (13 October 1917): 244.

101 Thurstan, *A Text Book of War Nursing*: 13.

102 Anon., Column, *BJN* (15 September 1917): 165; Anon., Column, *BJN* (22 September 1917): 181.

103 Walton, 'Nurse Violetta Thurstan': 8–9. There is an account of this incident in Anon., 'Miss Violetta Thurstan on Active Service in Spain'.

104 Norman Gooding, *Honours and Awards to Women* (London: Savannah Publications, 2013): 149–50; Anon., 'Nursing and the War', *BJN* (24 November 1917): 332.

105 Anon., 'Medal for a Nurse', *BJN* (1 December 1917): 351; Anon., Column, *BJN* (19 January 1918): 47; Anon., 'Nursing and the War', *BJN* (7 September 1918): 151. See also: Somerfield and Bellingham, *Violetta Thurstan*: 17–18; Walton, 'Nurse Violetta Thurstan': 6.

106 Anon., 'Miss Violetta Thurstan on Active Service in Spain'.

107 Walton, 'Nurse Violetta Thurstan': 10.

108 Anon., 'National Union of Trained Nurses' (31 July 1920); Anon., 'Miss Violetta Thurstan on Active Service in Spain'. See also: Walton, 'Nurse Violetta Thurstan': 10.

109 Thurstan's writings on weaving and dyeing include: Violetta Thurstan, *The Use of Vegetable Dyes for Beginners* (London: Dryad Press, 1930); Violetta Thurstan, *A Short History of Decorative Textiles and Tapestries* (Exeter: Papler and Sewell, 1934); Violetta Thurstan, *Weaving Patterns of Yesterday and Today* (London: Dryad Press, n.d.); Violetta Thurstan, *Weaving without Tears* (London: Museum Press, n.d.). See also: Anon., 'Our Fellows: What Are They Doing?', *BJN* (November 1927): 266; Violetta Thurstan, 'Art and Medicine', *BJN* (November 1927): 272; Anon., 'What Our Fellows Are Doing', *BJN* (April 1928): 85; Violetta Thurstan, 'Old English Handicrafts', *BJN* (April 1928): 101; Anon., 'Weaving Exhibition', *BJN* (July 1929): 179.

110 Violetta Thurstan, 'A Three Weeks' Journey in the Libyan Desert', *BJN* (February 1925): 42.

111 Anon., 'Miss Violetta Thurstan on Active Service in Spain'.

112 Walton, 'Nurse Violetta Thurstan': 10.

113 Walton, 'Nurse Violetta Thurstan': 10.

114 These were: the Military Medal, the Order of St George (Russia), the Ordre de la Reine Elisabeth (Belgium), the Mons Star with clasp and roses (Britain), the Allied Medal, the Companion of the Vatican, the British War Medal, and the Victory Medal: Walton, 'Nurse Violetta Thurstan': 11. See also: Somerfield and Bellingham, *Violetta Thurstan*: 91 (who actually list nine medals); and Gooding, *Honours and Awards to Women*: 149–50, who refers to two Russian medals.

115 Brian Abel-Smith, *A History of the Nursing Profession* (London: Heinemann, 1960); Eva Gamarnikow, 'Nurse or Woman: Gender and Professionalism in Reformed Nursing, 1860–1923', in Pat Holden and Jenny Littlewood (eds), *Anthropology and Nursing* (London: Routledge, 1991): 110–29; McGann, *The Battle of the Nurses*.

116 Sandra Gilbert, 'Soldier's Heart: Literary Men, Literary Women and the Great War', in Margaret Randolph Higonnet, Jane Jenson, Sonya Michel, and

Margaret Collins Weitz (eds), *Behind the Lines: Gender and the Two World Wars* (New Haven: Yale University Press, 1987): 197–226.

117 Margaret Higonnet and Patrice Higonnet, 'The Double Helix', in Higonnet, Jenson, Michel, and Weitz, *Behind the Lines*: 31–47; Joan Scott, 'Rewriting History', in Higonnet, Jenson, Michel, and Weitz, *Behind the Lines*: 21–30; Susan Grayzel, *Women's Identities at War: Gender, Motherhood, and Politics in Britain and France during the First World War* (Chapel Hill: University of North Carolina Press, 1999).

118 Gail Braybon and Penny Summerfield, *Out of the Cage: Women's Experiences in Two World Wars* (London: Routledge, 2012 [1987]).

Part III
Volunteer girls

Tens of thousands of women prepared themselves for war service as nurses in the years leading up to the First World War. A minority of these were fully trained. Others attached themselves to VADs, undertook short courses in sick-nursing, bandaging, invalid cookery, and hygiene, and held themselves in readiness for war. Still others came forward at the outbreak of war with no training at all, and began developing their skills in the heat and stress of the wartime emergency. Anne Summers has shown that British and Dominion women had been preparing themselves, at least mentally, for decades to play their part in an anticipated conflict; their very preparedness had made war more likely.[1] As nurses they knew that not only would they be in an ideal position to observe the events of war; they would also be 'in the thick of the action,'[2] and their eagerness to volunteer for overseas service can be understood as part of this desire to be an integral element of the war effort.

As nurses' memoirs began to be published during the war itself, it became evident that events were not meeting their expectations. Although war service was sometimes exciting and adventurous, it more often alternated between tedious and uncomfortable waits, and 'rushes' of overwhelming activity during which one watched men die, powerless to save them. In the first months of war, VADs served only in voluntary hospitals of the Red Cross or Order of St John of Jerusalem. In the spring of 1915, at the height of the emergency created by unsuccessful assaults on the Western Front at Ypres, Festubert, and Neuve Chapelle, the military medical services agreed to accept VADs in military hospitals both in Britain and overseas.[3]

The writings of VADs offer a different viewpoint from those of trained nurses. VADs had more time and less responsibility than professionals, and were therefore more able to observe and record the life of the military hospital. Their perspective was, furthermore, a simple one, undistorted by previous nursing experience. The very newness of their experience made their observations sharper and more focused – and yet more judgemental and simplistic – than those of trained nurses. In some volunteer writings, the VAD herself is the heroine, and the actions of other hospital personnel exist to create challenges for her. In others the professional nurse takes centre-stage, and the VAD is the all-seeing witness, capturing events, apparently without distortion. But such appearances are deceptive: VADs were far from dispassionate, and tensions between them and their professional supervisors resulted in a distortion of the historical record that has exaggerated the excess discipline of the military hospital and underplayed the emotional labour undertaken by nurses. A myth of wartime nursing has emerged, which places young, compassionate, and willing VADs at the centre of the action and invites audiences to watch as they grapple with the practical and emotional crises created by an inhuman military medical machine mediated by harsh and bitter spinster nurses.[4]

Romantic notions of journeying through extraordinary landscapes, of struggling, and of being tested also appear with remarkable regularity in the writings of VADs – as does the tendency to reduce the war to one enormous battle between good – represented by the British and their allies – and evil – represented by the central powers. It appears that volunteer nurses were more likely to use these old romantic literary tropes than their trained professional colleagues.[5] This may be because they, like their middle- and upper-class brothers, were steeped in the highly romantic literary canon of the day. It may also be that their motives for nursing the wounded had more to do with their desire more to be a part of the 'great struggle' of war than with any wish to develop their expertise as nurses.[6]

Notes

1 Anne Summers, *Angels and Citizens: British Women as Military Nurses, 1854–1914*, rev. edn (Newbury: Threshold Press, 2000).

2 Anon., *Twenty Months a VAD* (Sheffield: J. Northen, n.d.), 96/317: 13, Red Cross Archive Library, London.

3 The majority of VADs served on the 'Home Front'. On VADs, see: Sue Light, 'British Military Nurses and the Great War: A Guide to the Services', *The Western Front Association Forum* (7 February 2010): 4, available at www. westernfrontassociation.com (accessed 30 October 2012).

4 Christine E. Hallett, ' "Emotional Nursing": Involvement, Engagement, and Detachment in the Writings of First World War Nurses and VADs', in Alison S. Fell and Christine E. Hallett (eds), *First World War Nursing: New Perspectives* (New York: Routledge, 2013): 87–102; Christine E. Hallett, *Veiled Warriors: Allied Nurses of the First World War* (Oxford: Oxford University Press, 2014), introduction.

5 See, for example, the writings of Olive Dent, Mary Britnieva, and Florence Farmborough, considered later in this section: Olive Dent, *A VAD in France* (London: Grant Richards, 1917); Mary Britnieva, *One Woman's Story* (London: Arthur Baker, 1934); Florence Farmborough, *Nurse at the Russian Front: A Diary 1914–18* (London: Book Club Associates, 1974). On the 'romance pattern', see: Paul Fussell, *The Great War and Modern Memory* (Oxford: Oxford University Press, 2000 [1975]): 130–1.

6 Janet S. K. Watson, 'Wars in the Wards: The Social Construction of Medical Work in First World War Britain', *Journal of British Studies*, 41(2002): 484–510. See also: Janet S. K. Watson, *Fighting Different Wars: Experience, Memory and the First World War* (Cambridge: Cambridge University Press, 2004): *passim*.

7

American young women at war

Introduction: American women at war

American women participated in the First World War long before their nation entered the conflict. Wealthy and independent women who could afford to travel joined volunteer units or offered their services independently to the Committees of the French and Belgian Red Cross.[1] Their efforts were rewarded by admission into some of the most dramatic – and horrific – scenarios of the war. Nothing could have prepared them for the seriousness of the wounds they encountered. Industrial warfare was not a new phenomenon: the Second Anglo-Boer War (1899–1902) and the Russo-Japanese War (1904–5) had featured the use of machine guns and the deployment of heavy artillery. What was new, and (for most) unexpected, was the extent of the carnage. The unsuccessful assaults that characterised the first three-and-a-half years of the First World War led to massive numbers of casualties, sometimes numbering tens of thousands in one day. Typically, the wounded would arrive at field hospitals as 'rushes' – more than could be coped with by even the best-staffed hospital with the most highly trained clinical personnel.[2]

Many American volunteer nurses enlisted with the French Red Cross and found themselves posted to field hospitals where fully trained nurses were scarce. The development of a nursing profession in France had been slow and uneven. There were very few secular training schools, and much of the country's civilian nursing care was in the hands of religious nuns who, even though they were often highly competent carers, had very little technical training.[3] The outset of the war also saw the recruitment of large numbers of French 'lady volunteers', motivated more by patriotism than by a desire to nurse.

Disillusionment and despair: meeting the realities of war

The opportunity to cross the Atlantic and travel to the Old World of which they had heard so much fired the imaginations of many American women. Some freely admitted to having been driven by highly romantic fantasies. Shirley Millard described how she 'wanted to save France from the marauding enemy', adding that 'banners streamed in my blood; drums beat in my brain; bugles sounded in my ears'.[4]

Millard began her published memoir of the war with a foreword in which she described how, in the mid-1930s, she had rediscovered her diary: a 'record of the year 1918', wrapped in a small French tricolour. At this point, Europe seemed to be moving inexorably towards another war, and her fear that warfare would threaten the future of her five-year-old son prompted her to write a book, somewhat eccentrically entitled *I Saw Them Die*.[5] True to its title, the book contains numerous references to horrifying deaths in French military hospitals. Millard writes of the power of a long-forgotten diary to evoke the sights, sounds, and smells of another time. Her foreword resonates with nostalgia as she surveys the 'small pig-skin volume with a gilt clasp'. The memoir is clearly intended both to offer an eye-witness account of the horror of war – a record written with pacifist intentions – and to chronicle Millard's own development from naive adventuress to war-weary woman, made wise by her experience and unable to view with equanimity the approach of another conflict.

At the outset of war, Millard's fantasies had been driven by both the romance of nursing and a more focused romantic love for a particular object:

> I visualized myself driving an ambulance along the battle lines, aiding and comforting the wounded, or kneeling beside dying men in shell-torn No Man's Land. Or better still, gliding silently among hospital cots, placing a cool hand on fevered brows, lifting bound heads to moisten pain-parched lips with water ... Perhaps Ted, whom I was then regarding with some favour, would be brought back to the hospital – wounded. Oh, very slightly

wounded, of course. Gassed a bit perhaps. Or with a sprained ankle. He would open his eyes and find me bending over him, my white veil brushing his cheek.[6]

Composing her memoir almost twenty years after the events it describes, Millard is conscious of both the frustrated energy and the self-absorption of youth that drove so many women to volunteer as nurses. Upon arrival in France, Millard found herself in a temporary makeshift hospital in a chateau near Soissons. On 28 March 1918, she wrote in her diary of how different hospital work was from all that she had imagined. The hospital had 3,500 beds and the wounded seemed to pour in from a 'procession of ambulances'. Once the chateau was full, many had to sleep on stretchers outside, where 'from the black shadows under the trees came their moans, their cries and sobs'.[7] Millard offers a vivid impression of herself: a volunteer who was out of her depth, nursing – with neither training nor experience – seriously injured trauma casualties:

Some one thrust a huge hypodermic needle and a packet of something into my hands and told me hurriedly that every man who came in must have a shot against tetanus. The soil of the battlefields was impregnated with poisons from gas and explosives. After that I was to 'get them ready' for the operating table. 'Hurry! Fast as you can!' I looked about helplessly. How on earth did one give a hypodermic? I'd never even *had* one. And what did 'get them ready' mean?[8]

Millard describes how she learned injection technique by watching other nurses and attempting to mirror their practice, and how she received some basic tuition from a friendly orderly.

Although her nursing skills left much to be desired, Millard's writing skills cannot be doubted. While they are raw and unsophisticated, her precise and vivid descriptions of what she saw leave a deep impression on the mind of the reader:

Gashes from bayonets. Flesh torn by shrapnel. Faces half shot away. Eyes seared by gas; one here with no eyes at all. I can see down into the back of his head. Here is a boy with a grey, set face. He is hanging on … too far gone to make a sound. His stomach is blown wide open, and only held together by a few bands of sopping gauze which I must pull away. I do so, as gently as I can. The odour is sickening; the gauze is greenish yellow. Gangrene. He was wounded days ago and has been waiting in the grounds. He will die …

My hands get firmer, faster. I can feel the hardness of emergency setting in. Perhaps after a while I won't mind. Here is an unconscious lad with his head completely bandaged. The gauze is stiff with blood and dirt. I cut carefully and remove it, glad he is unconscious; much easier to work when they cannot feel the pain. As the last band comes off, a sickening mass spills out of the wide gash at the side of his skull. Brains! I am stunned. I cannot think what to do. No time to ask questions. Everyone around me is occupied with similar problems. Boldly I wrap my hand in sterile gauze and thrust the slippery mass back as best I can, holding the wound closed while I awkwardly tie a clean bandage around the head. It does not occur to me until afterwards that he must have been dead.[9]

Millard's diary is rare because it describes the experiences of an entirely untrained and inexperienced young woman. The policy of the Army Nurse Corps was to allow only fully trained nurses to accompany official medical units to Europe.[10] American volunteer units like the one Millard joined worked under the auspices of the American Red Cross. Their services were welcomed by the Belgian and French military medical services. Millard appears to have been unusual in having no nursing or first-aid training at all.[11] Most volunteer nurses equipped themselves with a range of basic skills and techniques – usually taught by trained nurses hired by the Red Cross. In Britain, where a war had long been anticipated, such training sessions were organised by VADs, and the preparation of volunteer nurses had attained a degree of sophistication. In the USA there was consensus among nurse leaders that it was not advisable to encourage the organised development of 'volunteer nursing' units. In May 1918, a year after America's entry into the war, leaders of the profession met at the Convention of the National Nursing Organizations in Cleveland, Ohio, to discuss the serious shortage of military nurses on the war front. They decided that the shortfall in the numbers of trained US military nurses should be made good, not by the employment of volunteers, but by the recruitment of probationer nurses via the Army School of Nursing, which had been formed in the previous year.[12]

The determination of US nurse leaders not to supplement their profession's numbers with semi-trained volunteers had two consequences. It brought a greater stability to nursing services on war fronts, but it also resulted in a lower investment of the professional nursing services' time and resources into the training of volunteer nurses. When American volunteer units did travel to Europe they were often accompanied by women with very little training or preparation of any kind.[13]

The mystery of *War Nurse*

The theme that war can damage women as well as men is taken up by feminist writer Rebecca West in her highly sensationalised *War Nurse*, a work that stands outside the influence of propaganda, offering a unique and highly individual perspective.[14] Like Millard's less conscious work, West's writing seems to derive from a compulsion to set out the horrific consequences of war. The anonymously published *War Nurse* is one of the most elusive texts of the First World War. Ghost-written by West from the diaries of an anonymous volunteer nurse, known only as 'Corinne Andrews', the text contains shocking accounts of the brutality of military surgery.[15] Its main purpose, however, is to convey a sense of how women, as well as men, could be irreparably damaged by war: the focus is on the destruction of the volunteer nurse herself. The book's main character is the daughter of a wealthy American who travels to Paris to work for the American Ambulance at the outset of war. The story traces her descent from optimistic-but-naive war worker, through disillusionment and flight into romance, to physical and emotional self-destruction through overwork and a damaging relationship. The sensationalist nature of the work may have led West – who, by the time it was published in book form, was a writer of some repute – to distance herself from the project. The book's main figure – the nurse – remains anonymous, leaving the reader with a sense of the unreality of what is nevertheless a powerfully told story.

The American Ambulance at Neuilly was an American volunteer hospital, operating under the auspices of the French Red Cross. It appears to have had a reputation as a quirky institution. An anonymous article, written, apparently, by two trained US nurses and published in the *American Journal of Nursing*, offers a light-hearted and amusing perspective on the work of its untrained volunteers:

> The majority of the volunteer workers were very splendid people, and without their good, honest, hard work the hospital could not have been run.

Mixed with those, however, were some who took the work less seriously and, although they gave the nurses some anxious moments and little help, they did furnish us with many a good laugh … I recall the words of the naïve young lady who, when asked how a certain patient was doing, said, 'Oh, he is getting along beautifully, his temperature goes up a little more each day!'.[16]

The 'American Ambulance' had been established in the grand buildings of the Lycée Pasteur in Neuilly-sur-Seine, a suburb of Paris.[17] Trained nurses Ellen La Motte and Agnes Warner both worked there for a short time.[18] The hospital appears to have been a largely effective, but highly eccentric, institution. 'Corinne Andrews', the heroine of *War Nurse*, appears to have spent several months there, working as a volunteer nurse.

War Nurse must be seen as having dual authorship. The publicity material produced by the publisher, the Cosmopolitan Book Corporation of New York, states that:

> 'Corinne Andrews' is not the real name of the woman whose war story is told here. But the story, transcribed from her diary, is authentic. The sheltered daughter of a staid New York family became a war nurse. In a new world that seemed to be built on contrasts and paradoxes, melodrama, irony and illicit romance became the stuff of matter-of-fact daily life, and with matter-of-fact sincerity she set the poignant story down.[19]

The two ideas that stand out from this piece of publicity are the idea that the account is 'authentic' and the claim that it has a 'matter-of-fact sincerity'. But what exactly are 'authenticity' and 'matter-of-fact sincerity', particularly when they are placed alongside 'paradoxes, melodrama, irony and illicit romance'? And, if the account is really transcribed from an anonymous nurse's diary, how could authorship have been attributed to Rebecca West? And can one know that the events related in the diary actually took place? The veracity of West's account is called into question not only because there is no way of knowing who 'Corinne Andrews' was, but also because the ghost-writer – West – is something of a ghost herself. Born Cicely Fairfield, West took her pen name from a character in Ibsen's play *Rosmersholm*. Not even Rebecca West was exactly who she claimed to be.[20] And the mystery of the book's authorship goes even further than this. Rebecca West's name was removed from the book when it was published in 1930. Biographer Victoria Glendinning has suggested that West's original work on the serialisation of the diary in 1926 was primarily motivated by financial need: West was a single mother.[21] It may be that, having achieved success and acclaim as an author by 1930, she no longer wanted to be associated with this unusual and avant-garde production of her earlier years. It may also be that she saw *War Nurse* as a less polished, less sophisticated piece of writing than her other works. The book's staccato passages and, at times, overwrought impressions contrast markedly with the beautiful and polished prose of her most famous early work, *The Return of the Soldier*,[22] and it never achieved the critical acclaim of later novels such as *The Fountain Overflows* and *The Birds Fall Down*.[23]

To understand *War Nurse* it is necessary to appreciate West's insistent feminism. A campaigner for women's rights in the popular press of her time, she allowed a sense of the injustices suffered by the women of the early twentieth century resonate through her writings, along with her belief that their contributions and sacrifices were not recognised.[24] This may be what drew her to the story of 'Corinne Andrews', whose health is said to have been irreparably damaged by the heavy lifting of patients to the extent that the war has left her disabled: physically and emotionally damaged and, significantly, unable to have children and fulfil her accepted role as a woman in 1920s society. 'Corinne Andrews' has been just as badly damaged as any soldier wounded by the war – just as disabled by her experience. Perhaps, then, the central message of *War Nurse* is that men do not have the right to claim a monopoly of suffering and sacrifice in time of war, just as they do not have the monopolistic right to claim the power to determine war's execution.[25]

There is no way of knowing whether the compelling style of *War Nurse* derives mainly from the intensity of 'Corinne Andrews''s original setting-down of her experiences in her diary or of 'Rebecca West''s skill with a pen in redrafting and developing those original experiences and ideas. The book has a remarkable intensity and verve. We learn of how 'Andrews' chose to travel to France rather than accept the stultifying life of a rich American wife; of her first encounters with the brutality at the heart of military surgery when an eye specialist hands her a shrapnel-filled eye he has just removed from a conscious patient, ordering her to 'find the piece of steel';[26] of the strange sense of 'exaltation and happiness' her work gave her;[27] of the

disillusionment that sets in, not only for her, but for her fellow workers, as the war drags on into its third year, when not even the triumph
of America's entry into the conflict can settle the nagging feeling that
life is meaningless. We learn of her flight (and that of many of her
fellow hospital workers) into romance, as she begins an affair with an
ambulance-driver-turned-air-force-pilot; of her wounding, her dramatic near-fatal collapse, and finally, the greatest disillusionment of
all: the return home to an empty world, which leaves only an impo-
tent desire to go back again to a wartime existence that can never be
recaptured.

The nurse writes of her early realisation that the world is not the
safe place she had assumed it to be:

> It was a hard knock realizing that we fool ourselves all the time about the
> mastery we have over nature; that there are thousands of ways pain and
> suffering can hit the body which medical science can barely alleviate, which
> simply have to be met with courage. The only consolation was that at the
> same time you found how much pain and suffering there is in the world,
> you found something else, too. It's the fashion to talk now as if the war was
> utterly squalid, as if everybody went to pieces under it, and there was noth-
> ing glorious there at all. That isn't how I found it. It was the most amazing
> thing I've ever known, how brave these soldiers were. They came up to the
> operating table without flinching. They made jokes about it, called it the
> billiard table.[28]

West's writing in the earlier part of the book mirrors that of more
traditionalist writers. The heroic motif is prominent. But later, when
'Andrews' has lost her own health and strength, we learn that even the
courage of her fellow sufferers cannot give her hope. On her return
to New York, she works as a hospital nurse for three months, yet she
realises that 'the procession of pallid, stunted human misfits which
passed through those wards would go on forever and ever. It just
seemed hopeless to me. So I weakened and quit. There are a lot of
things about which it can be said, "It was all right in the war, but it's
no use in peace."'[29]

Rebecca West's *War Nurse* was a hard-hitting exposé of the destructiveness of war, and of the naivety that had compelled young women –
as well as men – to expose themselves to its force. For Corinne
Andrews, as for many other nurses, the war was somehow a 'force of
nature', something that human beings were drawn into rather than

creating for themselves. West records an incident in which Andrews encounters a young patient who is about to undergo the torture of a sixth operation on an amputation stump:

> I said, 'Thank God, that kid will be going home soon.'
> The doctor said, 'But he won't. Dr Laroche intends to operate again on Thursday.'
> I was so mad I stopped the dressing-cart. 'But why?' I exclaimed. 'Why? I thought he was doing so beautifully. What do we want to operate for?'
> He shrugged his shoulders.
> 'C'est comme la guerre. Il ne faut pas chercher à comprendre.'
> 'It's like the war. You needn't try to understand it.'
> They used to say it about everything; I tell you, they all felt as I did. As if the war was a masterless thing like the tides, and it was coming right for you.[30]

Conclusion: the truth about the war

Rebecca West was not the only author who chose to describe the war as if it were a 'masterless thing like the tides'. The metaphor of the war as a vast ocean that drew men into its destructive core, and then cast up their damaged bodies onto the metaphorical beach that was the 'zone of the armies' finds echoes in the writings of Maud Mortimer, Mary Borden, and Ellen La Motte.[31] Describing the realities of war – particularly from the perspective of someone who was nursing its wounded – was a complex endeavour. The truth about the war was not a simple matter. And exposing the inadequacies of volunteer nursing services sometimes meant exposing one's own inadequacies – as Shirley Millard discovered. A writer such as Rebecca West could present the diaries of a volunteer nurse such as 'Corinne Andrews' as a succession of morality tales of war's corrosiveness; yet those diaries remain shrouded in mystery – weakening their power, and leaving the reader with a sense of not knowing whose voice is being heard.

British volunteer nurses – particularly those wealthy women who established their own volunteer hospitals – received significant positive publicity from the British national press. American volunteers were less celebrated in their own country, where, until 1917, there was ambivalence about whether Americans should be engaging in the war at all.[32] Personal feelings of support for the allies – particularly for the French – meant that numerous women did experience a powerful compulsion to offer their services to the wounded, through volunteer units acting under the auspices of the French and Belgian Societies of the Red Cross. Many were totally unprepared for nursing work. The memoir of an inexperienced and untrained volunteer such as Shirley Millard offers an oblique perspective on the intricacies and challenges of nursing, and illustrates, more vividly than any professional nursing treatise, the importance of formal training. Rebecca West's rendition of the diary of 'Corinne Andrews' is more complex. It has some of the qualities of feminist writings such as Mabel St Clair Stobart's *The Flaming Sword in Serbia and Elsewhere* and ironic, pacifist treatises such as Ellen La Motte's *The Backwash of War*. Yet its sensationalist style implies that one of its author's main purposes was simply to attract a wide readership and sell copy.

The women who wrote about volunteer war nursing during the First World War undoubtedly had multiple motives for doing so. A desire to promote the feminist project of demonstrating that women, as well as men, could play significant roles in the war effort was sometimes accompanied by a pacifist wish simply to expose the horror of war from the perspective of one who had witnessed its direst consequences. Most nurse writers seem also to have felt that their war nursing work was the most powerful experience of their lives – and one that must be shared.

Notes

1 On the involvement of American volunteers in the nursing services of the First World War, see: Christine E. Hallett, *Veiled Warriors: Allied Nurses of the First World War* (Oxford: Oxford University Press, 2014): 190; Jane Potter, '"I begin to feel as a normal being should, in spite of the blood and anguish in which I move": American Women's First World War Nursing Memoirs', in Alison S. Fell and Christine E. Hallett (eds), *First World War Nursing: New Perspectives* (New York: Routledge, 2013): 51–68.

2 Christine Hallett, *Containing Trauma: Nursing Work in the First World War* (Manchester: Manchester University Press, 2009): 194–8; Hallett, *Veiled Warriors*: 47–54.

3 Katrin Schultheiss, *Bodies and Souls: Politics and the Professionalization of Nursing in France, 1880–1922* (Cambridge, MA: Harvard University Press, 2001); Hallett, *Veiled Warriors*: 24–5.

4 Shirley Millard, *I Saw Them Die: Diary and Recollections of Shirley Millard*, ed. Adele Comandini (London: George G. Harrap, 1936): 12.
5 Millard, *I Saw Them Die*: 10.
6 Millard, *I Saw Them Die*: 12–13.
7 Millard, *I Saw Them Die*: 20–1.
8 Millard, *I Saw Them Die*: 23–4.
9 Millard, *I Saw Them Die*: 26–7.
10 Mary T. Sarnecky, *A History of the US Army Nurse Corps* (Philadelphia: University of Pennsylvania Press, 1999): 85.
11 Millard, *I Saw Them Die*: 15.
12 Sarnecky, *A History of the US Army Nurse Corps*: 85.
13 On the Army School of Nursing, and the decision of American nurse leaders not to introduce volunteer nurses into American military hospitals, see: Hallett, *Veiled Warriors*: 216–17.
14 Rebecca West, *War Nurse: The True Story of a Woman who Lived, Loved and Suffered on the Western Front* (New York: Cosmopolitan Book Corporation, 1930): *passim*.
15 West, *War Nurse*; most examples of surgical work are between 48 and 73.
16 Anon. [K. K. and M. E. H.], 'Experiences in the American Ambulance Hospital, Neuilly, France', *American Journal of Nursing*, 15.7 (April 1915): 549–54 (550).
17 Anon., 'The American Ambulance in Paris', *BJN* (10 October 1914): 281; Anon., 'Letters from the Front: From France', *BJN* (17 October 1914): 306–7; Anon., 'Book of the Week: *The Diary of a French Army Chaplain*', *BJN* (30 October 1914): 369.
18 Ellen La Motte wrote an article on her experiences at the American Ambulance: Ellen N. La Motte, 'An American Nurse in Paris', *The Survey*, 34 (10 July 1915): 333–6. On Ellen La Motte, see Chapter 3; on Agnes Warner, see Chapter 2.
19 West, *War Nurse*: dust jacket publicity material, 1st edn.
20 Victoria Glendinning, *Rebecca West: A Life* (London: Macmillan, 1988 [1987]): 36.
21 Glendinning, *Rebecca West*: 108.
22 Rebecca West, *The Return of the Soldier* (London: Virago, 1980 [1918]).
23 Rebecca West, *The Fountain Overflows* (London: Virago, 1984 [1957]); Rebecca West, *The Birds Fall Down* (London: Macmillan, 1966). See also West's masterpiece on Yugoslavia: Rebecca West, *Black Lamb and Grey Falcon: A Journey through Yugoslavia* (Edinburgh: Cannongate, 2006 [1942]).
24 Glendinning, *Rebecca West*: 30–2, 37–40.
25 This deliberately voiced view can also be found in the writings of early pacifist feminists. See, for example, Catherine Marshall, *Militarism versus Feminism* (London: Virago, 1987 [1915]); E. Sylvia Pankhurst, *The Home Front* (London: Hutchinson, 1987 [1932]).

26 West, *War Nurse*: 47.

27 West, *War Nurse*: 49.

28 West, *War Nurse*: 52.

29 West, *War Nurse*: 227.

30 West, *War Nurse*: 71–2.

31 Maud Mortimer, *A Green Tent in Flanders* (New York: Doubleday, Page, 1918); Mary Borden, *The Forbidden Zone* (London: William Heinemann, 1929); Ellen N. La Motte, *The Backwash of War: The Human Wreckage of the Battlefield as Witnessed by an American Hospital Nurse* (New York: G. P. Putnam's Sons and The Knickerbocker Press, 1916). For a discussion of these writings, see Chapters 2 and 3 of this book.

32 Potter, 'I begin to feel as a normal being should': 51–68.

8

The British 'VAD'

Introduction: becoming a VAD

The allied nursing workforce of the First World War was a complex, heterogeneous group of the trained, the semi-trained, and the almost completely untrained. In Britain, instruction for volunteer nurses (the so-called 'VADs') was administered by Voluntary Aid Detachments, acting under the auspices of the British Society of the Red Cross and the St John Ambulance Association, a branch of the Order of St John of Jerusalem. Most British VADs took courses, passed examinations, and obtained certificates in four aspects of nursing care: first aid and bandaging, sick-room cookery, hygiene, and home nursing. Voluntary Aid Detachments hired fully trained nurses to demonstrate skills and offer basic knowledge on these vital subjects to their volunteers.[1] In this way, fully trained professional nurses were able to ensure that the volunteers who would later act as their assistants had a good rudimentary knowledge, and were able to offer safe care to vulnerable patients.

Once they had acquired at least some relevant training certificates, most VADs underwent a further apprenticeship training – usually of about six months – in a local hospital to permit them to consolidate their skills. Most found themselves undertaking menial tasks, ranging from sweeping ward floors and cleaning out grates and ward stoves, to preparing breakfasts for whole wards of patients. The trained staff of most hospital wards treated VADs in the same way as they would treat new trainees, or probationer nurses, giving them simple, safe, and mundane work in order to allow them a period of 'settling-in', which could last several weeks or months. After this, the volunteers were permitted to come into direct contact with the care and clinical treatment of patients. Workloads on hospital wards were high; the wartime emergency meant that civilian wards were short-staffed, while military hospitals experienced high pressures of work. Hence, most VADs found themselves providing fundamental care to their patients – albeit under the close supervision of the ward staff – within a few months of their arrival. Over time, many became highly proficient in offering such care. For Lesley Smith, the environment of the hospital was like a 'new world', and the knowledge of infectious diseases she acquired in her local hospital's isolation block left her with hands like 'raw meat from constant soaking in perchloride'.[2]

Most VADs began their brief nursing 'careers' on civilian wards, and many found this a source of frustration, because their primary motivation for undertaking nursing work had been to offer direct assistance to the 'war effort'. Some offered their services to auxiliary hospitals belonging to the Red Cross or the Order of St John of Jerusalem. From the early spring of 1915, VADs were permitted to practise in military hospitals (including those overseas) and, from this time onwards, many consolidated their brief skills-training in the arduous environment of a territorial hospital. Overseas postings were usually reserved for those who had demonstrated exemplary skill in a hospital on the 'home front'. It appears, however, that some wealthier and more socially connected women were able to gain postings to northern France before having fully consolidated their skills. Trained nurses, some of whom found that they were not able to gain release from British hospitals to serve overseas, were deeply frustrated at the knowledge that semi-trained volunteers were working in base hospitals close to the Western Front, while they themselves were effectively trapped in civilian practice.[3]

Realising war's realities

Some works, such as Kate Finzi's *Eighteen Months in the War Zone* and Lesley Smith's *Four Years out of Life*, illustrate the extent to which, even whilst being influenced by war propaganda, volunteers could feel compelled to give faithful accounts of their experiences that actually undermined that propaganda.[4] The overriding sense gained from Finzi's account is of the extent to which some women felt compelled to contribute to the war effort. Beginning her wartime 'career' at the very outset of the war as a volunteer nurse, Finzi later found herself ousted from her position in a Boulogne base hospital by an influx of trained nurses. Declaring that she would do anything at all to be helpful, she spent many months running a YMCA rest hut – gruelling work that resulted in her becoming seriously ill.

Finzi's descriptions of the suffering of her wounded patients have a raw edge. Yet her main concern seems to be a desire to convey a sense of their heroism and stoicism. She writes of:

> fingerless hands, lungs pierced, arms and legs perfectly well gangrenous, others already threatening tetanus (against which they are now beginning to inoculate patients), mouths swollen beyond all recognition with bullet shots, fractured femurs, shattered jaws, sightless eyes, ugly scalp wounds; yet never a murmur, never a groan except in sleep. As the men come in they fall on their pallets and doze until roused for food.[5]

Eighteen Months in the War Zone contains two significant themes. It bears witness to the suffering of those injured by the war. And it points out that women as well as men might be damaged as a result of their war work – not so directly and obviously, perhaps, as men on active service, but insidiously, as a direct result of their heavy exhausting work, long hours, and poor living and working conditions.[6] Finzi's writing, perhaps unwittingly, undermines the imperialist propaganda that the women of the British Empire were part of an invincible force that was fighting for the right in a simple war in which good would defeat evil.

Lesley Smith's *Four Years out of Life* offers similar insights into the pressures faced by semi-trained and inexperienced VADs:

> Hour after hour day after day we cut down stinking bandages and exposed great gaping wounds that distorted the whole original plan of the body; human figures had become mere curious abortions. One man had both buttocks blown off and lay in a misshapen heap on his stomach, one arm had been amputated at the elbow and he had a host of smaller wounds from flying metal. Another man lay propped on sphagnum moss to absorb the

discharge from two large holes in each thigh where a bullet had cut a great furrow across his body. There were numberless buttock and shoulder cases, the result of men laying in the open on their faces. A small, wiry Scotsman had lost both legs and both arms and lay extended in iron splints as though he were crucified.[7]

Smith describes her work with ward sisters in various parts of a base hospital in northern France. Her memoir indicates that she – a semi-trained volunteer – enjoyed good relationships with senior, trained staff. But her style is unusual: other writers focus on conflict. Indeed, the tension between trained, professional nurses and VADs is one of the strongest themes to emerge from women's wartime writings. It is striking that this tension appears far more frequently and forcefully in VADs' writings than in those of professionals. The latter – as in, for example, the case of Kate Luard – seem intent on recording the suffering and resilience of their patients. But whilst trained nurses were observing their patients, it seems that VADs were observing *them* – often with fascination, sometimes with admiration for their skill and efficiency, and frequently with scorn for their excessive attention to hospital etiquette and discipline. Stories of bullying nurses and victimised VADs are manifold.[8] D. M. Richards writes of her work in a large hospital in Dorset. As junior probationer she made beds, swabbed the ward floor, wiped lockers, and emptied bed pans 'whilst the Sister's steely eyes looked on'.[9] Eventually, she 'disgraced' herself by responding to an enquiry by a surgeon during a ward round:

> At the end of the round, the Surgeon spoke to me personally, he was not young, but had a compassion for his patients, and staff. I would never have dared to speak to Him [sic], because to look at a Doctor above his feet was unheard of familiarity.
>
> All he said to me was: 'How are you settling down nurse? Are you happy in Hospital training?' I dared to look him straight in the eye, simply saying 'Oh yes Sir. I love the work.' He had scarcely left the ward, before Sister called me to her table, in the centre of the ward, 'How dare you make yourself obvious to the Surgeon – or Doctor? Disgusting behaviour and must on no account be repeated!'[10]

The portrayal of professional nurses exhibiting ridiculous behaviour was a common motif in the writings of VADs, as was the theme of hardship and suffering endured by young women, many of whom had never before engaged in menial work.[11] Eventually, Richards withdrew from nurse training and joined a VAD. She spent the last months of the war attached to a military hospital on Salisbury Plain, where the matron 'was just what folks dream about, as a matron commanding not demanding respect, human, perceptive, discriminating, the lot, and possessing two of the deepest blue eyes I have ever seen'.[12] This 'good' matron, unlike her 'bad' counterpart in Dorset, is not the subject of detailed description. The reader is offered no vignettes or narratives of her behaviour, and we never see her in action.

Other VADs wrote of poor living and working conditions. Few appear to have minded the hardship associated with 'active service'. Of much greater concern to them were the bureaucratic 'pettiness and red tape' that restricted their actions. One anonymous diary-writer expressed her indignation that many women who, with further training, would have made excellent nurses, were deflected into other careers.[13] She herself offered her services to the French Red Cross when, after several months of work on the 'home front', she was unable to get an overseas posting as a British VAD. After some time in a French military hospital, working with French doctors and orderlies and English volunteer nurses, she obtained a transfer to a British base hospital in northern France, 'right on top of the cliffs over looking the sea'.[14] One of her most powerful experiences was being placed in the ward for German prisoners. Here, she experienced conflict between her patriotic hatred for 'the enemy' and her sense of pity at the suffering of her young patients:

> Although I began by hating to nurse the Germans, after some weeks of it I got to like it. True, the work was harder than in the other wards, as we had more help in the British lines, but the VADs took more responsibility and did all the dressings in the German wards, thus giving us experience and making us independent. I always found the men very plucky (with a few exceptions) and very grateful for anything one did for them, and some of them were wonderfully nice, and in spite of their nationality one couldn't help getting fond of them.[15]

She goes on to describe the obnoxious behaviour of one German officer, who complains about hospital food and shouts as he leaves the ward: 'Deutschland über Alles!'.[16] This seems to ease her sense of tension and conflict, as she decides that it is the officers, not the ordinary German soldiers, who are responsible for prolongation of the war.

Ultimately, her experience of nursing German prisoners enables her to see war itself as a disaster into which ordinary people on both sides have been unwillingly drawn.

Memoirist Henrietta Tayler recounts a similar experience of serving with the French Red Cross in Italy. Having been placed on the 'prisoners' ward' because she could speak German, she soon discovered that hardly any of her patients actually were German. She found herself nursing 'a heterogeneous medley of Austrian subjects ... three Hungarians, one Bohemian, two Rumanians [sic] from Transylvania, two Bosnians, a Pole and the rest Croatians'.[17] Although the language she uses in describing these patients is quite patronising, she manages to convey a sense of the poignancy of her relationships with them:

> These sick men, mostly chest and heart cases, were in the lowest possible condition, almost starving, and we had great struggles to pull them through. One, who had intestinal troubles as well, had a temperature of 40 degrees Cent. (104 degrees Fahr.) for over a week ... but at length he began to yield to treatment; and later he embarrassed me by announcing daily that he owed his life only to 'Bogu e Gospodina' (God and the lady) and rubbing his forehead on my hand whenever he got the chance! He was a shepherd by trade, and strangely like a sheep. None of these men impressed one as being great warriors, nor as having much stomach for the present fight. They only longed to get home.[18]

Allied nurses and volunteers expressed a mixture of emotions towards their prisoner-patients. American volunteer Shirley Millard described how some of her German patients were 'sulky and arrogant', 'insolent, cocky and rude', and how she was afraid they might injure her or her hospital colleagues.[19] Yet she also describes how she nursed a German 'boy' of sixteen who spoke good English and had visited Milwaukee: 'I'm afraid I made quite a pet of him. I wonder if he ever did get back to America. I doubt it. His right leg was gone above the knee, and his right arm was so shattered he would never use it again. His eyes were large and gentle ... He ... often told me, very confidentially, that he hated the War.'[20]

Offering descriptions of well-behaved, polite, and clearly vulnerable German patients appears to have been used by some nurse writers as a deliberately pacifist device. Others may simply have felt compelled to write what they saw.

Vera Brittain's *Testament*

Probably the most forceful – and certainly the most famous – pacifist text of the First World War is Vera Brittain's *Testament of Youth*. Brittain's life has been well documented.[21] She was born in Buxton, the daughter of wealthy middle-class parents, and enjoyed a privileged and 'ladylike' upbringing. From an early age, she longed to be well educated like her much-loved brother, Edward, and persuaded her parents to allow her to be tutored for the entrance examination to Oxford University. Brittain's story has become part of the mythology of the First World War: the narrative of a golden summer followed by four years of hell.[22] As she was poised in 1914 to follow her brother and his friend Roland Leighton – with whom she was already falling in love – to Oxford, her country entered the First World War, and the lives of her generation were, at best disrupted, at worst blotted out. Brittain did begin her Oxford education, but felt compelled to leave after completion of her first year, unable to see her brother and his friends face danger and hardship at the front, while herself remaining safe at home. For a young, well-brought-up lady, nursing was the obvious choice of war work, and Brittain offered her services to the Devonshire Hospital in her home town of Buxton, starting her career as a VAD on 27 June 1915.[23] On 18 October, she transferred to the First London General Hospital at Camberwell.[24]

Brittain's writings offer a vivid illustration of the emotional trajectory followed by an intelligent young woman who, at the outset of war, engaged enthusiastically, anticipating challenge, but found horror and despair. When she first began nursing, she exclaimed in her diary: 'Oh! I love the British Tommy! I shall get so fond of these men I know. And when I look after any one of them, it is like nursing Roland by proxy.'[25] But, after Roland's death, she found that she hated the work. Claire Tylee has commented on the 'mental flannel' – the curious combination of innate innocence and susceptibility to propaganda that encouraged women like Brittain to romanticise the war until affected personally by its consequences.[26]

At both the Devonshire and the First London General, Brittain encountered distressingly overbearing nurses, who seemed intent on bullying young VADs, and at the latter hospital she judged the behaviour of the 'Bart's Sisters' harshly, referring to their 'bright immunity from pity'.[27] Her encounters in Malta during 'a short year of glamorous beauty and delight' were altogether friendlier.[28] But it was not until she was posted to Etaples on the Western Front, in August 1917,[29] that she experienced real friendship with a trained nurse. And it was in Etaples, too, that she began to believe that the war was nothing more than a futile waste of life – a belief that was strengthened by her experiences in the 'German Ward' – the ward reserved for wounded prisoners of war. Her first encounter with German patients was an uncomfortable one:

> it was somewhat disconcerting to be pitch-forked, all alone – since VADs went on duty half an hour before the Sisters – into the midst of thirty representatives of the nation which, as I had repeatedly been told, had crucified Canadians, cut off the hands of babies, and subjected pure and stainless females to unmentionable 'atrocities'. I didn't think I had really believed all those stories, but I wasn't quite sure.[30]

In this way, Brittain gently mocks the propaganda of war, leaving the reader uncertain of the extent to which she herself has been influenced by it. Lynne Layton has commented on the ambivalence of Brittain's attitude, arguing that 'not until war touched her personally did she begin a painful rebellion against the patriarchal values that had dominated her prewar life'.[31] In fact, as Layton argues, and as Brittain's own diaries demonstrate, Brittain was drawn to the war by a belief that it was a noble cause in which a heroic generation was sacrificing itself for the good of all.[32] It was only later that she realised that 'naïve idealism ... had been both the virtue and the fatal weakness of her generation'.[33] Brittain herself commented in her later autobiography, *Testament of Experience*, that her experience in the 'German Ward' had set her on the path to pacifism and work for the League of Nations.[34] In *Testament of Youth*, she recalled the vulnerability of her German prisoner-patients, and her sense of a common humanity with them. A young Prussian lieutenant, being discharged from the hospital for transport to Britain,

> held out an emaciated hand to me as he lay on the stretcher waiting to go, and murmured: 'I tank [*sic*] you, Sister.' After barely a second's hesitation I took the pale fingers in mine, thinking how ridiculous it was that I should be holding this man's hand in friendship when perhaps, only a week or two earlier, Edward up at Ypres had been doing his best to kill him. The world was mad and we were all victims; that was the only way to look at it. These

shattered, dying boys and I were paying alike for a situation that none of us had desired or done anything to bring about.[35]

No less surprising than Brittain's fellowship with her German patients is her friendship with a trained British nurse, to whom she gives the pseudonym 'Hope Milroy'. Brittain comments that such friendship would never have been tolerated at the First London General Hospital, but that here, in Etaples, 'the Q.A. Reserve Sisters had no such feeling of professional exclusiveness towards the girls who had helped them to fight so many forms of death'.[36] Brittain is clearly impressed by 'Hope Milroy', who is her intellectual equal: 'a highbrow in revolt against highbrows'.[37] She comments on the dedication of the staff in the 'German Ward' to their prisoner-patients. There can be no doubt that institutional prejudice was shown towards the Germans: they were given far fewer members of staff to care for them. But the effects of this prejudice were ameliorated by a dedicated staff, who worked long hours and gave up their breaks to ensure that their patients were cared for. The character of Hope Milroy is used to demonstrate this ambivalence. On one occasion, she is depicted as showing concern for a patient's exposed wound by commanding Brittain to 'get the iodoform powder and scatter it over that filthy Hun!'. Brittain describes how:

The staff of 24 General described [Milroy] as 'mental', not realising that she used her reputation for eccentricity and the uncompromising candour which it was supposed to excuse as a means of demanding more work from her subordinates than other Sisters were able to exact. At first I detested her dark attractiveness and sarcastic, relentless youth, but when I recognised her for what she was – by far the cleverest woman in the hospital, even if potentially the most alarming, and temperamentally as fitful as a weather-cock – we became constant companions off duty.[38]

Vera Brittain wrote one of her most moving poems about the 'German Ward', giving 'Hope Milroy' a central role, referring both to her 'tenderness' and to 'her scornful energy of will'.[39]

After the armistice, Brittain struggled to pick up the threads of her studies, finding herself strangely detached from life at Somerville College, Oxford, and feeling, at times, close to psychological collapse. She fought to make sense of her wartime experience while pursuing her literary career, and went on to write a number of novels, two of which, *The Dark Tide* and *Honourable Estate*, attempted to make sense of life for those who had committed totally to war and suffered enormous –and apparently unnoticed – loss.[40]

Vera Brittain's *Testament of Youth*, published in 1933 as Europe seemed to be edging towards another war, was a deliberate challenge to the jingoistic propaganda that had led the war generation to destruction. It was also an act of feminism. In her later memoir, *Testament of Experience*, Brittain described how she had read the war memoirs of Robert Graves, Richard Aldington, Erich Maria Remarque, Ernest Hemingway, Edmund Blunden, and Siegfried Sassoon, and wondered: 'Why should these young men have the war to themselves?'.[41] Women, too, had entered war with high ideals, suffered disillusionment, and then somehow found the courage to go on. Although *Testament of Youth* was written primarily in memory of the men Brittain had lost – her fiancé, her brother, and two close friends – it was also written for those women who had served in wartime, to ensure that the female voice would be heard, and that one particular feminine perspective would be understood.

Enid Bagnold: military medicine as part of the 'war machine'

If some wartime nurse writers may be viewed as 'heretics' – as individuals who attacked the received wisdom of their day – then Enid Bagnold is perhaps one of the most skilful and least openly aggressive of these. Her soft irony and quiet observations evoke a more muted form of horrified fascination than Shirley Millard's gory descriptions or Rebecca West's clinically precise accounts and grim surgical realities. And yet, her writing claws insistently at the reader's consciousness, presenting, every so often, an image that etches itself into the memory leaving a troubling scar. Bagnold's artistry creates vivid images that – quite intentionally – disturb the complacency of those who have never encountered war injury. And yet, even as her work impresses with its honesty and openness, it repels with its detachment.

Enid Bagnold was a relatively wealthy and privileged member of British society. She was, perhaps, typical of the young, upper-middle-class women who joined VADs in their thousands, eager to participate in the war by nursing its wounded.[42] Yet, in other ways, she was atypical. As an aspiring author, she was much more committed to writing than to nursing, and her wartime memoir, *A Diary without Dates*, appears to be designed to capture accurately, and yet also poetically, the realities of life in a military hospital. Her desire to recount her experience in an aesthetically beautiful way distorted the realities of hospital work. Many years after the war, she wrote an effusive letter to Virginia Woolf expressing both her admiration for Woolf's new novel *Orlando* and her own wish to be a better writer:

> It isn't only that I envy you, or that I admire you. Of course, I do both unstintingly. But you have found the one track that in my wildest dreams I dreamed of treading: you have found a method of spilling out all your metaphors and images … and above all, of being a poet and a novelist at the same moment … I have dreamt and lived and battled dimly towards a certain kind of writing, a sort of vase to hold poetry and prose together.[43]

In *A Diary without Dates* Bagnold seems to have wanted to capture the essence of the military hospital, rather than faithfully to chronicle its events and realities. Her desire to 'hold poetry and prose together' and to create something that transcended reality resulted in a book that is both a compelling record of her own perceptions and a highly impressionistic version of events. Ironically, Woolf's own initial reaction to *A Diary without Dates* was not favourable. She is said to have written caustically to her sister, Vanessa Bell, on 29 January 1918: 'did you ever meet a woman called Enid Bagnold – would be clever and also smart? … She has written a book, called, as you can imagine, "A Diary without Dates" all to prove that she's the most attractive and popular and exquisite of creatures.'[44]

Barbara Willard characterises Enid Bagnold as a woman who was 'fighting for a required fame' in a highly self-aware and deliberately 'bohemian' pre-war society.[45] Bagnold is said to have written for three hours a day every day, throughout her life. Her first novel, *Serena Blandish*, was published anonymously (by 'a Lady of Quality') in order to protect the sensibilities of her parents. She finally achieved the fame she desired in 1935, with the publication of her best-known book, *National Velvet*. An escapist children's novel about a butcher's daughter who wins the Grand National, the book was highly successful commercially; it made Bagnold's name on both sides of the Atlantic, and was produced as a film in 1944.[46]

Bagnold's *Diary without Dates* relates her impressions of the Royal Herbert Hospital in Woolwich, London, where she served as a volunteer nurse. Her experiences appear to have been very similar to those of other genteel volunteers, such as Vera Brittain and Irene Rathbone, differing only insofar as they did not involve the harsh 'living-in' conditions described by others.[47] In her autobiography, Bagnold writes of going on duty at the hospital and then returning to her friend Catherine's house, where she sleeps in a 'little room with gold stars on dark blue paper' and where grand parties continue throughout the war.[48] She also writes of her shock at the harshness of hospital discipline: at, for example, the way in which men are seen as 'malingerers', and beds are stripped and cleaned before the eyes of bereaved relatives.[49]

Bagnold's *Diary without Dates* emerged from this strangely disjointed lifestyle and was written as a gift for her friend, the Romanian diplomat Antoine Bibesco, who returned it with a note, saying: 'Why not keep something for yourself?'.[50] Bagnold approached William Heinemann, who agreed to publish the work and asked its author to dinner. 'We liked each other', she remarked in her autobiography,[51] and the progress of her book to and through the press illustrates the value of her social connections to her writing career.

Bagnold recounts that 'when *A Diary without Dates* was published, I was sacked from the hospital by the Matron in the first half-hour of my day'.[52] She joined the First Aid Nursing Yeomanry and went to France, where she served as an ambulance driver during the last months of the war. In the immediate post-war period she travelled through the war zone recording her impressions. Her writing from this phase of her life was very different from *A Diary without Dates*. Her novel *The Happy Foreigner* tells of a love affair between an English VAD and a French artillery captain, and is based, in part, on numbered letters, sent home to her mother.[53] Several successful novels followed.[54] In 1941 she wrote her first play, *Lottie Dundass*,[55] which was rapidly followed by others, including the highly successful *The Chalk Garden*, which ran for two years in London's West End.[56] In old age, she referred to herself as 'an old lady masking a sort of everlasting girl inside', and Nigel Nicolson describes her as 'an exhilarating companion ... ebulliently communicative', yet 'too fond of the great and grand to be taken seriously by the literary establishment'.[57] Perhaps it was not only the literary establishment that refused to take Enid Bagnold seriously. In the world of the military hospital, her insights into the experiences of her patients were seen as, at best, naive and, at worst, highly unprofessional and potentially damaging.

It is a feature of the published writings of volunteer nurses that they tended to focus on the harshness of hospital discipline, particularly as it was expressed through the actions and attitudes of trained professional nurses. The power and popularity of their writings was such that the detachment and inhumanity of some military hospital nurses has acquired the status of myth. Bagnold's own contribution to the myth is a particularly powerful one. The image she offers of the military discipline she encountered at the Royal Herbert Hospital is one that stays with the reader long after her laconic and deftly written text has been left behind. She writes of a new sister, who 'is absolutely without personality, beyond her medal. She appears to be deaf.'[58] Later she comments that '*My* Sister is afraid of death. She told me so. And not the less afraid, she said, after all she has seen of it. That is terrible. But the new Sister is afraid of life. She is shorter-sighted.'[59] By means of such terse sentences, Bagnold throws the full weight of her not-inconsiderable judgement against her professional nursing colleagues. She comments on how one sister sits by the fire with the medical officer drinking tea, 'a harmless amusement', while a patient suffers unbearable pain in a bed nearby. When she draws the patient's pain to the sister's attention, the latter merely comments 'quite decently' that 'He must stick it out.'[60] And there is the sister who has 'eternal youth, eternal fair hair, cold and ignorant judgments'.[61] Eventually, she observes:

> I shall never get to understand Sisters; they are so strange, so tricky, uncertain as collies. Deep down they have an ineradicable axiom: that any visitor, anyone in an old musquash coat, in a high-boned collar, in a spotted veil tied up at the sides, anyone with whom one shakes hands or takes tea, is more important than the most charming patient (except, of course, a warded M.O.).[62]

Yet, Angela Smith has identified a contradiction at the heart of Bagnold's text. Like many women's writings of the Great War, *A Diary without Dates* identifies the strange role reversal that permits female nurses to hold power over their male soldier-patients, and in which there is a 'constant dehumanization and infantilisation' of wounded combatants.[63] Bagnold both dissociates herself from this power and expresses a fascination with it.

Bagnold retains her sense of compassion for her patients – but only with difficulty. Alongside her terse representations of the unintentional callousness of the medical and nursing staff, she places some of the most extraordinary evocations of suffering to be found in war literature. We read of Mr Wickes, who paid a private specialist to cure his illness, yet lies helpless in a hospital bed staring at his 'haunted bedrail'; or of 'Smiff', whose 'foot is off' and who complains at being kept 'starin' at green walls … [for] nine blessed months'.[64] Or of Corrigan, who is given an anti-tetanus injection without being asked for his consent or even informed that a needle is about to be inserted into his arm.[65] We learn as much as it is possible to learn of pain by reading about Rees, who,

> when he wakes, wakes sobbing and says, 'Don't go away nurse' … holds my hand in a fierce clutch, then releases it to point in the air, crying, 'there's the pain!' as though the pain filled the air and rose to the rafters. As he wakes it centralizes, until at last comes the moment when he says, 'Me arm aches cruel', and points to it. Then one can leave him.[66]

Fear, too, is a focus for Bagnold. She tells the story of Gayner, who is convinced he has tetanus. He is unable to keep still, and feels that his 'jaws want to close'. Bagnold's text is pervaded with both Gayner's fear and her own. As a new and inexperienced VAD, she is terrified that her patient may actually be mortally ill. When his temperature proves to be normal, she feels unable to speak to him about his fears because he is 'one of those men so pent up, so rigid with some inner indignation, one cannot tamper with the locks'. The trained junior sister meets Bagnold's news of Gayner's symptoms with equanimity and the 'gimlet-eyed' doctor pronounces the diagnosis to be 'hysteria'. Bagnold's anxiety shifts. She no longer fears that her patient may actually die of tetanus; her attention now is on his immediate suffering and her own helplessness: '"Is no one going to reassure Gayner?" I wondered. And no one did. Isn't the fear of pain next brother to pain itself? Tetanus or the fear of tetanus – a choice between twin nightmares. Don't they admit that?'[67]

Bagnold's position as a relatively powerless figure in the hospital hierarchy is, perhaps, one of the reasons for her frustration and her latent hostility towards the qualified staff. In another episode, she promises a patient in pain that he will receive a sedative at eight o'clock. But the sister chooses not to give the drug, because 'he will want it more later in the night, and he can't have it twice'. Bagnold is honest about her own error: 'I ran back to tell him so quickly – but one cannot run back into the past'.[68]

Ultimately, Bagnold's message is that war dehumanises everyone: its victims; those who nurse them; and the civilians who remain at home, comfortable in their ignorance of its realities. Her ultimate anxiety is about her own process of dehumanisation. Her text is watchful; it logs not only what she sees, but her own reactions to those sights. We gain the impression that one of her purposes in writing her *Diary without Dates* is to prevent herself becoming hardened by her experience. And yet it is difficult not to sympathise also – at least to some extent – with the senior nursing staff of the Royal Herbert Hospital who reacted to the publication of her book by summarily dismissing her. Her observations are perhaps just a little too keen; her descriptions of her patients' lives, her recounting of their most private sayings and experiences, just a little too accurate. Her breach of confidentiality, her breaking of trust, is too obvious – obvious enough to become an act of bad faith. Her truth is just too fierce, her reality too harsh. And yet, these are also the qualities that give *A Diary without Dates* its power.

Needed by the country: Irene Rathbone's 'novel'

One of the best known women's memoirs of the First World War is Irene Rathbone's *We That Were Young*. First published in 1932 it quickly achieved popularity and remained in press for much of the twentieth century. Hugely readable, with engaging characters and dramatic (if not melodramatic) plotlines, it contains many of the tropes of popular mid-twentieth-century women's fiction: an attractive central heroine who suffers, yet stands by her ideals; a handsome and steadfast, but somewhat distant, hero, who provides a romantic interest without distracting the reader from the heroine's adventures; a group of female friends, whose fortunes provide sub-plots, adding interest to the broader narrative; and, as backdrop, the Great War, depicted as a dreadful force and lending an epic quality to the narrative. *We That*

Were Young appears to have been highly valued by a post-war generation brought up on both Bessie Marchant's novels of high adventure, and myths of the hardships and challenges faced by First World War VADs.[69] It depicts female wartime action in many guises: volunteer work in YMCA rest stations; dangerous and exhausting munitions work; and, of course, that classic female contribution to the war: nursing work in military hospitals.

Rathbone's purpose in writing the novel was undoubtedly to record the contributions of young women to the British nation during the First World War, and to inform a post-war generation of the significance of their service. A sense of the suffering endured by the war generation – both male and female – suffuses the book. In reading it, one senses that Rathbone felt compelled to record the sadness and horror behind the experiences of those who were young at the time of the war. In this sense, her novel is a classic example of the type of female war writing that emerged in the late 1920s and early 1930s. Works by men such as Erich Maria Remarque (*All Quiet on the Western Front*), Henri Barbusse (*Le Feu*), Robert Graves (*Goodbye to All That*), and Edmund Blunden (*Undertones of War*) had sought to find a language that would enable those who had fought to make sense of their experience – an experience that could never be shared by those who had remained at home. But a handful of women began to offer their own perspectives at around the same time.[70] Published in 1932, a year before Vera Brittain's *Testament of Youth*, Rathbone's novel was one of a small number of women's writings that offered witness testimony to the realities of female war service. A sense of outrage at the apparent indifference of those not directly involved in the conflict suffuses the novel, mirroring that expressed by male writers. On one occasion Rathbone's heroine, Joan, berates an uncle who claims to envy her generation, declaring: 'I think it's utterly damnable to be young at this particular time of history. The "splendid burden" as you call it will break us before we're through.'[71]

Rathbone's work, because of its rather melodramatic and often sentimental style, never became a part of the 'canon' of First World War writings. Rathbone clearly decided – for whatever reason – not to offer a straightforward memoir of her war years, writing, instead, a semi-fictionalised account, which, while safeguarding herself and friends whose experiences she may have depicted, leaves the reader unsure about what is real and what imagined. Rathbone's purpose may have been to touch the emotions of her readers, rather than to offer a faithful record of events. And yet, much of the detail of her book seems to be offered with realism in mind – as when she describes a typical day at the First London General Hospital, in which VADs sweep floors, dust lockers, empty bedpans, 'take down' dressings, cut up food, make swabs, pad splints, and rub patients' 'backs'.[72] Rathbone's work has contradiction at its core. On the one hand, its descriptions of hospital life are vivid and arresting, and contain sufficient detail to convince the reader that they are drawn from life. On the other, the book's narrative passages are full of melodrama and romance. Over the whole is placed the subtitle: *A Novel by Irene Rathbone*.

Rathbone depicts the trained, professional nurses of the First London General Hospital as stereotypes of unfeeling, middle-aged spinsters.[73] The discipline they mete out to VADs, orderlies, and patients is often harsh and invariably meaningless. In their working lives, they exhibit a marked lack of creativity and imagination; and they appear to have no personal or social lives at all. Indeed, they live their lives in 'bunks': small, narrow rooms beside their wards, which seem to symbolise their small, narrow minds.[74] The matron is depicted as an unthinking martinet, who places hospital discipline above patient care. Rathbone's image of Rachael Cox Davies, matron of the First London General Hospital, as 'a brute of a woman'[75] contrasts with the *BJN*'s presentation of her as a fine leader, who inspires an admirable 'esprit de corps' among her trained staff, the majority of whom are 'St Bartholomew's trained, and have great pride in their identity'.[76]

The novel traces the development of the VAD nurse's skills. Its heroine, Joan, first volunteers for hospital service in 1916, having served for some time in a YMCA rest hut in northern France. She finds herself working in a small hospital in Hampstead peeling potatoes and cutting 'stacks of bread'. Eventually, she moves from the kitchens to the wards, but still finds herself 'more of a housemaid than of a nurse'.[77] It is only when convoys of wounded begin 'pouring in' from the Somme battlefields in July 1916 that Joan is finally called up to the First London General Hospital as a volunteer nurse. Her relief is evident. Here, at last, are both recognition and action: 'The middle-class, home-sheltered girls of England felt, at last, that their existence was not wholly futile. How different from being merely "allowed to do things" was the fact of being definitely asked to come and do them. They were in the same position as their brothers now: needed by the country.'[78] Yet her pride is matched by her anxiety, as she finds work in a military hospital very different from her previous experience:

> It had been one thing to amble in and out of cosy little wards at the Hampstead hospital, carrying meals, doing housework, and even assisting at the mild dressings; it was quite another here, in Ward 33 of the 1st London General, to see limbs which shrapnel had torn about and swollen into abnormal shapes, from which yellow pus poured when the bandages were removed, which were caked with brown blood, and in whose gangrenous flesh loose bits of bone had to be sought for painfully with probes.[79]

At night, she dreams of horrific wounds. But by the end of a week, she has 'adjusted herself' and is able to face the horrors of the First London General with equanimity, pouring her energies into the task of doing her job well, infusing the mundane work with a sense of value – both practical and spiritual. Rathbone writes of the mental 'adjustments' made by Joan and other VADs in glowing terms – as a natural consequence of their endurance and fortitude. Of the adjustments made by trained, professional nurses, she is casually critical. We soon learn, for example, that the trained nurse in charge of Ward 33 is Sister Ewart, 'a gaunt, rather acid woman of few words but great efficiency'. Meanwhile, it seems an acknowledged fact that all nurses 'cringed to their superiors' and 'treated their subordinates with severity'.[80]

Alongside her deep interest in nurses and their work stands Rathbone's fascination with relationships between VADs and their patients. She comments on how she wondered, years later, why open flirtation between the two was so rare. Apart from the strict rules forbidding such flirtation, she chooses to attribute the preservation of professional distance to a combination of 'the hospital atmosphere … the decency of the men … and a certain English directness and innocence in her young self'.[81] And yet, she comments on how it gave her heroine, Joan, 'a peculiar soothing joy to take hold of a long white arm, to soap it, sponge it, and dry it; to wash a muscular young back'. She adds that, although a 'fixed and rigid' gulf existed between nurse and patient, 'across that gulf, unrecognized and certainly unheeded by either, stretched the faint sweet fingers of sex'.[82] And Rathbone does openly break the taboos of the nurse–patient relationship by depicting a somewhat overwrought love affair between one of her characters, Pamela, and a New Zealand officer, which ends in tragedy when the officer dies in action. This episode, along with numerous others in which VADs are depicted struggling with overwork, harsh living conditions, and loss, are clearly designed to give power to Rathbone's message: that women as well as men served their country and suffered during the Great War. Perhaps the most dramatic playing-out of this theme is Joan's near-fatal injury, which begins as a septic finger and ends as a life-threatening septicaemia.[83] And at the very end of the war – after the armistice has been signed – Joan loses a beloved brother to the 'Spanish Flu' epidemic, which sweeps a weakened population. Joan, just like any front-line soldier, risks her life, suffers pain and loss, and faces life at the end of the war experiencing 'at the roots of her being … a vast indifference'.[84]

Conclusion: the VAD as witness

Britain's 'VADs' achieved iconic status after the First World War. Because they personified the classic feminine traits of gentleness, compassion, and kindness, and yet worked under harsh conditions and exhibited both mental and physical strength, they became invested with notions of ideal British womanhood. They acted out this ideal, demonstrating a willingness both to comfort the wounded and to undertake heavy manual labour. They exhibited courage, endurance, and fortitude – qualities seen as highly desirable in a victorious nation with an empire to preserve. In post-war mythology, the trained nurses to whose supervision they owed so much of their skill and knowledge acted as foils to their courage and humanity – tough, working women who were somehow just part of the inhumanity of the military medical machine. The injustice of some VAD representations of trained nurses has only recently been exposed.[85] And yet, because of both their powerlessness and their relative detachment from the hospital hierarchy, VADs were also able to give vivid and arresting accounts of patients' experiences. Some of their writings have acted as significant witness statements about the suffering created by the First World War, by focusing on the realities of injury and trauma. And the focus of VADs on German prisoner-patients was, perhaps, one of the earliest and most tentative ways in which some women began to question the validity of warfare itself.

Thelka Bowser, advocate of the VAD movement, wrote in 1917: 'The Great War has revealed many national truths never even suspected before it burst upon the world, but amongst all its surprises none has been greater than that provided by the success of the Voluntary Aid Detachment movement.'[86] Each generation makes its own 'national truths', and these are modelled and moulded by the powerful writings of witnesses. The notion that the Great War was a catastrophe that 'burst upon the world' giving rise to a heroic response was only just beginning to be broken down when Irene Rathbone wrote of her heroine's sense of 'vast indifference', and Vera Brittain reflected on her encounters with the German lieutenant who held out his hand and said: 'I tank you, Sister.'[87]

Notes

1 On the work of VADs, see: Thelka Bowser, *The Story of British VAD Work in the Great War* (London: Imperial War Museum, 2003 [1917]); Sharon Ouditt, *Fighting Forces, Writing Women: Identity and Ideology in the First World War* (London: Routledge, 1994); Janet S. K. Watson, 'Wars in the Wards: The Social Construction of Medical Work in First World War Britain', *Journal of British Studies*, 41 (2002): 484–510; Audrey Cruse, 'The Diary of Alice Maud Batt', *Journal of Medical Biography*, 18.4 (2010): 205–10; Christine E. Hallett, '"Emotional Nursing": Involvement, Engagement, and Detachment in the Writings of First World War Nurses and VADs', in Alison S. Fell and Christine E. Hallett (eds), *First World War Nursing: New Perspectives* (New York: Routledge, 2013): 87–102; Christine E. Hallett, *Veiled Warriors: Allied Nurses of the First World War* (Oxford: Oxford University Press, 2014): 18–20.

2 Lesley Smith, *Four Years out of Life* (London: Philip Allan, 1931): 16–17.

3 For an exploration of their writings to professional journals on these issues, see: Hallett, 'Emotional Nursing'.

4 Kate Finzi, *Eighteen Months in the War Zone: The Record of One Woman's Work on the Western Front* (London: Cassell, 1916): *passim*; Smith, *Four Years out of Life*: *passim*. On tensions felt by these writers between patriotism and a desire to give a 'true' image of the realities of war, see: Angela Smith, *The Second Battlefield: Women, Modernism and the First World War*

(Manchester: Manchester University Press, 2000), Chapter 3, 'Accidental Modernisms': 70–101; Santanu Das, *Touch and Intimacy in First World War Literature* (Cambridge: Cambridge University Press, 2005), Chapter 5, '"The Impotence of Sympathy": Service and Suffering in the Nurses' Memoirs': 175–203, and Chapter 6, 'The Operating Theatre': 204–28.

5 Finzi, *Eighteen Months in the War Zone*: 30–4.

6 For a commentary on the emotional pressures faced by nurses in military hospitals, see: Das, *Touch and Intimacy*, Part III, 'Wounds': 175–228.

7 Smith, *Four Years out of Life*: 119.

8 Such narratives are told particularly powerfully in the writings of Irene Rathbone and Enid Bagnold, and are described in more detail later in this chapter. See: Irene Rathbone, *We That Were Young: A Novel* (New York: The Feminist Press, 1989 [1932]); Enid Bagnold, *A Diary without Dates* (London: Virago, 1978 [1918]); Enid Bagnold, *Enid Bagnold's Autobiography (from 1889)*, introduction by Barbara Willard (London: Century Publishing, 1985 [1969]): 112–13.

9 D. M. Richards, *Blues and Reds*, memoir, P328, Imperial War Museum, London, unpaginated.

10 Richards, *Blues and Reds*.

11 See, for example: Dorothy Potts, MS letters, 3246 Con Shelf, Imperial War Museum, London; Joyce M. Sapwell, 'The Reminiscences of a VAD', T2SAP, Red Cross Archive, London; Mary Schiff, papers and letters, 1788/1, Red Cross Archive, London.

12 Richards, *Blues and Reds*.

13 Anon., *Twenty Months a VAD* (Sheffield: J. Northen, n.d.), 96/317, Red Cross Archive, London: 13.

14 Anon., *Twenty Months a VAD*: 24.

15 Anon., *Twenty Months a VAD*: 29–30.

16 Anon., *Twenty Months a VAD*: 30.

17 Henrietta Tayler, *A Scottish Nurse at War: Being a Record of What One Semi-Trained Nurse Has Been Privileged to See and Do during Four and a Half Years of War* (London: John Lane, 1920): 75.

18 Tayler, *A Scottish Nurse at War*: 77.

19 Shirley Millard, *I Saw Them Die: Diary and Recollections of Shirley Millard*, ed. Adele Comandini (London: George G. Harrap, 1936): 37–8.

20 Millard, *I Saw Them Die*: 43.

21 The most complete and detailed biography of Vera Brittain is: Paul Berry and Mark Bostridge, *Vera Brittain: A Life* (London: Virago Press, 2001).

22 This notion of 'that last summer' is discussed by Paul Fussell, *The Great War and Modern Memory* (Oxford: Oxford University Press, 2000 [1975]): 24.

23 Vera Brittain, *Testament of Youth: An Autobiographical Study of the Years 1900–1925* (London: Virago, 2004 [1933]): 141.

24 Brittain, *Testament of Youth* (2004), 179.

25 Vera Brittain, *Chronicle of Youth* (London: Phoenix Press, 2000 [1981]): 230.

26 Claire Tylee, *The Great War and Women's Consciousness: Images of Militarism and Womanhood in Women's Writings, 1914–64* (Houndmills and London: Macmillan, 1990). See also: Carol Acton, 'Negotiating Injury and Masculinity in First World War Nurses' Writing', in Fell and Hallett, *First World War Nursing*: 123–38.

27 Brittain, *Testament of Youth*: 187.

28 Brittain, *Testament of Youth*: 263.

29 Brittain, *Testament of Youth*: 334.

30 These three stories were particularly current during the early years of the war, and Brittain undoubtedly chose them deliberately when recounting her experience in the early 1930s. Brittain, *Testament of Youth*: 340. On the use of these particular narratives as propaganda, see: Trudi Tate, *Modernism, History and the First World War* (Manchester: Manchester University Press, 1998): 43–6.

31 Lynne Layton, 'Vera Brittain's Testament(s)', in Margaret Randolph Higonnet, Jane Jenson, Sonya Michel, and Margaret Collins Weitz (eds), *Behind the Lines: Gender and the Two World Wars* (New Haven: Yale University Press, 1987): 70–83.

32 Vera Brittain's diaries were published in 1981: Brittain, *Chronicle of Youth*.

33 Lynne Layton, 'Vera Brittain's Testament(s)': 72.

34 Vera Brittain, *Testament of Experience: An Autobiographical Story of the Years 1925–1950* (London: Fontana, 1980 [1957]): 471.

35 Brittain, *Testament of Youth*: 343.

36 Brittain, *Testament of Youth*: 347.

37 Brittain, *Testament of Youth*: 341.

38 Brittain, *Testament of Youth*: 342. This quotation is also given in: Christine E. Hallett, ' "A very valuable fusion of classes": British Professional and Volunteer Nurses of the First World War', *Endeavour*, 38.2 (2014): 101–10.

39 Vera Brittain, *Because You Died: Poetry and Prose of the First World War and After*, ed. Mark Bostridge (London: Virago, 2008): 39.

40 Vera Brittain, *The Dark Tide* (New York: Macmillan, 1936 [1923]); Vera Brittain, *Honourable Estate: A Novel of Transition* (New York: Macmillan, 1936). See also: Layton, 'Vera Brittain's Testament(s)': 77–80; Berry and Bostridge, *Vera Brittain*: 129–52.

41 Brittain, *Testament of Experience*: 77.

42 Bagnold, *Autobiography*: *passim*. On the contribution of volunteer nurses to the war effort, see: Ouditt, *Fighting Forces, Writing Women*: 7–46.

43 Enid Jones, letter to Virginia Woolf (née Stephen), typescript copy, 1933; SxMs 18, Monks House Papers, Library of the University of Sussex, Brighton.

44 Angela Smith is here quoting: Anna Sebba, *Enid Bagnold: The Authorised Biography* (London: Weidenfeld and Nicholson, 1986): 61. See: Smith, *The Second Battlefield*: 73.

45 Barbara Willard, introduction to Bagnold, *Autobiography*.
46 Enid Bagnold, *National Velvet* (London: William Heinemann, 1935). The book was reprinted in 1939, 1946, 1954, 1958, 1962, 1978, 1984, and 1992. See: Willard, introduction to Bagnold, *Autobiography*.
47 Brittain, *Testament of Youth*; Rathbone, *We That Were Young*.
48 Bagnold, *Autobiography*: 112–13.
49 Bagnold, *Autobiography*: 128.
50 Bagnold, *Autobiography*: 128. See also: Smith, *The Second Battlefield*: 73–4.
51 Bagnold, *Autobiography*: 128.
52 Bagnold, *Autobiography*: 129.
53 Enid Bagnold, *The Happy Foreigner* (London: Virago Press, 1987 [1920]).
54 Enid Bagnold's novels include: Anon., *Serena Blandish; or, The Difficulty of Getting Married: By a Lady of Quality* (London: Heinemann, 1924); Enid Bagnold, *Alice, Thomas and Jane* (London: William Heinemann, 1930); Enid Bagnold, *The Squire* (London: William Heinemann, 1938); Enid Bagnold, *The Loved and Envied* (London: William Heinemann, 1951).
55 Enid Bagnold, *Lottie Dundass* (London: William Heinemann, 1941).
56 Enid Bagnold, *The Chalk Garden* (London: Willliam Heinemann, 1956). The play was reprinted in 1957, 1959, and 1970, and was translated into French in 1979. See: Nigel Nicolson, 'Bagnold, Enid Algerine [*Married Name* Enid Algerine Jones, Lady Jones] (1889–1981), Novelist and Playwright', in *Oxford Dictionary of National Biography* (Oxford: Oxford University Press, 2004).
57 Nicolson, 'Bagnold, Enid Algerine'.
58 Bagnold, *A Diary without Dates*: 12.
59 Bagnold, *A Diary without Dates*: 18.
60 Bagnold, *A Diary without Dates*: 23–4.
61 Bagnold, *A Diary without Dates*: 67.
62 Bagnold, *A Diary without Dates*: 29.
63 Smith, *The Second Battlefield*: 76–7.
64 Bagnold, *A Diary without Dates*: 57, 85.
65 Bagnold, *A Diary without Dates*: 86–7.
66 Bagnold, *A Diary without Dates*: 89–90.
67 Bagnold, *A Diary without Dates*: 105–6.
68 Bagnold, *A Diary without Dates*: 112.
69 Michelle Smith, 'Adventurous Girls of the British Empire: The Pre-War Novels of Bessie Marchant', *The Lion and the Unicorn*, 33.1 (2009): 1–25.
70 The best known texts are by Vera Brittain, Mary Borden, and Irene Rathbone herself: Brittain, *Testament of Youth*; Mary Borden, *The Forbidden Zone* (London: William Heinemann, 1929); Rathbone, *We That Were Young*.
71 Rathbone, *We That Were Young*: 126.
72 Rathbone, *We That Were Young*: 208–14.
73 The one exception – who seems to prove the rule – is Sister Muir, who was 'brimming with kindliness': Rathbone, *We That Were Young*: 284.

74 Rathbone, *We That Were Young*: 196, 210, 221–3.
75 Rathbone, *We That Were Young*: 224.
76 Anon., Column, *BJN* (16 June 1917): 415.
77 Rathbone, *We That Were Young*: 123, 128.
78 Rathbone, *We That Were Young*: 194.
79 Rathbone, *We That Were Young*: 194.
80 Rathbone, *We That Were Young*: 196, 210.
81 Rathbone, *We That Were Young*: 213.
82 Rathbone, *We That Were Young*: 213.
83 Rathbone, *We That Were Young*: 237–45.
84 Rathbone, *We That Were Young*: 449.
85 Ouditt, *Fighting Forces, Writing Women*; Sharon Ouditt, *Women Writers of the First World War: An Annotated Bibliography* (London: Routledge, 2000); Watson, 'Wars in the Wards'; Christine Hallett, *Containing Trauma: Nursing Work in the First World War* (Manchester: Manchester University Press, 2009); Hallett, 'Emotional Nursing'; Hallett, *Veiled Warriors: passim*.
86 Thelka Bowser, *The Story of British VAD Work*: Introduction.
87 Rathbone, *We That Were Young*: 449; Brittain, *Testament of Youth*: 343.

9

Epic romance on Western and Eastern Fronts

Introduction: the romance of volunteer work

Most volunteer nurses of the First World War were female, young, and – within the limits of their time – well educated. They were more likely than trained nurses to publish memoirs of the war. Somewhat paradoxically, they were also more likely to write about the intricacies of nursing practice. While the writings of trained nurses focused on the courage and endurance of patients, those of volunteers emphasised the drama of nursing itself. Chapter 8 explored the ways in which some British VADs observed the work of their professional colleagues and reflected on their own struggle to acquire competence without becoming emotionally detached from their patients' sufferings. But, for many volunteer nurses, the 'romance' of nursing went beyond the execution of nursing skills.

Cultural historian Paul Fussell has suggested that the 'romantic' trope was a familiar one to the young men of the early twentieth century, and was the result of their exposure to romances such as William Morris's *The Well at the World's End* and John Bunyan's *Pilgrim's Progress.*[1] The romantic, narrative trope involved the testing of a (male) hero, through the 'ordeal' of his experience. If he could withstand this test, he would be transformed through 'apotheosis' – a process that mirrored religious ideas of transcendence. The hero was, therefore, not just courageous, but also saintly: morally and spiritually pure. For the young men of the war generation, combat was their ordeal; surviving it with 'honour' would result in self-transformation.

211

Such 'myths' were exploded, after the war, by writers such as Siegfried Sassoon, Edmund Blunden, Henri Barbusse, and Erich Maria Remarque, who exposed the contrast between the romance trope and the ugly realities of modern, industrial warfare.

Volunteer nurses were mostly drawn from the middle or upper classes of their societies; they, too, were likely to write in ways that drew upon the 'high culture' of their time. Young, female nurses were exposed to many of the same romantic ideals that held such power over their brothers. But, for them, the romance trope was a complex one. Women in traditional, western romance had been portrayed as either passive victims, to be rescued from danger by male heroes, or as villainesses against whom the hero must battle. Rarely had they been actors at the centre of their own adventures. Now a new generation of young women was beginning to develop a new perspective: volunteer nurses found ways in which to view themselves as heroines. A new genre of female adventure-writing, with popular authors such as Bessie Marchant at its vanguard,[2] was already influencing girls to believe that they could situate themselves at the centre of their own stories: that they could even, through their own courage and adaptability, be the makers of their own futures. A new feminine myth was emerging, and volunteer nurses were determined to enact it. They were not to know that the realities of industrial warfare were soon to expose it as a hollow fiction.

Ordeals on the Western Front

Not all British volunteer nurses were 'VADs'. Henrietta Tayler, a keen volunteer who offered her services to the Anglo-French Red Cross, appears to have embarked on – but been unable to complete – a formal course of training. She clearly considered herself to be as skilled and knowledgeable as most fully trained nurses, and was chagrined at her lack of a formal qualification, commenting that she had 'had to bear the stigma of the semi-trained; a stigma that I have tried, as we all do, to rub off with extra hard work'.[3]

In 1916, after eighteen months' experience of running a VAD hospital in Scotland, Tayler was posted by the 'Anglo-French section of the British Red Cross' to L'Hôpital de l'Océan, in La Panne, Belgium. She was probably there for some months before Violetta Thurstan's arrival as matron. She considered service at L'Hôpital de l'Océan a privilege and wrote of the prestige of being sent to 'Dr Depages famous ambulance ... a splendid organization'.[4] She commented on the level of innovation and specialisation within the institution, which had units devoted to patients with abdominal, chest, head, and eye wounds, as well as wards for fracture cases, for patients with 'nerve lesions', and 'one especially devoted to experimental treatment of complicated cases with all the newest therapeutic discoveries'.[5] She pointed out that almost all wounds were treated using the most up-to-date method – irrigation using the Carrel Dakin technique – declaring that L'Hôpital de l'Océan shared with the Rockefeller Institute at Compiègne 'the distinction of being the best exponents of the system'.[6] Tayler seems to have taken great delight in being at the vanguard of clinical practice. If she had a 'romance quest' it was, clearly, to prove herself a good nurse and, in pursing her goal, she underwent ordeals of both a clinical and a personal nature. The work was onerous, and she found herself burdened by responsibility:

> I shall never forget one lurid night I passed with three [French North African patients] and ten other patients, the Sister in charge being engaged elsewhere; one brown man had to have injections of *huile camphrée* hourly, another morphia whenever his pain became unbearable, and the third was coughing up his lungs all night, and died before morning. The other two lived to be moved to another ward, but not much longer.[7]

She comments, in the dry and somewhat patronising language of the British imperialist, on how 'one Frenchman, belonging to the famous Algerian regiment of Joyeux, who gave us a great deal of trouble, desired me to write to his father that he had died the death of a hero and, when I pointed out "Nous ne sommes pas encore à ce point-là" was quite hurt. Him, I did manage to see again, being very noisy in another ward.'[8] Another patient, who 'was proud of his command of the English language, kept crying pathetically for hours: "Seestair, seestair, elevate me – I cannot respire."' Tayler explained to him that the nature of his wound meant that he must lie flat, but it took some time to convince him of this.[9]

Overwork and proximity to infection meant that Tayler contracted pneumonia, and was sent to the 'sick house', where she listened to the sounds of military funerals outside her window, wondering if she, too, would soon die, and writing, in somewhat dramatic tones, of how she had made 'the one person I really trusted promise to tell me when that moment seemed imminent, while holding fast to her hand, to combat the ghastly sensation of falling, falling, falling through the floor of the world!'[10]

Volunteer nurses did not have to endure near-death experiences to find themselves on perilous journeys or enduring ordeals that would change their perceptions of life. Olive Dent, in her prosaically titled *A VAD in France*, offers the following account of night duty in a base hospital:

> Naturally, we have had nights never-to-be-forgotten ... all the devlish [*sic*] horror and wracking torture of living again the eternal age with its waiting, waiting, waiting in No Man's Land, nights when a dying man on whom morphia has had no effect has persistently cackled ragtime while another, – one of the very, very few who have realised they are in the Valley of the Shadow, – reiterated again and again 'I'm dying, I'm dying, I'm dying' ... tense moments when we have fought for a life with strychnine, morphia, salines, nutrients, and hot-water bottles, crowded moments when, our lamps throwing Rembrandt shadows and gleams around the dark tent with its rows of huddled, maimed forms, there has been plugged and stemmed a haemorrhage from a place where the surgeon could not ligature ... One's eyes smart and feel filled with salt as a man with life ebbing – oh! so painfully quickly, – grasps one's hand and says 'Sister, God bless you.' The full meaning of the remark arrests one, its sanctity, its solemnity, the benedictory significance of the words spoken under such circumstances engulf one.[11]

Dent's extraordinary writing contains all the motifs of the romance quest: the strange eeriness of the lamp-lit base hospital ward with its 'Rembrandt shadows'; the 'devlish horror and wracking torture'; the reverential moments when men pass through 'the Valley of the Shadow'; the apotheosis – the moment of spiritual transformation, when the dying patient says 'God bless you'. The episodes described by Dent suggest that night duty was filled with moments of spiritual truth. For most nurses, its reality probably had much to do with cups of cocoa, the carrying of bedpans and vomit bowls, and the regular medicine-round. But Dent may have been speaking for her generation when she infused such meaning into her work. And the motif she used was one that her generation would have recognised.

An anonymous American writer, who entitled her memoir of the war *Mademoiselle Miss*, wrote of her 'unique and inexpressible life' in a French Red Cross hospital.[12] At the outbreak of war she served as 'helper in a small French hospital on the Riviera' and then in an English hospital at Mentone.[13] Eventually, however, she decided to take the examination for a 'nurse's diploma in the French Red Cross' and joined a French military hospital on the Marne.[14] On 20 September 1915, she described her first experience of enemy shelling: 'It is a sensation so vast and lonely and crowded and cosmic all at once that one seems born into a new phase of existence where the old ways of feeling do not answer any longer.'[15] Part of her purpose in writing seems to be to present the French military hospital as the strange, spellbinding place of legend and romance: 'It is all like a weird dream, laughter (for they laugh well, the soldiers) and blood and death and funny episodes, and sublime also, all under the autumn stars.'[16]

Most volunteer nurses had had minimal prior experience of ward work; their entry into the military hospital was preceded by only a few months' nursing work in a civilian or auxiliary hospital. It is probably because of their naivety and inexperience that their writings are, typically, filled with a sense of wonder at being in the presence of suffering patients and staff who are taking life-or-death decisions. The disjointed, strange, and contradictory qualities of memoirs such as *A VAD in France* and *Mademoiselle Miss* lure the reader into a sense of unreality – a feeling that one has entered a dream-world: a spiritual realm. Their authors juxtapose fantasy with horror.

'Wide open world': the adventures of Florence Farmborough

Stored in the Imperial War Museum, London, are seventeen reels of tape recording a conversation between memoirist Florence Farmborough and interviewer Margaret Brooks. In the first reel, Farmborough, in the high, cultured voice of a gentlewoman, tells of her childhood. Her narration is slow and deliberate, filled with certainty and self-belief, never faltering, offering what sounds almost like a recitation. She is conscious of the importance of her story, and therefore of her life. Her interview is not just a record; it is a piece of self-composure.[17] Florence Farmborough retold the story of her life and nursing work several times, through memoirs and interviews, each time capturing a sense that her life in Russia was a romantic mission – a journey into the unknown and a quest for discovery.[18]

215

Florence Farmborough's original diary was almost certainly written contemporaneously with the events it describes. Containing extended passages relating to specific events, it offers a vivid insight into her wartime nursing experiences; but it is disjointed, lengthy, and difficult to navigate. Her memoir offers a more reflective account, in which time has been foreshortened, apparent irrelevances are omitted, and events are ordered. Although it still often relates scenes of chaos and confusion, the text itself is carefully arranged and adjusted to permit the reader to follow Farmborough's spiritual journey as a neophyte nurse, as well as her geographical one first as a member of a Russian flying column and then as a British subject escaping from revolutionary Russia. The oral history interviews Farmborough gave to Margaret Brooks and Peter Liddle were conducted soon after she had published *Nurse at the Russian Front*, and both are strongly influenced by the memoir. It is as if, by this time, her life has ceased to be a succession of events and has become a carefully constructed recitation based on those events.

Florence Farmborough was born in 1887 at Steeple Claydon, Buckinghamshire, close to the Claydon estate of Florence Nightingale's brother-in-law, Sir Harry Verney. She was, in fact, named after Nightingale,[19] and this may have influenced her later decision to nurse the Russian wounded – although her narrative depicts her being swept into war service by the enthusiastic patriotism of her Moscow circle.

One of Farmborough's primary motivators was the desire to travel: 'I had decided', she says in her 1975 interview, 'long, long before anyone else knew it that I was going to be a traveller'.[20] This desire became 'a tremendous objective', which was fulfilled when, at the age of nineteen (but claiming to be twenty-one), she went to East Galicia to be a governess. She speaks of a 'tremendous feeling of wonderment – a tremendous thrill' upon first seeing the Carpathian Alps, followed by a desire 'to climb and see where [they] ended and what was beyond those enormous peaks'.[21] Her quest was to take a form that not even she could have imagined.

Farmborough first went to Russia in 1908. Her post was in Kiev, a city that she found exhilarating and moving: both 'splendid' and deeply spiritual.[22] She then travelled to Moscow, where she took a position as governess to the two daughters of renowned heart specialist Dr Pavel Sergeyevitch. Her Russian employers were kind and treated her as a part of their family; and her experience of Moscow was remarkably similar to that of Violetta Thurstan. Like Thurstan, she was fascinated by Russia's bells: 'It was said in those days that there were 40 times 40 churches and holy shrines in Moscow, and so you can imagine [on holy days] 40 times 40 bells rang out from all these great and small beautiful architectural edifices. And the whole city was resounding with the music of bells.'[23] Hearing Farmborough's voice, as she recounts her early experiences of Kiev and Moscow, a listener cannot help but be struck by her deep sense of nostalgia. With the hindsight of sixty years, and speaking in a world still fractured by the cold war, in which Eastern Europe and Russia were concealed behind an 'Iron Curtain', she was profoundly aware of 'her' Russia as a lost place that could never be recaptured: a place of myth, legend, and enchantment, where there were cities with '40 times 40 bells'.

In Moscow, Farmborough came to identify herself with her Russian family. She decided to play her part in Russia's war by enrolling, along with her two young charges, as a volunteer nurse.[24] In early-twentieth-century Russia, there were few nurse training schools; most civilian nursing was undertaken by Sisters of Mercy. Following a six-month Red Cross training, and a series of examinations, Farmborough was considered a fully qualified surgical nurse. Her experience casts light upon the findings of Violetta Thurstan, who was struck, during her time in Poland, both by the technical precision of the Russian 'nurses', and by their lack of wider nursing knowledge and skill.[25]

Farmborough enrolled in the 10th Surgical Unit of the all-Russian *Zemski Soyuz*, and was delighted to find herself posted to a *letuchka*, or 'flying column' – a rapidly moving mobile field hospital – based on the Eastern Front in the Carpathian Mountains.[26] She narrated her experiences not only in her remarkable memoir, *Nurse at the Russian Front*, but also in her *Russian Album*, her remarkable pictorial record of a vanished world. Her photographs capture a series of tantalising images of pre-war, wartime, and revolutionary Russia. From them stare the people of a lost generation, and alongside stands a clear and precise narration of events, interrupted with the occasional deliberately loaded comment. In the opening chapter, Farmborough announces: 'I went to Russia in 1908. I was twenty-one, with an urge to travel that had been with me since my earliest years. Reflecting now upon my travels, I have said that I loved Russia the most because she taught me the meaning of the word "suffering".[27]

In *Nurse at the Russian Front*, Farmborough relates her story in romantic terms: it consists of an epic journey through a vast, enchanted yet dangerous landscape in which both courage and resolve are tested. Transformation, or 'apotheosis', is reached on a final long, slow journey through Siberia with the realisation that even the cataclysm of the Russian Revolution cannot touch Russia's 'wide, changeless spaces', which 'bring only comfort and peace'.[28] Much of the book reads as a traveller's tale,[29] and its mood is loaded with the excitement of adventure, as its heroine faces danger and holds her nerve. On one occasion, Farmborough finds herself in acute danger, as a 'folvark' (an inn) in which she and her colleagues are spending a night is shelled. Her description is infused with dramatic tension: 'The noise was deafening; the house rocked as in an earthquake; a crash of timber splitting, falling; a cascade of broken glass spilling from a height.'[30]

Although she describes with care the episodes in which she finds herself in physical danger, it is the intensity of her moral, nursing dilemmas that Farmborough seems most keen to transmit to her readers. In one episode, she describes how she is forced to choose between rejoining her departing column, or remaining with a dying man who has begged her not to leave him.[31] In another, she describes how she resolves the ethical dilemma of caring for a soldier with self-inflicted wounds, by deciding to cover the 'dark tell-tale stain of a wound received at close quarters' with iodine and a bandage and despatching the man to base before his 'cowardice' can be discovered and punishment meted out.[32] One of the most moving passages in her 'diary', however, is the one in which she describes 'hastening a soldier's death through my disobedience'.[33] Having been told not to give any food or fluid to a 'stomach case' who has had surgery the previous night, she is confronted by a man who is clearly desperate for water. She is certain that he is dying:

His cries for water were insistent; he was beseeching, imploring; his thirst must have been agonising. Near one of the other men, a mug of water was standing. He had seen it and, raising an arm, pointed towards it. His eyes challenged mine; they were dying eyes, but fiercely alight with the greatness of his thirst. I reasoned with myself: if I give no water, he will die tormented by his great thirst; if I give him water, he will die, but his torment will be lessened. In my weakness and compassion, I reached for the mug; his burning eyes were watching me; they held suspense and gratitude. I put the mug to his lips, but he seized my arm and tilted the mug upwards. The water splashed into his open mouth, sprayed his face and pillow, but he was swallowing it in noisy gulps. When I could free my arm from his grasp, the mug was empty. I was deeply distressed and knew that I was trembling. I wiped his face dry and he opened his eyes and looked at me; in them, I saw a great thankfulness, an immense relief. But, before I could replace the mug, a strange gurgling sound came from him, and out of his mouth, there poured a stream of thick, greenish fluid; it spread over the stretcher-bed and flowed on to the floor. His eyes were closed and … he had stopped breathing.[34]

Farmborough's writing skilfully draws out the reader's emotions: horror at the man's death; relief that the nurse has granted his wish; fear that she has failed to obey an order; suspense at what the final outcome will be. Farmborough comes to understand the impossibility of achieving perfect solutions to the ethical dilemmas of nursing practice, and the peace of knowing that she has prioritised the easing of suffering over obedience to orders. She concludes that 'all my life I should have the grievous memory of hastening a soldier's death through my disobedience; but, at the same time, there would be another less grievous memory: that of a pair of dying eyes looking at me with infinite gratitude'.[35] In volunteer nurses' writings, episodes such as these represent the trials or tests that must be passed. If the male test is 'ordeal by combat' with its life-or-death outcome, then the female test is 'ordeal by suffering' – her own and that of others.

Broken spell: war and revolution in the writings of Mary Britnieva

Little is known about the experiences of Russian nurses – particularly those of the Sisters of Mercy, who relinquished their civilian practice for war service. Yet the memoirs of war-trained volunteer nurses can fill some of the gaps in the historical record, as well as offering insight into the experiences of middle- and upper-class women, who chose to serve as nurses.[36] Mary Britnieva was a member of the Anglo-Russian gentry at the outbreak of war in 1914. Her memoir of war and revolution, covering the period from 1914 to 1930, is a blend of one highly

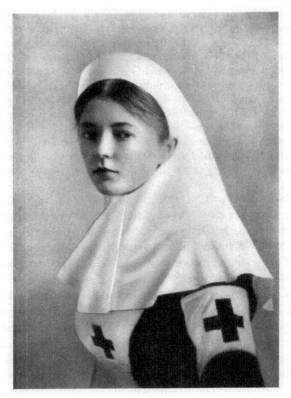

Figure 10 Portrait of Mary Britnieva

personal and tragic life-story with a sweeping, epic retelling of a turbulent period in Russian history.[37] Her narrative begins with the departure for the Eastern Front of the flying column to which she is attached. It ends with her narrow escape from the Soviet Union following an unsuccessful attempt to rescue her doctor-husband from the Stalinist purge of the 'intelligentsia'. The book's tone resonates with a sincere attachment to everything she considers to represent the 'old Russia' – a dying nation, which is being ruthlessly purged and rapidly replaced by a soulless and heartless bureaucracy. She avidly records any experience that suggests that the spiritual life of Russia and its people still lives and cannot be extinguished, and her book is clearly a deliberate attempt to keep alive the memory of everything that was ruthlessly wiped out by war and revolution.

Britnieva's memoir is pervaded by a feeling of nostalgia. It was written in the early 1930s when her feeling of loss and grief must still have been raw. Episodes in which she was happy – many of which took place at the height of war when the Russian army was retreating with huge losses – are recollected with warmth and pleasure. Ultimately, the book is a reflection on the destruction of Russian society and culture. Britnieva conveys a sense that the Russian people were, in the second and third decades of the twentieth century, 'sleepwalking' to their own destruction, unable to see what was happening to them until it was too late. In fact, the phrase 'too late' becomes Britnieva's meditation. She puts the words into the mouth of Russian intellectual Anatoli Feodorovitch: 'It seems to me that the most terrible, the most tragic thing that can befall one in life is to be *too late*. "Pozdno" (too late), what a cruel, what a relentless word! In its finality it is far more terrible than *Death* itself, and, being irrevocable, far, far worse than *Never!*'[38]

Mary Britnieva had enjoyed a privileged childhood as part of a wealthy Anglo-Russian family living in Petrograd. Towards the end of her book, she compares her former self with the children of the newly emerged Bolshevik elite, recognising that, in her youth, she had been spoiled, 'unconscious and blissfully ignorant' of the lives and conditions of the impoverished Russian proletariat.[39] A powerful sense of patriotism pervades her thinking and she describes how her first instinct at the outbreak of war was to train as a 'war nurse'.[40] Her training was probably very similar to that of Florence Farmborough. She was delighted to learn that she was to be appointed to a flying column, which operated under the patronage of the Russian Council of State. At this early point in the book, the reader is introduced to the man who is to become Britnieva's husband, although we never learn his name.[41] He is 'the head doctor', 'a well-known surgeon and a brilliant organizer'.[42]

For Britnieva, as for Florence Farmborough, the greatest trials she describes in this early part of her book are those associated with the care of the dangerously ill. Yet, her descriptions of her work resonate with an almost childish sense of excitement and adventure: the care of the wounded is a challenging game; winning brings the thrill of achievement:

> How excited I was when my first patient was brought! He was a German prisoner called Koppe and had peritonitis, being very seriously wounded in the stomach. Our head doctor had operated on him, extracting several bullets from his liver, which was (he found) practically in pieces. Koppe was hardly expected to live, his condition being almost hopeless, but thanks to his wonderful patience and amazing stoicism, he pulled through. For nine days after his operation he was not allowed to drink – only having his tongue moistened now and again with a drop of water.[43]

Although she gives credit to the patient for his 'wonderful patience and amazing stoicism', Britnieva seems also to be experiencing an unspoken sense of achievement in her own work. The outcome for Koppe is very different from the terrible death experienced by Farmborough's patient in her *Nurse at the Russian Front*. Britnieva's lack of enmity towards her German patient is also striking, particularly in view of her intense patriotism. Her writing conveys a sense that wartime nursing is a humanitarian endeavour, not very different from Red Cross work in times of natural disaster such as earthquake or epidemic.

Britnieva's war can be read through her memoir as a great adventure and an epic journey. Her descriptions of long and romantic treks through beautiful Eastern European landscapes are typical of Eastern Front nursing memoirs.[44] In December 1914, during the German advance into Poland, the flying column to which Britnieva was attached spent several weeks occupying an old and beautiful palace named Teresino. Here, the unit cared for some of the most horrifically wounded patients, including the victims of gas attacks. Yet, Britnieva remembers this time as one of the happiest of her life. Her description of arrival in Teresino is redolent of an episode in a fairy tale:

> It was a beautifully clear moonlit night and the frost had formed a soft crust on the snow's surface which crunched pleasantly under our feet as we crossed the field and entered the wood … our excitement reaching its culminating point at the magic sight that met our eyes when we reached a clearing in the park. A real fairy palace with turrets and galleries, gleaming white and dazzling in the moonlight, stood before us … We stood spellbound.[45]

The words 'spellbound', 'magic', and 'fairy palace' infuse Britnieva's account with a feeling of enchantment – almost as if she wants to convey a sense that she was living in a dream. If so, she soon brings the reader back to reality, as she describes how 'a steady stream of ambulances' arrived at the hospital, and the nurses found themselves 'up to their necks' in work. Patients arrived with 'shockingly' infected wounds and many died, in spite of the hospital's reputation for having the highest survival rate on that part of the Eastern Front.[46]

Following her return home on leave, Britnieva takes another journey, this time to her mother's estate in Chistopol, in the Government of Kazan. Her fiancé meets her there, and once again, she conveys a sense that she is living in a fantasy world: 'A feeling of peace reigned everywhere. The War seemed something unreal, remote, untrue. It seemed unbelievable that somewhere men were fighting and killing one another, when the world was so unspeakably lovely.'[47] Britnieva's determined exaggeration – her concern to convey how 'unspeakably lovely' her world was – undoubtedly reflects her sense of loss, as she writes her book in exile, in Britain, sensing that she will never return to her homeland. She writes of 'how infinitely beautiful' her country was, and of 'how little we guessed the dark terrible tragedy that was to befall her in a year's time'.[48] As the world of her childhood slipped away, Britnieva's real ordeal was beginning. And yet, her narrative itself does not become dark. It may be that her determined focus on all that remained beautiful in her world was part of a deliberate project to bring her sense of the spirit of Russia into the minds of a western readership. No less than those of British writers such as Millicent Sutherland or Sarah Macnaughtan, Britnieva's project was a patriotic one. For her western audience, Russia was another world – entirely out of reach – and Britnieva plays upon this notion of a 'lost world' by infusing her writing with a dreamlike quality. But this dream is both fantastic and utopian: and the Russia she creates owes as much to her own powerful and creative writing as to reality.

Britnieva married at the beginning of 1918, 'almost a year after the abdication of the Tsar and several months after the Bolsheviks had seized power'.[49] She conveys a sense that, even as her personal life is taking a new and satisfying course, the life of her nation is gradually being strangled by the Bolshevik Revolution, the decline into civil war, and the New Economic Policy.[50] At the end of the 1920s, Stalin's 'revolution from above', incorporating the collectivisation of agriculture, the industrial drive of the first Five Year Plan, and the 'Cultural Revolution' directed against the old intelligentsia, swept away the last remnants of Britnieva's 'old Russia'. It is only with hindsight that one can view these events as episodes in a tragic – albeit temporary – process of social, economic, and cultural devastation. Sheila Fitzpatrick has commented that the twenty-first century has chosen to view the Russian Revolution as 'a wrong turning that took Russia off course for seventy-four years'.[51] For those living through these events, there was always the hope that stability would return. For Britnieva, 'these new-fangled persons who called themselves Bolsheviks' had created 'complete chaos in every single branch of life which was the only visible consequence of their advent to power'.[52] As members of the so-called 'intelligentsia' – an inchoate group of highly educated and skilled individuals – Britnieva's family were under threat. Although the Russian intelligentsia held 'passive liberal attitudes rather than active revolutionary commitment to political change',[53] they were identified as the 'class enemies' of the new state, and as such were subjected to the 'totalitarian terror' meted out first by the radicalised Bolsheviks and then by Stalin's autocracy. Britnieva traces the tragic destruction of this group.[54] Although Britnieva herself, with a claim to British citizenship, was able to escape from Bolshevik Russia with her children, her husband remained behind. Britnieva made several visits, but on the final one she was unable to trace her husband, learning only weeks after his death that he had been executed in prison. Returning home and looking through his possessions, she found a letter stamped 'Chistopol – May 1916'. Her words express the nostalgia that infuses her entire book: 'The glittering Kama in the distance … How long ago! How far away…'.[55]

Conclusion: 'ordeal' and 'apotheosis'

For many of those who nursed the wounded of the First World War, their experiences were more extraordinary than anything they could have imagined. In writing of those experiences, they drew upon cultural conceptions of 'the extraordinary', 'the magical', and 'the amazing', to fit their own narratives into a romantic trope that was only just beginning to be recognised as dangerous. Their perspectives would, by the end of the twentieth century, be regarded as archaic and naive. Their stories contain 'ordeals' in which they battle death, and often resolve into 'apotheoses' in which 'suffering' somehow becomes the highest spiritual truth. The romantic narrative trope was especially powerful in the memoirs of volunteer nurses, and was particularly likely to be applied to experience on the Eastern Front. Individuals such as Florence Farmborough and Mary Britnieva produced stories of their own lives, which take notions of 'self-composure' to the highest level, presenting the nurse writer as the heroine of her own adventure. Yet, these are not works of deliberate propaganda or self-promotion; their writers seem to want only to bear witness to the extraordinary times through which they lived.

One of the most frequently cited reasons for publishing a war diary was the compulsion to bear witness to the horrors of war. Authors wrote of their desire to tell the truth. Yet the truth differed depending upon background, perspective, and experience; it was coloured by cultural and ideological influences. For VADs, their backgrounds as genteel middle- and upper-class ladies of the British Empire brought a strong element of patriotism to their writings, even as they began to realise that the war was not the simple crusade against a marauding Teutonic horde they had believed it to be. It also inclined them to express a remarkable level of confidence in their own natural abilities as nurturers of the wounded.[56] A project that they embraced with particular eagerness was the presentation of nursing itself as an ordeal, through which only the strongest could pass unscathed. The 'truth' that most seemed anxious to convey was that nursing work was a transformative process, which, if approached with a genuine desire to alleviate suffering, could have a profoundly positive effect not only on the patient, but on the nurse herself.

Notes

1 Paul Fussell, *The Great War and Modern Memory* (Oxford: Oxford University Press, 2000 [1975]): 135–44. See also: Benedict Anderson, *Imagined Communities: Reflections on the Origin and Spread of Nationalism* (London: Verso, 1991).

2 Michelle Smith, 'Adventurous Girls of the British Empire: The Pre-War Novels of Bessie Marchant', *The Lion and the Unicorn*, 33.1 (2009): 1–25.

3 Henrietta Tayler, *A Scottish Nurse at War: Being a Record of What One Semi-Trained Nurse Has Been Privileged to See and Do during Four and a Half Years of War* (London: John Lane, 1920): 15.

4 Tayler, *A Scottish Nurse at War*: 29–30. On L'Hôpital de l'Océan, see Christine E. Hallett, *Veiled Warriors: Allied Nurses of the First World War* (Oxford: Oxford University Press, 2014): 40–3.
5 Tayler, *A Scottish Nurse at War*: 30.
6 Tayler, *A Scottish Nurse at War*: 30.
7 Tayler, *A Scottish Nurse at War*: 39.
8 Tayler, *A Scottish Nurse at War*: 39.
9 Tayler, *A Scottish Nurse at War*: 40.
10 Tayler, *A Scottish Nurse at War*: 42.
11 Olive Dent, *A VAD in France* (London: Grant Richards, 1917): 282–7.
12 Anon., *Mademoiselle Miss* (Liskeard: Diggory Press, 2006 [1916]): 31.
13 Anon., *Mademoiselle Miss*: preface.
14 Anon., *Mademoiselle Miss*: preface.
15 Anon., *Mademoiselle Miss*: 14.
16 Anon., *Mademoiselle Miss*: 28–30.
17 Florence Farmborough: oral history interview conducted by Margaret A. Brooks, 1975, 17 reels, Imperial War Museum, London, Reel 1. On 'self-composure', see: Penny Summerfield, *Reconstructing Women's Wartime Lives* (Manchester: Manchester University Press, 1998): 16–23.
18 Farmborough gave another interview – to Peter Liddle – Florence Farmborough: oral history interview conducted by Peter Liddle at Abbeyfield House, The Mount, Heswall, 1975, Liddle Collection, Brotherton Library, University of Leeds. Farmborough's original diaries are held at the Imperial War Museum, London: Florence Farmborough, diaries, private papers, 1381. Her memoir, *Nurse at the Russian Front*, was published in 1974; and her *Russian Album*, a collection of her own photographs, in 1979. Florence Farmborough, *Nurse at the Russian Front: A Diary, 1914–18* (London: Book Club Associates, 1974), later republished in a new edition: Florence Farmborough, *With the Armies of the Tsar: A Nurse at the Russian Front in War and Revolution, 1914–1918* (New York: Cooper Square Press, 2000); Florence Farmborough, *Russian Album 1908–1918*, ed. John Jolliffe (Wilton: Michael Russell, 1979). See also: Peter Liddle, *Captured Memories 1900–1918: Across the Threshold of War* (Barnsley: Pen and Sword, 2010), Chapter 16, 'Florence Farmborough F.R.G.S.': 231–44.
19 Farmborough, *Russian Album*: 7.
20 Oral history interview conducted by Margaret A. Brooks: Reel 1.
21 Oral history interview: conducted by Margaret A. Brooks: Reel 1.
22 Farmborough, *Russian Album*: 9; Oral history interview conducted by Margaret A. Brooks: reel 1.
23 Oral history interview conducted by Margaret A. Brooks: reel 2.
24 Farmborough, *Russian Album*: 27.
25 See Chapter 6.

26 Farmborough, *Russian Album*: 27–8. On the work of British nurses in fly-ing columns, see: Christine Hallett, 'Russian Romances: Emotionalism and Spirituality in the Writings of "Eastern Front" Nurses', 1914–1918, *Nursing History Review*, 17 (2009): 101–28.
27 Farmborough, *Russian Album*: 9.
28 Farmborough, *Nurse at the Russian Front*: 396.
29 On the tradition of British travel writing in Russia, see: Anthony Cross, 'From the Assassination of Paul I to Tilsit: The British in Russia and Their Travel Writings (1801–1807), *Journal of European Studies*, 42.1 (2012): 5–21. See also: Katya Hokanson, 'Russian Women Travellers in Central Asia and India', *Russian Review*, 70.1 (2011): 1–19.
30 Farmborough, *Nurse at the Russian Front*: 128.
31 Farmborough, *Nurse at the Russian Front*: 130–1.
32 Farmborough, *Nurse at the Russian Front*: 131.
33 Farmborough, *Nurse at the Russian Front*: 230.
34 Farmborough, *Nurse at the Russian Front*: 229–30.
35 Farmborough, *Nurse at the Russian Front*: 230.
36 Susan Grant, 'Nursing in Russia and the Soviet Union, 1914–41: An Overview of the Development of a Soviet Nursing System', *Bulletin of the UK Association for the History of Nursing*, 2 (2012): 21–33; Laurie Stoff, 'The "Myth of the War Experience" and Russian Wartime Nursing in World War I', *Aspasia: The International Yearbook of Central, Eastern, and Southeastern European Women's and Gender History*, 6 (2012): 96–116; Hallett, *Veiled Warriors*: Chapter 3.
37 Mary Britnieva, *One Woman's Story* (London: Arthur Baker, 1934).
38 Britnieva, *One Woman's Story*: 209.
39 Britnieva, *One Woman's Story*: 258.
40 Britnieva, *One Woman's Story*: 9–13.
41 At one point, she refers to him briefly as 'Sasha': Britnieva, *One Woman's Story*: 89.
42 Britnieva, *One Woman's Story*: 10.
43 Britnieva, *One Woman's Story*: 15.
44 Both Violetta Thurstan and Florence Farmborough write of long treks through forests and farmland: Violetta Thurstan, *Field Hospital and Flying Column: Being the Journal of an English Nursing Sister in Belgium and Russia* (London: G. P. Putnam's Sons, 1915); Farmborough, *Nurse at the Russian Front*. See also: Hallett, 'Russian Romances'.
45 Britnieva, *One Woman's Story*: 27.
46 Britnieva, *One Woman's Story*: 31.
47 Britnieva, *One Woman's Story*: 51.
48 Britnieva, *One Woman's Story*: 64.
49 Britnieva, *One Woman's Story*: 67.

50 On the Russian Revolution, see: Orlando Figes, *A People's Tragedy: The Russian Revolution, 1891–1924* (London: Pimlico, 1997 [1996]); Sheila Fitzpatrick, *The Russian Revolution*, 3rd edn (Oxford: Oxford University Press, 2008). On the New Economic Policy of 1921, see: Chris Ward, *Russia's Cotton Workers and the New Economic Policy: Shop Floor Culture and State Policy, 1921–1929* (Cambridge: Cambridge University Press, 2002).

51 Fitzpatrick, *The Russian Revolution*: 1. See also: Figes, *A People's Tragedy*.

52 Britnieva, *One Woman's Story*: 69.

53 Fitzpatrick, *The Russian Revolution*: 22.

54 'They had all committed the same crime, the crime of being educated and cultured': Britnieva, *One Woman's Story*: 237.

55 Britnieva, *One Woman's Story*: 279.

56 Claire Tylee, *The Great War and Women's Consciousness: Images of Militarism and Womanhood in Women's Writings, 1914–64* (Houndmills and London: Macmillan, 1990).

Conclusion

Remembering and memorialising

Memory is fallible; and, because the reader of any memoir knows this, no memoir is fully believed. Yet, some are more convincing than others. Some are taken as faithful renditions of experience; others are recognised as close approximations to 'the truth'; still others have clearly identifiable fictional elements. An author such as Edmund Blunden could write with authority of the terrors of the trenches: of how a lance corporal was reduced by a shell to 'gobbets of blackening flesh', of how an 'excellent sentry' was shot through the head while staring through a loophole.[1] Nurses, too, could write with authority. Although only a combatant like Blunden could faithfully describe a sudden death or the emotional turmoil of trench life, a nurse such as Alice Fitzgerald could write of the horror of witnessing slow death from wound sepsis or the anxiety of lying in a bell tent during a bombardment with a steel helmet over her face.

Some nurse writers were careful observers and relentless truth-tellers. Others wrote with purpose, some with pacifist intent – to show that war was horrific, not heroic. In this way, their work bore some similarities to those of male writers who wanted to draw society's attention to the realities of the trenches.[2] Yet, in some ways, the writings of nurses were starker, because they bore witness to the suffering that followed battle injury. Rebecca West insisted on demonstrating the way in which war debased those involved in it. Enid Bagnold exposed the dehumanising effects of the military medical system. Ellen La Motte – the most shocking of all – offered an exposé of the brutality of war itself, demonstrating how, beneath the surface of its apparent heroism, lurked fear and degradation. Mabel St Clair Stobart interspersed her powerful story with brief reflective homilies on the nature of warfare, while Lesley Smith simply described her patients' injuries with raw immediacy. These writers were, it seems, driven by a need to tell the truth as they saw it. For most, their project appears to have been to remember rather than to memorialise – to show how things really were rather than to cover reality with a heroic gloss. Or perhaps, for them, the truth (as they saw it) was the most honourable memorial to the suffering of their fellow countrymen.

In writing of their nursing work during the First World War, nurses were also composing portraits of themselves. Whilst some seem to have wanted to remain shadowy figures in the background, foregrounding the courage and resilience of their patients, others chose to depict themselves as actors on a world stage.[3] When they wrote, British women such as the Baroness de T'Serclaes, Sarah Macnaughtan, and Millicent Sutherland were drawing upon narrative tropes current in their own culture. The adventure novels of G. A. Henty and Henry Rider Haggard had long provided a template for male action within the field of enterprise that formed the British Empire.[4] But girls read these novels too. And if this created a sense of dissonance – because all the heroes were boys – they could turn to a small but burgeoning corpus of 'girl's own adventure' writings. Although limited, this included the novels of Bessie Marchant, whose heroines faced challenge and hardship and experienced 'heroic adventure'.[5] While her plot resolutions often involved marriage, Marchant's heroines frequently displayed the same courage, toughness, and endurance as boys. And although her heroines only 'engaged in adventure out of necessity' to preserve life or prevent crime, they displayed 'physicality and resourceful capability'.[6] When Millicent, Duchess of Sutherland wrote in her diary during the bombardment of Namur that she 'felt as if I were actually *living* some book of adventure, such as I had read in my youth',[7] she was undoubtedly drawing upon such powerful cultural influences. For American women, a pioneering cultural trope was dominant. Women such as Julia Stimson and Helen Dore Boylston portrayed themselves as intrepid pioneers, who could meet any challenge with calmness and capability.

Dutiful daughters of the allied cause

Those who nursed the allied wounded of the First World War came from a range of backgrounds. Yet most would have viewed themselves as 'genteel' or 'middle class'. The prestige of army nursing meant that places within elite corps such as the QAIMNS and the ANC were reserved for women who were able to afford a good education, and a sound professional training. At the outset of the war it had been impossible to become a volunteer nurse unless one had sufficient funds to pay for a uniform, a minimal training, and one's own travel; these expenses naturally excluded women of lower class.[8] Hence, many of those who nursed the wounded during the First World War viewed themselves as 'ladies'; and, as such, they were constrained by the expectation that they would be 'ladylike' in their behaviour as well as being steeped in the patriarchal values of their times. It would not have occurred to most female writers to question the masculine authority that dictated their respective governments' entries into the First World War. Nor would it have occurred to them to question the authority of the Army Medical Services, which mobilised their efforts and transferred them – sometimes at a few hours' notice – from one treatment scenario to another.

British and North American nurses had much in common. As Sidonie Smith and Julia Watson observe: 'remembering has a politics'.[9] Nurses who would not have viewed themselves as 'politically minded' wrote memoirs that both reveal a stark reality about the wounding and maiming brought about by warfare, and conceal a political truth about its nature and origin. Kate Luard and Julia Stimson were born several thousand miles and eleven years apart. Yet their backgrounds were remarkably similar. Both belonged to large, middle-class families, with fathers who were prominent clergymen and significant public figures in their localities.[10] Both were dutiful daughters. Luard's actions, in resigning early from her position within the QAIMNS Reserve, were dictated by the needs of a sick father at home. Stimson's own father, Henry A. Stimson, wrote the foreword to her compilation of letters, and may have been instrumental in securing their publication. Both women, in common with the vast majority of their colleagues, placed themselves very firmly as subordinates within a patriarchal society. Yet both were powerful. Stimson became a leading female figure in an essentially masculine wartime world, while the force of Luard's writing ensured that her work was noticed by the military establishment. When published in 1930, *Unknown Warriors* was preceded by a preface by Field-Marshall Viscount Allenby, formerly Commander of the Third Army. Allenby's words may explain why Luard's earlier work, published in 1915 at one of the most difficult and uncertain periods of the war – a time when the British Government was careful to suppress any writing that could be seen to endanger morale – was allowed to remain in print.[11] 'I look back', Allenby wrote, 'with admiration on the amazing endurance and self-sacrificing devotion of those Nursing Sisters in their work of mercy'.[12] The writing of nurses such as Luard and Stimson – like their practice – was placed carefully into a humanitarian category, which permitted their readers to view the First World War as one might view a natural disaster – a tidal wave or earthquake. They did not question the wisdom of political or military leaders. Instead, they consciously emphasised both the heroism of soldiers and the redemptive qualities of nursing: a work that, through its devotion, its inherent goodness, and its spirit of self-sacrifice, might rescue humanity from war's horror and degradation.

American nurse Alice Fitzgerald appears to have paid a high personal price for her attachment to duty and her devotion to her soldier patients. She found herself – as a coopted member of the BEF – more or less entrapped within the bounds of her military service. This sense of being confined – of being unable to act with autonomy or determine one's own fate – seems to have been typical of members of the 'official' military nursing services, particularly when on active service overseas.[13] As a guest member of the BEF in France, Fitzgerald commented on the restrictions of military service, observing that any individual who joins the army 'weaves himself or herself into a cocoon of red tape from which it is impossible to emerge as an individual'.[14] Fitzgerald embraced military service as an opportunity and endured great hardship as a result – and yet appears to have felt the reward that came with the fulfilment of her 'mission'. Eventually, though, she sought the greater freedom of Red Cross service.

Nurses such as Fitzgerald were able to make choices because they were among the most highly trained technical nurses of their day. Their skills and knowledge were in high demand, enabling the pursuit of their goals. Fitzgerald desired – above everything else – to make use of her expertise. Nursing itself was her reward, and, for her, the greatest stressors associated with active service were those pressures that prevented the perfect execution of her work. When she retired and moved into the Peabody Home in New York City she sent all her medals and decorations to the Johns Hopkins School of Nursing in Baltimore, declaring that they were 'more properly a credit to her profession than to her personal merit'.[15]

Intrepid travelling nurses

Service, duty, endurance, courage: such concepts resonate through the writings of women who served as nurses during the Great War. The grand ideas that fed those writings, and the exemplars on which they were modelled, suffused the culture of the British and Allied nations in the decades prior to 1914 and provided the fuel that drove whole nations to participate in one of the most destructive conflicts of modern times. They were the ideas of empire, and, for women, they found an outlet in nursing.[16]

Some nurses' narratives are full of danger and adventure. Some involve freedom of movement on a scale previously unknown for most women; and here they differ from male narratives. While the writings of men tell of being led up to the war front and held there either to survive or to be dragged into and destroyed by the war machine, for those female writers not attached to 'official' services, flight was possible and could occur at almost any time. Memoirs such as Violetta Thurstan's *Field Hospital and Flying Column* have this tone. They are about freedom, not captivity. Nurses who avoided 'official' enlistment, and offered their services, instead, to 'freelance' hospital units or to Red Cross Societies in countries where fully trained nurses were scarce, found that the war afforded them a level of freedom they had never previously experienced. Thurstan's professional training became, effectively, a ticket to travel – to enjoy the opportunities afforded by a qualification from one of London's most prestigious nursing schools. She 'flew' in and out of war nursing, as a bird might fly in and out of a storm. Thurstan appears to have been immensely comfortable with her nursing expertise – to the point at which she felt able to write one of the few technical manuals of wartime nursing to be published during the First World War.[17] After her death, she was buried with her eight medals – clasping to herself forever the reward and honour with which they were infused.

On the Western Front, certain geographical locations took on a symbolic significance, becoming inextricably entangled with narratives of the war itself. Vera Brittain found Etaples a sad place filled with camp hospitals and 'crosses grey'.[18] Even before her arrival in France, by about 1916, certain places had begun to take on a mythic status. At Ypres the ruined Cloth Hall symbolised the destruction of the old civic values.[19] When Ellen La Motte saw it from a distance, she stood transfixed, commenting later on her sense of awe and dread at finding herself in such proximity to one of the epicentres of war's destruction.[20] On the Somme, another symbolic structure captured the imagination: a massive gilded statue of the Virgin and Child, dislodged by shelling, which hung from the top of the ruined basilica at Albert. Anxious to attach meaning to what was really only an 'accidentally damaged third rate gilded metal statue', those who saw it chose to believe that it symbolised suffering and sacrifice, and that the war would end when it fell to the ground.[21] After the war, it was possible to take a 'Cook's Tour' of the affected areas, or to buy a series of *Illustrated Michelin Guides to the Battlefields (1914–1918)*, and visit the devastated zones for oneself.[22] Writers such as Enid Bagnold and Vera Brittain did spend time touring and recording their experiences.[23]

For Elsie Knocker, the war was an opportunity both to prove her own worth and – ultimately – to test some of her ideas about the treatment of trauma. Her efforts in establishing – with Mairi Chisholm – her advanced field dressing station on the Belgian Front won her acclaim and recognition as one of the 'Heroines of Pervyse'. The experience of other adventurous women was – ultimately – altogether bleaker. For Sarah Macnaughtan, her desire to serve on the Persian war front led to her own destruction.

At the outbreak of war, the British Empire was at the height of its powers, and the British people were – as a nation – at the height of their confidence. For a population accustomed to conquering the globe, the war may have presented itself as just another challenge. There had, it seemed, been many wars in the previous five decades: the Zulu War, the Egyptian Crisis, and the Boer Wars, to name a few. Yet, the British project of expanding not only its own empire but also 'the known world' itself, had often ended in misery and fail-ure. Ernest Shackleton had been acclaimed a hero following the failed Trans-Antarctic Expedition of 1914–17, when a dramatic escape from the doomed ship *Endurance* had made his name. Yet Antarctica was to claim his life when, despite suffering from heart failure, he insisted on returning to the continent in 1920, only to die of a myocardial infarction on board his ship *Quest*.[24] For Captain Robert Scott, his achievement in reaching the South Pole on 17 January 1912 was to turn to tragedy when he discovered that not only had he been beaten to his objective by Norwegian Roald Amundsen, but he had also left it too late in the season to be able to return to safety. He and his team died on the return journey.[25] And on 6 June 1924, two men, George Mallory and Sandy Irvine, set out from a camp on Mount Everest's North Col and were never seen again.[26] This tendency to test oneself beyond the limits of one's own powers, to attain heroic status while destroying one's own life – although not a peculiarly British trait – does seem to have been expressed most powerfully by the British dur-ing the early twentieth century. When Sarah Macnaughtan reached home in May 1916, she is said to have remarked to her maid: 'Russia has killed me.'[27] She might as soon have remarked 'The war has killed me'; her determination to be present wherever her experience of war could be at its most intense had led to her destruction. Her death illustrates the fact that women, as well as men, could value a patriotic cause beyond their own lives.

Heretical nurses

Not all nurse writers saw themselves in uncomplicated terms as part of a civilising force, siding with good against evil. Some wrote with the deliberate intention of destroying the false heroic myths of the First World War and revealing what they saw as its squalid and hor-rific truths.[28] Two of the most insistently pacifist writers of the Great War – Mabel St Clair Stobart and Ellen La Motte – were also two of the most highly educated women of their day. Stobart, a member of the British upper-middle class, was wealthy enough to fund her own unit – the Women's Sick and Wounded Convoy Corps – and to travel independently to Serbia. Ellen La Motte was a fully qualified profes-sional nurse; an alumna of the prestigious nurse training school at the Johns Hopkins Hospital in Baltimore, she was one of the most independent and radical American nurses of her day. Stobart and La Motte wrote in very different styles, yet they conveyed a similar message: modern warfare was not heroic; it was debasing and destructive to both the physical and moral fibres of its protagonists.

Millionaire philanthropist Mary Borden, who founded and directed a field hospital, 'L'Hôpital Chirurgical Mobile No. 1', published her *The Forbidden Zone* ten years after the armistice. She declared her writings to be the 'fragments of a great confusion',[29] and appears to have had no intention of presenting events in tidy chronological order, wishing, rather, to get close to a fragmentary and inchoate 'truth'.

These writers were 'heretics' because they pushed against the received wisdom of their own time. Most were volunteers rather than trained, professional nurses (with the obvious exception of La Motte); and all were women.[30] They came from a range of national and social class backgrounds.[31] And yet there are significant similarities among them. All chose to write in ways that were likely to cause shock or offence and all attacked their readership with a relentless insistence that one must not turn away from the realities of war, which are in actual fact disgusting, not heroic.

Some of their works met – not surprisingly – with negative responses in their own times. Enid Bagnold was summarily dismissed from her post as a volunteer nurse soon after the appearance of her *Diary without Dates*.[32] La Motte's *The Backwash of War* was suppressed by the censors in combatant nations soon after its publication.[33] Rebecca West's *War Nurse* met with perhaps the most interesting and mysterious fate. Disowned by its own author, it appeared for the first time as a complete piece in 1930 as an anonymous text.[34] It was only in the last three decades of the twentieth century that these memoirs came to be highly valued. Their rediscovery by women's historians and scholars of literary modernism has assured them a place in the modern 'canon' of the First World War.

The writings of 'heretics' such as Mabel St Clair Stobart and Ellen La Motte contrast with those of better-known authors such as Vera Brittain and Irene Rathbone, who chose to depict both the wounded soldier and the volunteer nurse in a heroic light. Although pacifist in intent and powerful in their effects, the latter refrain from exposing the reader to the more brutal and degrading elements of warfare, preferring to emphasise, in Brittain's case, its poignancy and, in Rathbone's, its drama and pathos.[35] Although, in many ways, the writings of women such as La Motte and Stobart were produced from very similar motives, their deliberate intention to disrupt and disturb the – perhaps rather complacent – beliefs of their readership sets them apart from the more traditionalist writings of their contemporaries.

'Heroism' was a contentious notion for nurse writers. Most of those who questioned the validity of war distrusted it as an ideological concept. Although individuals such as Kate Finzi and Stobart chose to recognise it in the way their patients endured pain and suffering, others – notably La Motte – refused to see it as anything other than a false ideology. This refusal is part of an uncompromising attitude to 'the truth', which pervades all of La Motte's writings – from the earliest part of her career, to her latest campaigns against the opium trade. In *The Tuberculosis Nurse*, when discussing the fact that nurses must inform patients of their diagnosis, she expresses what seems to be an article of faith: 'people are never really injured by being told the truth'.[36] In 'A Joy Ride' she compares soldiers in their hutted encampments to animals in sheds, passively awaiting slaughter, oblivious to the truth about their fate. She is struck by the helpless, driven horses on the Poperinghe-to-Ypres road, with rope over their eyes, protected from shrapnel, but unable to see. When she takes shelter with the Canadians in a 'flimsy hut' she too is protected from stray shrapnel, yet blinded by the darkness; and in that darkness nobody speaks of their fear.[37] Later, while travelling in the Far East, she develops the metaphor of the Buddha trapped under a wine glass, representing the man who has lost his spirit.[38] For La Motte only two things mattered: to see clearly and to write the truth.

Autonomy and agency

Few writers were as uncompromising as La Motte. Many found it difficult to see the conflict as something that had been created and prolonged by human beings. It was easier to regard it as a force of nature, which no-one could have prevented or curtailed. It was, perhaps, for this reason that metaphors of standing close to a great ocean and watching its waves bring in the shattered remnants of soldiers occur frequently. Margaret Deland had the feeling, in the early months of war, that 'in Europe the Peoples of all nations [were] rising – rising – rising on the crest of its awful Wave!'.[39] In a similar vein, Sarah Macnaughtan wrote: 'My own experience was much like that of persons who stand on the beach while others put out to sea, and at whose feet pieces of wreck and corpses are thrown up by the tide.'[40]

For Maud Mortimer, although the war may be a 'force of nature', its combatants are not merely passively waiting for destruction; their involvement requires an effort of will. For her, the field hospital seems like a sanctuary on the edge of a fierce ocean. Its reception hut catches 'the spindrift of [a] shattered endeavour'.[41] For Mary Borden, in her reception hut on the Somme Front, 'the dying men on the floor were drowned men cast up on the beach, and there was the ebb of life pouring away over them, sucking them away, an invisible tide'.[42] She and her 'old orderlies, like old sea-salts out of a lifeboat' worked to save lives.[43] Ellen La Motte saw a similar scene from a very different vantage point: L'Hôpital Chirurgical Mobile No. 1 lay in the 'backwash' of war, but into it seeped 'the slime in the shallows'.[44] For most of these nurses, the war was a force against which individual agency was powerless. And yet, all come across in their writings as active, not passive: exercising a limited autonomy. Sarah Macnaughtan – like Violetta Thurstan and Henrietta Tayler – travelled where she chose, endeavouring to save life where she thought she might be most needed. Borden used her wealth to create hospitals and took pride in their low mortality rates. Mabel St Clair Stobart established a mobile unit and placed herself at its head: 'The Lady of the Black Horse'. Her desire was, paradoxically, both to equal the martial prowess of men, and to expose the ultimate worthlessness of their military exploits. Ellen La Motte's desire was equally ambitious – to expose the realities of war. But her work was suppressed and she exercised her own freedom by leaving the continent that was being laid waste and travelling to another, where her campaigning zeal could have an effect.

In June 1917, a column in the *BJN* asserted that:

> never have our nurses been in such danger to life in any previous war, and their calmness and courage will for all time, we hope, disabuse men's minds of the fallacy that British women are devoid of our finest national qualities. Indeed, the women of every nation in every war zone have risen to the sublime heights of valour and daring ... deny them the vote if you dare![45]

It was not only as nurses that women were able to claim such rights. Yet it was as nurses that they pushed forward their claims most forcibly, because nursing gave them a role in warfare that was both acceptable as a feminine pursuit and advantageous as a heroic and intrepid one. Some were able to use nursing as a vehicle that would give them influence and a place in the world at a time when they would, otherwise, have been confined to the domestic scene on the 'home front'.[46] War represented an opportunity for women 'to escape domestic restrictions, to get "out of the cage"'.[47]

In discussing the cultural changes of the late nineteenth and early twentieth centuries, Sheila Rowbotham has commented that the women who worked to transform both their own lives and the world around them were 'dreamers and adventurers, for they explored with only the sketchiest of maps and they headed towards the unknown courageously'.[48] Nurse writers, more than any other women, moved into the unknown: not only did they enter the 'forbidden zone' of war; they also invented new ways of describing what they found there.

It has been argued that the First World War strengthened nursing through the winning of both female suffrage (in 1918) and a professional register for Britain (in 1919).[49] Their nursing work, and the experience it offered them, enabled women to take their places among the finest writers of the war – to become part of the literary canon of the twentieth century. It was one of the levers with which they thrust open the doors to civic and political participation, bringing them to prominence and giving them a place and a voice.

The truth about the war

To capture both the essence and the full reality of what they witnessed was the primary project of most nurse writers. Yet, the existence of both pro-war propaganda and fierce censorship often prevented the fulfilment of that project.[50] Women such as Millicent Sutherland, whose thinking was deeply influenced by the imperialist values of their time, could write of the heroism and adventure of war without experiencing conflict. Others wrote with difficulty of what they saw; their desire to capture accurately the courage and resilience of their patients was confounded by uncomfortable truths about the war's realities. Some, such as Alice Fitzgerald, entered war believing that they were fighting for a noble cause, and came out of it convinced that it had been a horrific waste. Only a few opposed both the patriarchal system and the propaganda of war from the start. Of all the writers discussed in this book, Ellen La Motte is the only one who did so with total confidence, writing incisively about the debasing qualities of warfare. What is most remarkable is the fact that she first published her *The Backwash of War* in 1916, more than ten years before the powerful witness statements of men such as Erich Maria Remarque, Henri Barbusse, and Robert Graves.

Vera Brittain wrote that 'the truth is so often one of the most difficult things to discover, let alone to impress upon others'.[51] Yet, in Rebecca West's view, truth was not what mattered. Only experience mattered, and Corinne Andrews' experience was that the war was, quite simply, incomprehensible: 'Ç'est comme la guerre. Il ne faut pas chercher à comprendre: It's like the war. You needn't try to understand it.'[52] Some nurses reflected on how naively and innocently they – like their male counterparts – had entered the most destructive conflict that had ever been fought. After her experiences in Belgium, Sarah Macnaughtan recollected the way she and other volunteer nurses had learned their bandaging skills on 'little messenger boys' with 'convenient fractures'. These pseudo-patients had never 'screamed and writhed or prayed for morphia when they were being bandaged'.[53]

Nurse writers chose to use their privileged position as part of the military medical machine to compose powerful witness statements about the nature of war. In using this opportunity, grasping it, and transforming it into something more than just a sentimental account of the suffering and bravery of the wounded, these women pushed at the boundaries of their existing social roles, and confounded society's expectations. Their work can be viewed as a statement about the power of women – and more particularly the power of nurses – to see with clarity and write with precision about subjects that had previously been exclusively within the domain of men. The fact that women could write the most vivid accounts of wounds, despair, and suffering – that they could, themselves, be endangered and sometimes damaged by war – was a statement about their right to act as participants in the political decision-making that might lead to war.[54]

Going much further than witness statements, these works depict the horror of the First World War: not just the gore and blood, but also the existential suffering. Nurse writers clearly wanted the world to share their insights. Some went so far as deliberately to expose propagandist myths. The fact that war was not noble – that it produced horrific outcomes – had come as an unexpected shock to many of them and created a sense of outrage that demanded an emotional outlet. And many appear also to have had a desire to express their sense of the self-transformation that their experiences had brought about. Their writings were about war; they were also about nursing; but, ultimately, they were about the self: as engaged participant, as observing witness, as suffering victim, as powerful and autonomous agent. The nurses of the First World War were the first female generation of the twentieth century: the generation whose experience was forged in the greatest man-made catastrophe of modern times. As such, they were also the generation whose insights would transform the lives not only of their daughters and granddaughters, but of their sons and grandsons too.

Notes

1   Edmund Blunden, *Undertones of War* (London: Penguin, 2010 [1928]): 46.
2   Paul Fussell, *The Great War and Modern Memory* (Oxford: Oxford University Press, 2000 [1975]). On soldiers' writings, see also: Frank Field, *British and French Writers of the First World War* (Cambridge: Cambridge University Press, 1991); Samuel Hynes, *A War Imagined: The First World War and English Culture* (London: Pimlico, 1992); Samuel Hynes, *The Soldier's Tale: Bearing Witness to a Modern War* (London: Penguin, 1998).
3   Sidonie Smith and Julia Watson have observed that life-writing is, in itself, a 'performative act': Sidonie Smith and Julia Watson, *Reading Autobiography: A Guide for Interpreting Life Narratives* (Minneapolis: University of Minnesota Press, 2010): 61. See also their Chapter 3: 63–102.
4   See, for example: Henry Rider Haggard, *King Solomon's Mines* (New York: Longmans, Green, 1901 [1885]); Henry Rider Haggard, *She* (London: Harper and Bros, 1886). G. A. Henty wrote over 100 adventure stories, with overall sales exceeding 25 million: Michelle Smith, 'Adventurous Girls of the British Empire: The Pre-War Novels of Bessie Marchant', *The Lion and the Unicorn*, 33.1 (2009): 1–25; Claire Tylee, *The Great War and Women's Consciousness: Images of Militarism and Womanhood in Women's Writings, 1914–64* (Houndmills and London: Macmillan, 1990): 33.
5   Smith, 'Adventurous Girls': 1–25.
6   Smith, 'Adventurous Girls': 3.

7 Millicent, Duchess of Sutherland, *Six Weeks at the War* (London: *The Times*, 1914): 37–8.

8 Anne Summers, *Angels and Citizens: British Women as Military Nurses, 1854–1914* (London: Routledge and Kegan Paul, 1988). On the social class backgrounds of military nurses, see 228; on VADs, see 237–70.

9 Smith and Watson, *Reading Autobiography*: 24.

10 On Julia Stimson's family background and the position of her father as a 'prominent New York clergyman', see: Kimberly Jensen, *Mobilizing Minerva: American Women in the First World War* (Urbana and Chicago: University of Illinois Press, 2008): 136.

11 On the censorship of writing during the First World War, see: Tylee, *The Great War and Women's Consciousness*: 53.

12 Kate Luard, *Unknown Warriors: Extracts from the Letters of K. E. Luard, R.R.C., Nursing Sister in France* (London: Chatto and Windus, 1930), preface by Field-Marshall Viscount Allenby: vii–ix.

13 Christine Hallett, *Containing Trauma: Nursing Work in the First World War* (Manchester: Manchester University Press, 2009): 209.

14 Alice Fitzgerald, 'Memoirs', MS987, Box 2, Maryland Historical Society Archives, Baltimore, Maryland; Alice Fitzgerald, unpublished memoirs incorporating war diary, c. 1936, Alice Fitzgerald Papers, Md HR M2633, Md HR M2634, Maryland Historical Society, Baltimore, Maryland.

15 Alice Howell Friedman, 'Fitzgerald, Alice Louise Florence', in Martin Kaufman (ed.), *Dictionary of American Nursing Biography* (New York: Greenwood Press, 1988): 123. Friedman points out that Fitzgerald had been awarded medals by the governments of Great Britain (Victory Medal), Italy, Poland, Serbia, Hungary, Russia, France (Campaign and Victory Medal, and Médaille d'honneur with rosette), and China. She had also been awarded the International Florence Nightingale Medal (122–3). Friedman omits to mention the Royal Red Cross, second class, which was also awarded by the British Government: Fitzgerald, unpublished memoirs, Chapter 10, unpaginated. Alice Fitzgerald's medals are now held by the Alan Mason Chesney Archives, Johns Hopkins Medical Institutions, Baltimore, Maryland.

16 Anne Marie Rafferty and Diana Solano have shown how these aspirations led nurses to join the Colonial Nursing Association in the early years of the century: Anne Marie Rafferty, 'The Seductions of History and the Nursing Diaspora', *Health and History: Journal of the Australian and New Zealand Society for the History of Medicine*, 7.2 (2005): 2–6; Anne Marie Rafferty and Diana Solano, 'The Rise and Demise of the Colonial Nursing Service: British Nurses in the Colonies, 1896–1966', *Nursing History Review*, 15 (2007): 147–54.

17 Violetta Thurstan, *A Text Book of War Nursing* (London: G. P. Putnam's Sons, 1917). Only two others are extant: Minnie Goodnow, *War Nursing*

(Philadelphia: W. B. Saunders, 1917); M. N. Oxford, *Nursing in War Time: Lessons for the Inexperienced* (London: Methuen, 1914).

18 Vera Brittain, *Testament of Youth: An Autobiographical Study of the Years 1900–1925* (London: Virago Press, 2004 [1933]): 329.

19 Fussell, *The Great War and Modern Memory*: 40.

20 Ellen N. La Motte, 'A Joy Ride', *The Atlantic Monthly*, 118 (October 1916): 481–90 (484).

21 Fussell, *The Great War and Modern Memory*: 131–3 (quote at 131).

22 Fussell, *The Great War and Modern Memory*: 69; Juliet Nicholson, *The Great Silence: 1918–1920. Living in the Shadow of the Great War* (London: John Murray, 2009): 122.

23 Enid Bagnold, *The Happy Foreigner* (London: Virago Press, 1987 [1920]); Brittain, *Testament of Youth*: 481–2. In Brittain's case, she was visiting her brother Edward's grave in Italy. On travel literature, see: Barbara Brothers and Julia Gergits, *British Travel Writers, 1910–1939* (Detroit: Gale, 1998); Angela Jones, 'Romantic Women Travel Writers and the Representation of Everyday Experience', *Women's Studies*, 26.5 (1997): 497–522; Daniel Kilbride, 'Travel Writing as Evidence with Special Attention to Nineteenth-Century Anglo-America', *History Compass*, 9.4 (2011): 339–50. On travel writing as part of an imperial project, see Arash Khazeni, 'Across the Black Sands, and the Red: Travel Writing, Nature and the Reclamation of the Eurasian Steppe circa 1850', *International Journal of Middle East Studies*, 42.4 (2010): 591–614.

24 Frank Hurley, *South with Endurance: Shackleton's Antarctic Expedition 1914–1917* (London: Bloomsbury, 2004); Hugh Robert Mill, *The Life of Sir Ernest Shackleton* (London: William Heinemann, 2006).

25 Edward Ratcliffe Garth Russell Evans, *South with Scott* (London: Collins, 1949); David Crane, *Scott of the Antarctic: A Life of Courage and Tragedy in the Extreme South* (London: HarperCollins, 2005).

26 Wade Davies, *Into the Silence: The Great War, Mallory, and the Conquest of Everest* (New York: Alfred A. Knopf, 2011): 537–54.

27 Sarah Macnaughtan, *My War Experiences in Two Continents*, ed. Mrs Lionel Salmon [Betty Keays-Young] (London: John Murray, 1919): 257.

28 On the creation of heroic myths of warfare, see: Michael Paris, *Warrior Nation: Images of War in British Popular Culture, 1850–2000* (London: Reaktion Books, 2000), *passim*; Graham Dawson, *Soldier Heroes: British Adventure, Empire and the Imagining of Masculinities* (London: Routledge, 1994), *passim*.

29 Mary Borden, *The Forbidden Zone* (London: William Heinemann, 1929): preface.

30 On the significance of the gendered nature of nursing during the war, see: Miriam Cooke and Angela Woollacott (eds), *Gendering War Talk* (Princeton, NJ: Princeton University Press, 1993); Helen M. Cooper, Adrienne Auslander Munich, and Susan Merrill Squier (eds), *Arms and the Woman: War, Gender and Literary Representation* (Chapel Hill: University of

North Carolina Press, 1989). On nursing and gender, see: Eva Gamarnikow, 'Nurse or Woman: Gender and Professionalism in Reformed Nursing, 1860–1923', in Pat Holden and Jenny Littlewood (eds), *Anthropology and Nursing* (London: Routledge, 1991): 110–29.

31 Although it should be noted that all were, in some sense, 'middle class', individuals such as Borden, Bagnold, and Stobart were undoubtedly much wealthier than La Motte and West. Most of the writers considered in this section were British, though a few – notably La Motte and Borden – were American. Rebecca West was a British writer, who ghost-wrote the diary of an American nurse.

32 Enid Bagnold, *Enid Bagnold's Autobiography (from 1889)*, introduction by Barbara Willard (London: Century Publishing, 1985 [1969]): 129.

33 Margaret Higonnet, *Nurses at the Front: Writing the Wounds of the Great War* (Boston, MA: Northeastern University Press, 2001), introduction: xiv; Angela Smith, *Women's Writings of the First World War: An Anthology* (Manchester: Manchester University Press, 2000): 330.

34 Victoria Glendinning, *Rebecca West: A Life* (London: Macmillan, 1988 [1987]): 108.

35 Brittain, *Testament of Youth, passim*; Irene Rathbone, *We That Were Young: A Novel* (New York: The Feminist Press, 1989): *passim*.

36 Ellen N. La Motte, *The Tuberculosis Nurse: Her Function and Her Qualifications. A Handbook for Practical Workers in the Tuberculosis Campaign. By Ellen N. La Motte, R.N., Graduate of Johns Hopkins Hospital; Former Nurse-in-Chief of the Tuberculosis Division, Health Department of Baltimore*, introduction by Louis Hamman, M.D., Physician in Charge, Phipps Tuberculosis Dispensary, Johns Hopkins University (New York and London: G. P. Putnam's Sons and The Knickerbocker Press, 1915): 125.

37 La Motte, 'A Joy Ride'.

38 Ellen N. La Motte, 'Under a Wine Glass', *The Century Magazine* (December 1918): 150–4.

39 Margaret Deland, *Small Things* (New York: D. Appleton, 1919): 57.

40 Sarah Macnaughtan, *A Woman's Diary of the War* (London: Thomas Nelson and Sons, 1915): 158–9.

41 Maud Mortimer, *A Green Tent in Flanders* (New York: Doubleday, Page, 1918): 198.

42 Borden, *The Forbidden Zone*: 143–4.

43 Borden, *The Forbidden Zone*: 144.

44 Ellen N. La Motte, *The Backwash of War: The Human Wreckage of the Battlefield as Witnessed by an American Hospital Nurse* (1916): vi.

45 Anon., 'French Flag Nursing Corps', *BJN* (30 June 1917): 452. See also: Christine E. Hallett, *Veiled Warriors: Allied Nurses of the First World War* (Oxford: Oxford University Press, 2014): Conclusion.

46 On the significance of women's participation in the war through the VAD movement, see: Sharon Ouditt, *Fighting Forces, Writing Women: Identity and Ideology in the First World War* (London: Routledge, 1994): 7–46; Summers, *Angels and Citizens*.

47 Tylee, *The Great War and Women's Consciousness*: 243. Tylee is drawing upon the work of Gail Braybon and Penny Summerfield, *Out of the Cage: Women's Experiences in Two World Wars* (London: Routledge, 2012 [1987]).

48 Sheila Rowbotham, *Dreamers of a New Day: Women who Invented the Twentieth Century* (London: Verso, 2010): 3.

49 Susan McGann, *The Battle of the Nurses: A Study of Eight Women who Influenced the Development of Professional Nursing, 1880–1930* (London: Scutari Press, 1992); Hallett, *Veiled Warriors*: Conclusion.

50 On censorship, see: Tylee, *The Great War and Women's Consciousness*: 53. On propaganda, see: Trudi Tate, *Modernism, History and the First World War* (Manchester: Manchester University Press, 1998): 41–62.

51 Paul Berry and Mark Bostridge, *Vera Brittain: A Life* (London: Virago Press, 2001): frontispiece.

52 Rebecca West, *War Nurse: The True Story of a Woman who Lived, Loved and Suffered on the Western Front* (New York: Cosmopolitan Book Corporation, 1930): 71–2.

53 Macnaughtan, *A Woman's Diary of the War*: 22–3.

54 On the risks taken by nurses, see: Hallett, *Containing Trauma*: 194–223; Hallett, *Veiled Warriors*: *passim*.

Bibliography

Primary sources

Archives consulted

The Alan Mason Chesney Medical Archives of the Johns Hopkins Medical Institutions, Baltimore, Maryland, USA

Alice Fitzgerald, handwritten diary
Alice Fitzgerald, medals
Ellen La Motte, biographical file

Archives of the Hypatia Trust at the Jamieson Library, Penzance, Cornwall, UK

Copies of Violetta Thurstan's diaries (originals held at Magdalene College, Cambridge)
Letters and papers of Violetta Thurstan, including unpublished manuscripts of unfinished novels: *The Lucky Mary*; *The Demon*; *The Three Miss Trotts of Polperi*; *Moussa, The Snake Charmer*; *Lunch with the Sheikh*

Archive of the Nursing and Midwifery Council, London, UK

Register for Nurses, 1923, General Part: entries for Kate Evelyn Luard and Anna Violet Thurstan

The Archives of Saint John, New Brunswick, Canada

File on Agnes Warner
Holdings of local Saint John Newspapers
  Saint John Globe
  Daily Telegraph
  Saint John Standard
  Telegraph Journal

Archives of the Royal London Hospital, Aldgate, London, UK

Register of Probationers, no. 7, entry for Anna Violet Thurstan
Register of Probationers, no. 8, entry for Anna Violet Thurstan
Ward reports: report by the sister on 'Mellish Ward' for the week ending
    1 February 1902

Army Medical Services Museum Archives, Aldershot, UK

Dame Sidney Browne Papers, Queen Alexandra's Royal Army Nursing Corps
    (QARANC) Collection, Box I

The Churchill Archives, Churchill College, Cambridge, UK

Letters, January 1917–February 1918, SPRS files 1–3: Mary Borden, letter to
    Edward Spears, SPRS 11/1/1

*Claude Moore Health Sciences Library, University of Virginia,
Charlottesville, USA*

Anon., *The University of Virginia Base Hospital Forty-One* (unpublished account,
    1925), box-folder 001-001, Historical Collection

Essex Record Office, Colchester, UK

Luard family papers, files 55/13/1–4

Imperial War Museum, London, UK

Miss Bickmore, MS essay, 3814, 85/51/1
Mrs I. Edgar (née Layng), letters and diary, P211
Florence Farmborough, diaries, private papers, 1381
Florence Farmborough: oral history interview conducted by Margaret A. Brooks,
    1975, 17 reels
Miss Elizabeth Agnes Greg, letters, 01/17/1
H. M. Harpin, MS letters, 3051 Con Shelf
Lady Leila Paget, *With Our Serbian Allies* (printed for private circulation,
    1916), 34602
Dorothy Potts, MS letters, 3246 Con Shelf
D. M. Richards, *Blues and Reds*, memoir, P328
Baroness de T'Serclaes, MS diary, 9029-2

Liddle Collection, Brotherton Library, University of Leeds, UK

Florence Farmborough: oral history interview conducted by Peter Liddle at
    Abbeyfield House, The Mount, Heswall, 1975

Maryland Historical Society Archives, Baltimore, Maryland, USA

Alice Fitzgerald, 'Memoirs', MS987, Box 2
Alice Fitzgerald, unpublished memoirs incorporating war diary, *c.* 1936, Alice
   Fitzgerald Papers, Md HR M2633, Md HR M2634

Monks House Papers, Library of the University of Sussex, Brighton, UK

Enid Jones, letter to Virginia Woolf (née Stephen), typescript copy, 1933, SxMs 18

The National Archives, Kew, London, UK

Kate Luard War Office file, WO 399/5023
Kate Luard, Record of service in South Africa: register no. 4862/Reserve/3387

Red Cross Archive, London

Anon., *Twenty Months a VAD* (Sheffield: J. Northen, n.d), 96/317
Joyce M. Sapwell, 'The Reminiscences of a VAD', T2SAP
Mary Schiff, papers and letters, 1788/1

The Royal College of Nursing Archives, Edinburgh, UK

Holdings of *BJN* (also available online at www.rcn.org.uk/development/library_
   and_heritage_services/library_collections/rcn_archive/historical_nursing_
   journals)

Articles and columns published anonymously in the *British Journal of Nursing*

Account of a meeting of the Matrons' Council, *BJN* (8 February 1913): 106
'Appointments', *BJN* (8 February 1913): 108–9
'Nurses of Note: Miss Violetta Thurstan', *BJN* (15 February 1913): 130
Column, *BJN* (15 February 1913): 130
Column, *BJN* (12 April 1913): 288
'The Dublin Nursing Conference and Exhibition', *BJN* (26 April 1913): 329
'The Spezia Hospital', *BJN* (10 May 1913): 367
'Nursing Echoes', *BJN* (31 January 1914): 89
'Coming Events', *BJN* (9 May 1914): 424
'League News', *BJN* (27 June 1914): 584
'Is It Just?', in 'Letters to the Editor', *BJN* (4 July 1914): 22
'Active Service', *BJN* (22 August 1914): 158
Column, *BJN* (19 September 1914): 224
'The American Ambulance in Paris', *BJN* (10 October 1914): 281
'Letters from the Front: From France', *BJN* (17 October 1914): 306–7
Column, *BJN* (24 October 1914): 324

Bibliography

'Book of the Week: *The Diary of a French Army Chaplain*', *BJN* (30 October 1914): 369
'Letters to the Editor' *BJN* (19 December 1914): 497
Column, *BJN* (13 February 1915): 130–3
Column, *BJN* (20 February 1915): 146
M.B., [probably Margaret Breay], ' "With a Flying Column of the Russian Red Cross": Miss Violetta Thurstan', *BJN* (13 March 1915): 207–10
'The National Council of Trained Nurses', *BJN* (13 March 1915): 210
'National Union of Trained Nurses', *BJN* (3 April 1915)
'Coming Events', *BJN* (17 April 1915): 330
'Book of the Week', *BJN* (24 April 1915): 352
Column, *BJN* (1 May 1915): 371, 377
Column, *BJN* (8 May 1915): 385
Column, *BJN* (5 June 1915): 489
Column, *BJN* (19 June 1915): 526
Column, *BJN* (26 June 1915): 550
Column, *BJN* (24 July 1915): 78
Column, *BJN* (7 August 1915): 118–19
Column, *BJN* (6 October 1915): 317
Column, *BJN* (23 October 1915): 340
Column, *BJN* (6 November 1915): 385
Column, *BJN* (27 November 1915): 445
Column, *BJN* (11 December 1915): 481
Column, *BJN* (8 January 1916): 29
Column, *BJN* (5 February 1916): 115–16
'An Edith Cavell Memorial Nurse', *BJN* (4 March 1916): 214
Column, *BJN* (4 March 1916): 214
Column, *BJN* (11 March 1916): 224
Column, *BJN* (18 March 1916): 243
Review of Violetta Thurstan, *The People who Run*, *BJN* (8 April 1916): 327–8
'French Flag Nursing Corps', *BJN* (29 April 1916): 378
'A School for Mothers in Petrograd', *BJN* (6 May 1916): 411
'French Flag Nursing Corps', *BJN* (27 May 1916): 458
'Refugees in Russia', *BJN* (27 May 1916): 462
'National Union of Trained Nurses', *BJN* (17 June 1916): 525
Review of Violetta Thurstan, *The People who Run*, *BJN* (1 July 1916): 13
'The Horrors of Deportation', *BJN* (12 August 1916): 134
'Hôpital Mobile No. 1', *BJN* (16 September 1916): 232–3
'Nursing and the War', *BJN* (30 September 1916): 269
'National Union of Trained Nurses', *BJN* (14 October 1916): 315
'National Union of Trained Nurses' *BJN* (21 October 1916): 335
'National Union of Trained Nurses', *BJN* (28 October 1916): 355
Column, *BJN* (4 November 1916): 377

Column, *BJN* (11 November 1916): 387

Column, *BJN* (9 December 1916): 477

Review of Sister Martin-Nicholson, *My Experiences on Three Fronts*, *BJN* (30 December 1916): 527

Column, *BJN* (20 January 1917): 41

'Nursing at La Panne', *BJN* (10 March 1917): 169

'Care of the Wounded', *BJN* (14 April 1917): 253

Column, *BJN* (14 April 1917): 254

'French Flag Nursing Corps', *BJN* (14 April 1917): 254

'French Flag Nursing Corps', *BJN* (26 May 1917): 361, 362

Column, *BJN* (16 June 1917): 415

'Croix de Guerre for Sister Jaffray', *BJN* (16 June 1917): 416

'French Flag Nursing Corps', *BJN* (23 June 1917): 434

'Decorations for Nurses', *BJN* (30 June 1917): 452

'French Flag Nursing Corps', *BJN* (30 June 1917): 452

Column, *BJN* (14 July 1917): 21

Column, *BJN* (15 September 1917): 165

Column, *BJN* (22 September 1917): 181

Review of Violetta Thurstan, *A Text Book of War Nursing*, *BJN* (13 October 1917): 244

'Nursing and the War', *BJN* (24 November 1917): 332

'Medal for a Nurse', *BJN* (1 December 1917): 351

Column, *BJN* (19 January 1918): 47

'French Flag Nursing Corps', *BJN* (16 February 1918): 113

'French Flag Nursing Corps', *BJN* (3 August 1918): 80–1

Column, *BJN* (6 April 1918): 241

'Nursing and the War', *BJN* (7 September 1918): 151

'French Flag Nursing Corps', *BJN* (19 October 1918): 234

'French Flag Nursing Corps: En Avant', *BJN* (14 December 1918): 363

'French Flag Nursing Corps', *BJN* (4 January 1919): 6–7

'Praise for Unit 16/21', *BJN* (1 February 1919): 66

'National Union of Trained Nurses', *BJN* (31 July 1920)

'Our Fellows: What Are They Doing?', *BJN* (November 1927): 266

'What Our Fellows Are Doing', *BJN* (April 1928): 85

'Weaving Exhibition', *BJN* (July 1929): 179

'Miss Violetta Thurstan on Active Service in Spain', *BJN* (March 1937): 79

Books and journal articles published between 1890 and 1946

Aldington, Richard, *Death of a Hero* (London: Hogarth, 1984 [1929])

Aldridge, Olive M., *The Retreat from Serbia through Montenegro and Albania* (London: Minerva, 1916)

Bibliography

Anon., Announcement, *Saint John Globe* (2 May 1894)

Anon., Notation, *New York Presbyterian Hospital Alumni Quarterly*, 1 (July 1906)

Anon., 'The Nursing Outlook: War Fever and War Spirit', *The Nursing Mirror and Midwives Journal*, 19 (22 August 1914): 397

Anon., 'Red Cross Nurse from Front on Visit Here Tells of War's Horrors', *Daily Telegraph* (26 December 1914): 12

Anon., Society Page, *Daily Telegraph* (26 December 1914): 6

Anon., *Diary of a Nursing Sister on the Western Front 1914–1915* (Edinburgh and London: William Blackwood and Sons, 1915)

Anon., 'Miss Warner on Her Way Back to the Front', *Daily Telegraph* (14 January 1915): 10

Anon., Society Page note, *Daily Telegraph* (16 January 1915): 10

Anon., Society Page, *Daily Telegraph* (16 January 1915): 10

Anon., Article, *Daily Telegraph* (19 January 1915)

Anon. [K. K. and M. E. H.], 'Experiences in the American Ambulance Hospital, Neuilly, France', *American Journal of Nursing*, 15.7 (April 1915): 549–54

Anon., *Mademoiselle Miss* (Liskeard: Diggory Press, 2006 [1916])

Anon., Supplement to the *London Gazette* (1 January 1916): 69

Anon., Article, *Saint John Globe* (12 July 1916): 3

Anon., Society Page note, *Daily Telegraph* (7 October 1916): 12

Anon., Article, *Daily Telegraph* (23 December 1916): 9

Anon., *My Beloved Poilus* (Saint John, NB: Barnes, 1917)

Anon. (ed.), *The Edith Cavell Nurse from Massachusetts: A Record of One Year's Personal Service with the British Expeditionary Force in France; Boulogne–the Somme, 1916–1917. With an Account of the Imprisonment, Trial and Death of Edith Cavell* (Boston, MA: W. A. Butterfield, 1917)

Anon., Society Page article about *My Beloved Poilus*, *Daily Telegraph* (24 February 1917): 9

Anon., 'General Warner', *Saint John Globe* (27 February 1917): 4

Anon., 'General D. B. Warner, War Veteran', *Saint John Globe* (27 February 1917): 10

Anon., obituary for General Darius B. Warner, *Daily Telegraph* (28 February 1917): 7

Anon., Society Page note, *Daily Telegraph* (10 March 1917): 12

Anon., 'First Nursing Unit over Hindenburg Line', *Saint John Globe* (7 December 1918): 5

Anon., *A War Nurse's Diary: Sketches from a Belgian Field Hospital* (New York: Macmillan, 1918)

Anon., 'Miss Warner Gets Croix de Guerre', *Saint John Globe* (11 January 1919): 12

Anon., Note, *Daily Telegraph* (6 February 1919): 7

Anon., Column, *Daily Telegraph* (1 March 1919): 2

Anon., 'Miss Agnes Warner Is Expected Soon', *Daily Telegraph* (3 March 1919): 4

Anon., 'Spent Five Years of Nursing among the French Soldiers', *Saint John Standard* (31 March 1919): 3

Anon., 'Nursing Sister Agnes Warner Was Entertained', *Saint John Standard* (5 April 1919)

Anon., 'Nursing Sister Agnes Warner Highly Honoured', *Daily Telegraph* (5 April 1919): 5

Anon., 'Returned Nursing Sister Entertained at Luncheon', *Saint John Standard* (8 April 1919)

Anon., 'Miss Warner Speaks at Reception', *Daily Telegraph* (8 April 1919): 7

Anon., 'Miss Warner Gave Splendid Lecture', *Saint John Standard* (11 April 1919)

Anon., 'War's Lessons Should Not Soon Be Forgotten: Miss Warner Tells New Phases of Her Work in France', *Daily Telegraph* (11 April 1919): 3

Anon., Society Page, *Daily Telegraph* (12 April 1919): 12

Anon., Column, *Daily Telegraph* (25 April 1919): 3

Anon., *History of the Pennsylvania Hospital Unit (Base Hospital No. 10, USA) in the Great War* (New York: Paul B. Hoeber, 1921)

Anon. (ed.), *Reminiscent Sketches, 1914–1919 by Members of Her Majesty Queen Alexandra's Imperial Military Nursing Service* (London: John Bale, Sons, and Danielsson, 1922)

Anon., *Serena Blandish; or, The Difficulty of Getting Married: By a Lady of Quality* (London: Heinemann, 1924)

Anon., 'Death Notice', *Saint John Globe* (23 April 1926): 10

Anon., 'Agnes Warner Death Notice and Obituary', *Telegraph Journal* (24 April 1926)

Anon., 'Obituary', *Saint John Globe* (26 April 1926): 3

Bagnold, Enid, *A Diary without Dates* (London: Virago, 1978 [1918])

Bagnold, Enid, *The Happy Foreigner* (London: Virago Press, 1987 [1920])

Bagnold, Enid, *Alice, Thomas and Jane* (London: William Heinemann, 1930)

Bagnold, Enid, *National Velvet* (London: William Heinemann, 1935)

Bagnold, Enid, *The Squire* (London: William Heinemann, 1938)

Bagnold, Enid, *Lottie Dundass* (London: William Heinemann, 1941)

Bagnold, Enid, *The Loved and Envied* (London: William Heinemann, 1951)

Bagnold, Enid, *The Chalk Garden* (London: William Heinemann, 1956)

Bagnold, Enid, *Enid Bagnold's Autobiography (from 1889)*, introduction by Barbara Willard (London: Century Publishing, 1985 [1969])

Barbusse, Henri, *Under Fire* (London: Penguin Classics, 2003 [1917])

Binyon, Laurence, *For Dauntless France: An Account of Britain's Aid to the French Wounded and Victims of the War. Compiled for the British Red Cross Societies and the British Committee of the Red Cross* (London: Hodder and Stoughton, 1918)

Blunden, Edmund, *Undertones of War* (London: Penguin, 2010 [1928])

Borden, Mary, *The Romantic Woman: By Bridget Maclagan – Mary Borden Turner* (London: Constable, 1924 [1916])

Borden, Mary, *Jane – Our Stranger: A Novel* (London: William Heinemann, 1923)

Borden, Mary, *Jericho Sands: A Novel* (London: William Heinemann, 1925)

Borden, Mary, *Four O'Clock and Other Stories* (London: William Heinemann, 1926)

Borden, Mary, *Flamingo; or, The American Tower* (London: William Heinemann, 1927)

Borden, Mary, *Jehovah's Day* (London: William Heinemann, 1928)

Borden, Mary, *The Forbidden Zone* (London: William Heinemann, 1929)

Borden, Mary, *The Forbidden Zone*, ed. Hazel Hutchison (London: Hesperus Press, 2008 [1929])

Borden, Mary, *The Woman with White Eyes* (London: William Heinemann, 1930)

Borden, Mary, *Sarah Gay* (London: William Heinemann, 1931)

Borden, Mary, *The Technique of Marriage* (London: William Heinemann, 1933)

Borden, Mary, *Mary of Nazareth* (London: William Heinemann, 1933)

Borden, Mary, *The King of the Jews* (London: William Heinemann, 1935)

Borden, Mary, *Action for Slander: A Novel* (London: William Heinemann, 1936)

Borden, Mary, *The Black Virgin: A Novel* (London: William Heinemann, 1937)

Borden, Mary, *Passport for a Girl* (London: William Heinemann, 1939)

Borden, Mary, *Journey down a Blind Alley* (London: Hutchinson, 1947 [1946])

Borden, Mary, *No. 2 Shovel Street: A Novel* (London: William Heinemann, 1949)

Borden, Mary, *For the Record* (London: William Heinemann, 1950)

Borden, Mary, *Martin Merriedew* (London: William Heinemann, 1952)

Borden, Mary, *Margin of Error* (London: William Heinemann, 1954)

Borden, Mary, *The Hungry Leopard* (London: William Heinemann, 1956)

Borden-Turner, Mary, 'At the Somme', *The English Review* (August 1917): 97–102

Bowser, Thelka, *The Story of British VAD Work in the Great War* (London: Imperial War Museum, 2003 [1917])

Boylston, Helen Dore, 'Sister': *The War Diary of a Nurse* (New York: Ives Washburn, 1927)

Boylston, Helen Dore, *Clara Barton: Founder of the American Red Cross* (New York: Random House, 1955)

Britnieva, Mary, *One Woman's Story* (London: Arthur Baker, 1934)

Brittain, Vera, *The Dark Tide* (New York: Macmillan, 1936 [1923])

Brittain, Vera, *Testament of Youth* (Glasgow: Collins and Sons, 1980 [1933])

Brittain, Vera, *Testament of Youth: An Autobiographical Study of the Years 1900–1925* (London: Virago Press, 2004 [1933])

Brittain, Vera, *Honourable Estate: A Novel of Transition* (New York: Macmillan, 1936)

Cator, Dorothy, *In a French Military Hospital* (New York: Longmans, Green, 1915)

Davies, Ellen Chivers, *A Farmer in Serbia* (London: Methuen, n.d.)

Deland, Margaret, *Small Things* (New York: D. Appleton, 1919)

Dent, Olive, *A VAD in France* (London: Grant Richards, 1917)

Dock, Lavinia L., column published in the *American Journal of Nursing*, quoted verbatim in *BJN* (7 August 1915): 119

Dock, Lavinia L, Sarah E. Pickett, Clara D. Noyes, Fannie F. Clement, Elizabeth
G. Fox, and Anna R. Van Meter, *History of American Red Cross Nursing*
(New York: Macmillan, 1922)

Ellison, Grace, 'Nursing at the French Front', in Gilbert Stone (ed.), *Women War
Workers: Accounts Contributed by Representative Workers of the Work Done by
Women in the More Important Branches of War Employment* (London: George
G. Harrap, 1917): 155–80

Finzi, Kate, *Eighteen Months in the War Zone: The Record of One Woman's Work
on the Western Front* (London: Cassell, 1916)

Gleason, Arthur and Helen Hayes Gleason, *Golden Lads: A Thrilling Account of
How the Invading War Machine Crushed Belgium* (New York: A. L. Burt, 1916)

Goldman, Emma, *Living My Life* (New York: Alfred A. Knopf, 1931), available at
http://theanarchistlibrary.org/library/Emma_Goldman_Living_My_Life.html
(accessed 14 December 2012)

Goodnow, Minnie, *War Nursing* (Philadelphia: W. B. Saunders, 1917)

Goodnow, Minnie, *Outlines of Nursing History* (Philadelphia: W. B. Saunders, 1923)

Graves, Robert, *Goodbye to All That* (London: Jonathan Cape, 1929)

Gilman, Charlotte Perkins, *Herland* (New York: Pantheon, 1979 [1915])

Haggard, Henry Rider, *King Solomon's Mines* (New York: Longmans, Green, 1901
[1885])

Haggard, Henry Rider, *She* (London: Harper and Bros, 1886)

Hemingway, Ernest, *A Farewell to Arms* (London: Arrow, 1994 [1929])

Inglis, Elsie, 'The Tragedy of Serbia', *The Englishwoman*, 30 (1916): 166

La Motte, Ellen N., *The Tuberculosis Nurse: Her Function and Her Qualifications.
A Handbook for Practical Workers in the Tuberculosis Campaign. By Ellen N. La
Motte, R.N., Graduate of Johns Hopkins Hospital; Former Nurse-in-Chief of the
Tuberculosis Division, Health Department of Baltimore*, introduction by Louis
Hamman, M.D., Physician in Charge, Phipps Tuberculosis Dispensary, Johns
Hopkins University (New York and London: G. P. Putnam's Sons and The
Knickerbocker Press, 1915)

La Motte, Ellen N., 'An American Nurse in Paris', *The Survey*, 34 (10 July
1915): 333–36

La Motte, Ellen N., 'Under Shell-Fire at Dunkirk', *The Atlantic Monthly*, 116
(November 1915): 692–700

La Motte, Ellen N., 'Heroes', *The Atlantic Monthly*, 118 (August 1916): 208–10

La Motte, Ellen N., 'A Joy Ride', *The Atlantic Monthly*, 118 (October 1916): 481–90

La Motte, Ellen N., *The Backwash of War: The Human Wreckage of the Battlefield
as Witnessed by an American Hospital Nurse* (New York: G. P. Putnam's Sons
and The Knickerbocker Press, 1916)

La Motte, Ellen, N., 'Under a Wine Glass', *The Century Magazine* (December
1918): 150–4

La Motte, Ellen N., *Civilization: Tales of the Orient* (New York: Books for Libraries
Press, 1919)

La Motte, Ellen N., *Peking Dust* (New York: Century, 1919)

La Motte Ellen N., *The Opium Monopoly* (New York: Macmillan, 1920)

La Motte, Ellen N., *The Ethics of Opium* (New York: Century, 1924)

La Motte, Ellen N., *'Snuffs and Butters' and Other Stories* (New York: Century, 1925)

La Motte, Ellen N., *Opium at Geneva; or, How the Opium Problem Is Handled by the League of Nations* (New York: The Nation, 1929)

La Motte, Ellen N., 'A Desert Owl', *The Atlantic Monthly* (January 1927): 81–6

La Motte, Ellen N., 'The Three Widows: The True Story of an International Crisis', *Harper's Magazine* (March 1931): 428–35

La Motte, Ellen N., *The Backwash of War: The Human Wreckage of the Battlefield as Witnessed by an American Hospital Nurse* (New York: G. P. Putnam's Sons, 1934)

Luard, Kate, *Unknown Warriors: Extracts from the Letters of K. E. Luard, R.R.C., Nursing Sister in France* (London: Chatto and Windus, 1930)

Maclagan, Bridget, *Collision* (London: Duckworth, 1913)

Maclagan, Bridget, *The Mistress of Kingdoms; or, Smoking Flax: A Novel* (London: Duckworth, 1912)

Maclagan, Bridget, *The Romantic Woman* (New York: Alfred A. Knopf, 1920)

Maclean, Hester, *Nursing in New Zealand: History and Reminiscences* (Wellington, NZ: Tolan, 1932)

Macnaughtan, Sarah, *My War Experiences in Two Continents*, ed. Mrs Lionel Salmon [Betty Keays-Young] (London: John Murray, 1919)

Macnaughtan, Sarah, *A Woman's Diary of the War* (London: Thomas Nelson and Sons, 1915)

Marshall, Catherine, *Militarism versus Feminism* (London: Virago, 1987 [1915])

Martin-Nicholson, Sister, *My Experiences on Three Fronts* (London: George Allen and Unwin, 1916)

Millard, Shirley, *I Saw Them Die: Diary and Recollections of Shirley Millard*, ed. Adele Comandini (London: George G. Harrap, 1936)

Millicent, Duchess of Sutherland, *Six Weeks at the War* (London: The Times, 1914)

Mitton, G. E. (ed.), *The Cellar-House of Pervyse: A Tale of Uncommon Things from the Journals and Letters of the Baroness de T'Serclaes and Mairi Chisholm* (London: A. and E. Black, 1916)

Mortimer, Maud, *A Green Tent in Flanders* (New York: Doubleday, Page, 1918)

Nutting, M. Adelaide and Lavinia L. Dock, *A History of Nursing: The Evolution of Nursing Systems from the Earliest Times to the Foundation of the First English and American Training Schools for Nurses*, 4 vols (New York and London: G. P. Putnam's Sons, 1907–12)

Oxford, M. N., *Nursing in War Time: Lessons for the Inexperienced* (London: Methuen, 1914)

Paget, Lady Leila, *With Our Serbian Allies* (printed for private circulation, 1916), 34602, Imperial War Museum, London

Pankhurst, E. Sylvia, *The Home Front* (London: Hutchinson, 1987 [1932])

Rathbone, Irene, *We That Were Young: A Novel* (New York: The Feminist Press, 1989 [1932])

Remarque, Erich Maria, *All Quiet on the Western Front*, trans. Brian Murdoch (London: Random House, 1996 [1929])

Sandes, Flora, *The Autobiography of a Woman Soldier: A Brief Record of Adventure with the Serbian Army, 1916–1919* (New York: Frederick A. Stokes, n.d.)

Sandes, Flora, *An English Woman-Sergeant in the Serbian Army* (London: Hodder and Stoughton, 1916)

Sassoon, Siegfried, *Memoirs of a Fox-Hunting Man* (London: Faber and Gwyer, 1928)

Sassoon, Siegfried, *Memoirs of an Infantry Officer* (London: Faber and Faber, 1930)

Sassoon, Siegfried, *Sherston's Progress* (London: Faber and Faber, 1936)

Smith, Lesley, *Four Years out of Life* (London: Philip Allan, 1931)

Stein, Gertrude, *The Autobiography of Alice B. Toklas* (London: Penguin, 2001 [1933])

Stimson, Julia, *Finding Themselves: The Letters of an American Army Chief Nurse at a British Hospital in France* (New York: Macmillan, 1927)

Stobart, Mabel St Clair, *The Flaming Sword in Serbia and Elsewhere* (London: Hodder and Stoughton, 1916)

Tayler, Henrietta, *A Scottish Nurse at War: Being a Record of What One Semi-Trained Nurse Has Been Privileged to See and Do during Four and a Half Years of War* (London: John Lane, 1920)

Thurstan, Violetta, 'The British Red Cross Society', *BJN* (24 January 1914): 65–6

Thurstan, Violetta, 'Letters from the Front', *BJN* (26 September 1914): 246–7

Thurstan, Violetta, 'From Brussels', *BJN* (10 October 1914): 286–7

Thurstan, Violetta 'An International Welcome', *BJN* (24 October 24 1914): 322

Thurstan, Violetta, *Field Hospital and Flying Column: Being the Journal of an English Nursing Sister in Belgium and Russia* (London: G. P. Putnam's Sons, 1915)

Thurstan, Violetta, 'From Warsaw', *BJN* (9 January 1915)

Thurstan, Violetta, *The People who Run: Being the Tragedy of the Refugees in Russia* (London: G. P. Putnam's Sons, 1916)

Thurstan, Violetta, 'ABC of State Registration', *BJN* (6 May 1916): 404

Thurstan, Violetta, 'Russian Red Cross Sisters', *BJN*, (27 January 1917): 62

Thurstan, Violetta, *A Text Book of War Nursing* (London: G. P. Putnam's Sons, 1917)

Thurstan, Violetta 'A Three Weeks' Journey in the Libyan Desert', *BJN* (February 1925): 42

Thurstan, Violetta 'Art and Medicine', *BJN* (November 1927): 272

Thurstan, Violetta, 'Old English Handicrafts', *BJN* (April 1928): 101

Thurstan, Violetta, *The Use of Vegetable Dyes for Beginners* (London: Dryad Press, 1930)

Thurstan, Violetta, *A Short History of Decorative Textiles and Tapestries* (Exeter: Papler and Sewell, 1934)

Thurstan, Violetta, *Stormy Petrel* (Falmouth: Violetta Thurstan, 1964)

Thurstan, Violetta, *The Foolish Virgin* (Marazion: Wordens of Cornwall, 1966)

Thurstan, Violetta, *The Hounds of War Unleashed* (St Ives, Cornwall: United Writers Publications, 1978)

Thurstan, Violetta, *Weaving Patterns of Yesterday and Today* (London: Dryad Press, n.d.)

Thurstan, Violetta, *Weaving without Tears* (London: Museum Press, n.d.)

Tilton, May, *The Grey Battalion* (Sydney: Angus and Robertson, 1933)

West, Rebecca, *The Return of The Soldier* (London: Virago, 1980 [1918])

West, Rebecca, *War Nurse: The True Story of a Woman who Lived, Loved and Suffered on the Western Front* (New York: Cosmopolitan Book Corporation, 1930)

West, Rebecca, *Black Lamb and Grey Falcon: A Journey through Yugoslavia* (Edinburgh: Cannongate, 2006 [1942])

Books and journal articles published between 1947 and 2014

Abel-Smith, Brian, *A History of the Nursing Profession* (London: Heinemann, 1960)

Acton, Carol, 'Negotiating Injury and Masculinity in First World War Nurses' Writing', in Alison S. Fell and Christine E. Hallett (eds), *First World War Nursing: New Perspectives* (London: Routledge, 2013): 123–38

Aiston, Sarah Jane, 'Women, Education and Agency, 1600–2000', in Jean Spence, Sarah Jane Aiston, and Maureen M. Meikle (eds), *Women, Education and Agency, 1600–2000* (London: Routledge, 2010): 1–8

Amoia, Alba and Bettina Knapp, *Women Travel Writers: From 1750 to the Present* (New York: Continuum, 2005)

Anderson, Benedict, *Imagined Communities: Reflections on the Origin and Spread of Nationalism* (London: Verso, 1991)

Anderson, Linda, *Autobiography (The New Critical Idiom)* (London: Routledge, 2010)

Anon., *The Johns Hopkins Nurses Alumnae Magazine*, 7 (1908)

Atkinson, Diane, *Elsie and Mairi Go to War: Two Extraordinary Women on the Western Front* (London: Preface Publishing, 2009)

Babini, Elisabetta, 'Nursing, Britishness and the War: The Cinematic Representation of British Nurses in Biopics', *Women's History Magazine*, 65 (2011): 26–32

Barker, Marianne, *Nightingales in the Mud: The Digger Sisters of the Great War 1914–1918* (Sydney: Allen and Unwin, 1989)

Bassett, Jan, *Guns and Brooches: Australian Army Nursing from the Boer War to the Gulf War* (Melbourne and Oxford: Oxford University Press, 1992)

Bendall, Eve and Elizabeth Raybould, *A History of the General Nursing Council for England and Wales, 1919–1969* (London: H. K. Lewis, 1969)

Berry, Paul and Mark Bostridge, *Vera Brittain: A Life* (London: Virago Press, 2001)

Bishop, Alan and Mark Bostridge, *Letters from a Lost Generation: First World War Letters of Vera Brittain and Four Friends* (London: Abacus, 1999)

Booth, Allyson, *Postcards from the Trenches: Negotiating the Space between Modernism and the First World War* (Oxford: Oxford University Press, 1996)

Booth, Howard and Nigel Rigby (eds), *Modernism and Empire* (Manchester: Manchester University Press, 2000)

Bostridge, Mark, *Florence Nightingale: The Woman and Her Legend* (London: Viking, 2008)

Bourdieu, Pierre, 'Cultural Reproduction and Social Reproduction', in R. Brown (ed.), *Knowledge, Education and Social Change: Papers in the Sociology of Education* (Tavistock: Tavistock Publications, 1973)

Bourdieu, Pierre, *Distinction: A Social Critique of the Judgement of Taste* (Cambridge, MA: Harvard University Press, 1984)

Bradshaw, Ann, *The Nurse Apprentice, 1860–1977* (Aldershot: Ashgate, 2001)

Brake, Laurel and Marysa Demoor, *Dictionary of Nineteenth-Century Journalism* (London: Academic Press and the British Library, 2009)

Braybon, Gail, *Women Workers in the First World War: The British Experience* (London: Croom Helm, 1981)

Braybon, Gail and Penny Summerfield, *Out of the Cage: Women's Experiences in Two World Wars* (London: Routledge, 2012 [1987])

Brittain, Vera, *Testament of Experience: An Autobiographical Story of the Years 1925–1950* (London: Fontana, 1980 [1957])

Brittain, Vera, *Chronicle of Youth* (London: Phoenix Press, 2000 [1981])

Brittain, Vera, *Because You Died: Poetry and Prose of the First World War and After*, ed. Mark Bostridge (London: Virago, 2008)

Brooks, Jane, 'Structured by Class, Bound by Gender: Nursing and Special Probationer Schemes, 1860–1939', *International History of Nursing Journal*, 6.2 (2001): 13–21

Brothers, Barbara and Julia Gergits, *British Travel Writers, 1910–1939* (Detroit: Gale, 1998)

Brush, Barbara, Joan Lynaugh, Geertje Boschma, Anne Marie Rafferty, Meryn Stuart, and Nancy J. Tomes, *Nurses of All Nations: A History of the International Council of Nurses, 1899–1999* (Philadelphia: Lippincott, Williams, and Wilkins, 1999)

Buhler-Wilkerson, Karen, *No Place like Home: A History of Nursing and Home Care in the United States* (Baltimore: Johns Hopkins University Press, 2001)

Buitenhuis, Peter, *The Great War of Words: Literature as Propaganda, 1914–18 and After* (London: B. T. Batsford, 1989 [1987])

Buller, Erin Bartels, 'Vouching for Evidence: The New Life of Old Writing in Lillian Hellman's Memoirs', *Arizona Quarterly*, 70.1 (2014): 109–34

Butler, Janet, 'Journey into War', *Australian Historical Studies*, 37.127 (2006): 203–17

Cabello, Juanita, 'On the Touristic Stage of 1920s and '30s Mexico: Katherine Anne Porter and a Modernist Tradition of Women Travel Writers', *Women's Studies*, 41.4 (2012): 413–35

Cardinal, Agnès, Dorothy Goldman, and Judith Hattaway, *Women's Writing on the First World War* (Oxford: Oxford University Press, 1999)

Chesnut, Mary Boykin, *Mary Chesnut's Diary*, with introduction by Catherine Clinton (New York: Penguin, 2011)

Clark, Alan, *The Donkeys* (London: Pimlico, 1991 [1961])

Clayden, Stephen R., 'Hay, George Upham', in George Williams Brown, David M. Hayne, Francess G. Halpenny, and Ramsay Cook (eds), *Dictionary of Canadian Biography*, Vol. XIV (Toronto: Toronto University Press, 1998)

Clendon, Jill, 'New Zealand Military Nurses' Fight for Recognition: World War I–World War II', *Nursing Praxis in New Zealand*, 12.1 (March 1997): 24–8

Connolly, Cynthia, '"I am a trained nurse": The Nursing Identity of Anarchist and Radical Emma Goldman', *Nursing History Review*, 18 (2010): 84–99

Conway, Jane, *Mary Borden: A Woman of Two Wars* (Chippenham: Munday Books, 2010)

Cooke, Miriam and Angela Woollacott (eds), *Gendering War Talk* (Princeton, NJ: Princeton University Press, 1993)

Cooper, Helen M., Adrienne Auslander Munich, and Susan Merrill Squier (eds), *Arms and the Woman: War, Gender and Literary Representation* (Chapel Hill: University of North Carolina Press, 1989)

Cooperman, Stanley, *World War I and the American Novel* (Baltimore: Johns Hopkins University Press, 1967)

Coroban, Costel, 'The Scottish Women's Hospitals in Romania during World War I', *Valahian Journal of Historical Studies*, 14 (2010): 53–68

Crane, David, *Scott of the Antarctic: A Life of Courage and Tragedy in the Extreme South* (London: HarperCollins, 2005)

Cross, Anthony, 'From the Assassination of Paul I to Tilsit: The British in Russia and Their Travel Writings (1801–1807), *Journal of European Studies*, 42.1 (2012): 5–21

Cruse, Audrey, 'The Diary of Alice Maud Batt (1889–1969)', *Journal of Medical Biography*, 18.4 (2010): 205–10

D'Antonio, Patricia, *American Nursing: A History of Knowledge, Authority and the Meaning of Work* (Baltimore: Johns Hopkins University Press, 2010)

Darrow, Margaret, 'French Volunteer Nursing and the Myth of War Experience in World War I', *American Historical Review*, 101.1 (1996): 80–106

Darrow, Margaret, *French Women and the First World War: War Stories from the Home Front* (New York: Berg, 2000)

Das, Santanu, *Touch and Intimacy in First World War Literature* (Cambridge: Cambridge University Press, 2005)

Davidoff, Leonore and Catherine Hall, *Family Fortunes: Men and Women of the English Middle Class, 1780–1850*, rev. edn (London: Routledge, 2002 [1987])

Davies, Wade, *Into the Silence: The Great War, Mallory, and the Conquest of Everest* (New York: Alfred A. Knopf, 2011)

Davin, Anna, 'Imperialism and Motherhood', *History Workshop*, 5 (1978): 9–65

Dawson, Graham, *Soldier Heroes: British Adventure, Empire and the Imagining of Masculinities* (London: Routledge, 1994)

Deacon, Prue, 'Australian Nurses at War', *Health and History: Journal of the Australian and New Zealand Society for the History of Medicine*, 14.1 (2012): 199–203

De Ritter, Richard, 'Reading "Voyages and Travels": Jane West, Patriotism and the Reformation of Female Sensibility', *Romanticism*, 17 (2011): 240–50

Dingwall, Robert, A. M. Rafferty, and C. Webster, *An Introduction to the Social History of Nursing* (London: Routledge, 1988): 69–70

Doyle, Brian (ed), *The Who's Who of Children's Literature* (New York: Schocken Books, 1968)

Dubois, Ellen Carol, *Woman Suffrage and Women's Rights* (New York: New York University Press, 1998)

Eaton, Harriet, *This Birth Place of Souls: The Civil War Nursing Diary of Harriet Eaton*, ed. Jane E. Schultz (Oxford: Oxford University Press, 2010)

Ecksteins, Modris, *Rites of Spring: The Great War and the Birth of the Modern Age* (Boston, MA: Houghton Mifflin, 1989)

Evans, Edward Ratcliffe Garth Russell, *South with Scott* (London: Collins, 1949)

Evans, Jonathan, *Edith Cavell* (London: London Hospital Museum, 2008)

Farmborough, Florence, *Nurse at the Russian Front: A Diary, 1914–18* (London: Book Club Associates, 1974)

Farmborough, Florence *Russian Album 1908–1918*, ed. John Jolliffe (Wilton: Michael Russell, 1979)

Farmborough, Florence, *With the Armies of the Tsar: A Nurse at the Russian Front in War and Revolution, 1914–1918* (New York: Cooper Square Press, 2000)

Fell, Alison S. and Ingrid Sharp (eds), *The Women's Movement in Wartime: International Perspectives 1914–1918* (Basingstoke: Palgrave, 2007)

Ferguson, Niall, *The Pity of War* (London: Allen Lane, 1998)

Ferro, Marc, *The Great War, 1914–1918* (London: Routledge, 1973 [1969])

Field, Frank, *British and French Writers of the First World War* (Cambridge: Cambridge University Press, 1991)

Fielding, Dorothie, *Lady under Fire: The Wartime Letters of Lady Dorothie Fielding M.M., 1914–1917, ed. Andrew* Hallam and Nicola Hallam (Barnsley: Pen and Sword Books, 2010)

Figes, Orlando, *A People's Tragedy: The Russian Revolution, 1891–1924* (London: Pimlico, 1997 [1996])

Fitzpatrick, Sheila, *The Russian Revolution*, 3rd edn (Oxford: Oxford University Press, 2008)

Freedman, Ariela, 'Mary Borden's *Forbidden Zone*: Women's Writing from No-Man's Land' *Modernism/Modernity*, 9.1 (2002): 109–24

Friedman, Alice Howell, 'Fitzgerald, Alice Louise Florence', in Martin Kaufman (ed.), *Dictionary of American Nursing Biography* (New York: Greenwood Press, 1988)

Friedman, Alice Howell, 'Stimson, Julia Catherine', in Martin Kaufman (ed.), *Dictionary of American Nursing Biography* (New York: Greenwood Press, 1988)

Friedman, Susan Stanford, 'Women's Autobiographical Selves: Theory and Practice', in Sidonie Smith and Julia Watson (eds), *Women, Autobiography, Theory* (Madison: University of Wisconsin Press, 1998): 72–82

Fussell, Paul, *The Great War and Modern Memory* (Oxford: Oxford University Press, 2000 [1975])

Gamarnikow, Eva, 'Nurse or Woman: Gender and Professionalism in Reformed Nursing, 1860–1923', in Pat Holden and Jenny Littlewood (eds), *Anthropology and Nursing* (London: Routledge, 1991): 110–29

Gilbert, Sandra, 'Soldier's Heart: Literary Men, Literary Women and the Great War', *Signs*, 8.3 (1983): 422–50

Gilbert, Sandra, 'Soldier's Heart: Literary Men, Literary Women and the Great War', in Margaret Randolph Higonnet, Jane Jenson, Sonya Michel, and Margaret Collins Weitz (eds), *Behind the Lines: Gender and the Two World Wars* (New Haven: Yale University Press, 1987): 197–226

Gilbert, Sandra and Susan Gubar, *No Man's Land: The Place of the Woman Writer in the Twentieth Century* (New Haven: Yale University Press, 1988)

Glendinning, Victoria, *Rebecca West: A Life* (London: Macmillan, 1988 [1987])

Goldman, Dorothy, *Women and World War I: The Written Response* (New York: St Martin's Press, 1993)

Gooding, Norman, *Honours and Awards to Women* (London: Savannah Publications, 2013)

Goodman, Rupert, *Our War Nurses: The History of the Royal Australian Army Nursing Corps, 1902–1988* (Brisbane: Boolarong Publications, 1988)

Gordon, Iain, *Lifeline: A British Casualty Clearing Station on the Western Front, 1918* (Stroud: History Press, 2013)

Gould, Jenny, 'Women's Military Services in First World War Britain', in Margaret Randolph Higonnet, Jane Jenson, Sonya Michel, and Margaret Collins Weitz (eds), *Behind the Lines: Gender and the Two World Wars* (New Haven: Yale University Press, 1987): 114–25

Grant, Susan, 'Nursing in Russia and the Soviet Union, 1914–41: An Overview of the Development of a Soviet Nursing System', *Bulletin of the UK Association for the History of Nursing*, 2 (2012): 21–33

Grayzel, Susan, *Women's Identities at War: Gender, Motherhood, and Politics in Britain and France during the First World War* (Chapel Hill: University of North Carolina Press, 1999)

Gregory, Adrian, *The Last Great War: British Society and the First World War* (Cambridge: Cambridge University Press, 2008)

Griffon, D. P., '"Crowning the Edifice": Ethel Fenwick and State Registration', *Nursing History Review*, 3 (1995): 201–12

Hagood, Thomas Chase, '"Literature to him was a recreation": A Life of Writing on the Southwestern Frontier', *Alabama Review*, 67.4 (2014): 374

Hallett, Christine, 'The Personal Writings of First World War Nurses: A Study of the Interplay of Authorial Intention and Scholarly Interpretation', *Nursing Inquiry*, 14.4 (2007): 320–9

Hallett, Christine, *Containing Trauma: Nursing Work in the First World War* (Manchester: Manchester University Press, 2009)

Hallett, Christine, 'Russian Romances: Emotionalism and Spirituality in the Writings of "Eastern Front Nurses", 1914–1918', *Nursing History Review*, 17 (2009): 101–28

Hallett, Christine, 'Portrayals of Suffering: Perceptions of Trauma in the Writings of First World War Nurses and Volunteers', *Canadian Bulletin of Medical History*, 27.1 (2010): 65–84

Hallett, Christine E., 'Nursing 1830–1920: Forging a Profession', in Anne Borsay and Billie Hunter (eds), *Nursing and Midwifery in Britain since 1700* (London: Palgrave, 2012)

Hallett, Christine E., '"Intelligent interest in their own affairs": The First World War, *The British Journal of Nursing* and the Pursuit of Nursing Knowledge', in Patricia D'Antonio, Julie A. Fairman, and Jean C. Whelan (eds), *Routledge Handbook on the Global History of Nursing* (London: Routledge, 2013): 95–113

Hallett, Christine E., '"Emotional Nursing": Involvement, Engagement, and Detachment in the Writings of First World War Nurses and VADs', in Alison S. Fell and Christine E. Hallett (eds), *First World War Nursing: New Perspectives* (New York: Routledge, 2013): 87–102

Hallett, Christine E., *Veiled Warriors: Allied Nurses of the First World War* (Oxford: Oxford University Press, 2014)

Hallett, Christine E., '"A very valuable fusion of classes": British Professional and Volunteer Nurses of the First World War', *Endeavour*, 38.2 (2014): 101–10

Hallett, Christine E. and Alison S. Fell, 'Introduction: New Perspectives on First World War Nursing', in Alison S. Fell and Christine E. Hallett, *First World War Nursing: New Perspectives* (New York: Routledge, 2013): 1–14

Hardie-Budden, Melissa, 'Thurstan, Anna Violet (1879–1978)', in *Oxford Dictionary of National Biography* (Oxford: Oxford University Press, 2008)

Harris, Kirsty, 'In the "Grey Battalion": Launceston General Hospital Nurses on Active Service in World War I', *Health and History: Journal of the Australian and New Zealand Society for the History of Medicine*, 10. 1 (2008): 21–40

Harris, Kirsty, 'Red Reflections on the Sea: Australian Army Nurses Serving at Sea in World War I, *Journal of Australian Naval History*, 6.2 (2009): 51–73

Harris, Kirsty, *More than Bombs and Bandages: Australian Army Nurses at Work in World War I* (Newport, NSW: Big Sky Publishing, 2011)

Harris, Kirsty, 'Girls in Grey: Surveying Australian Military Nurses in World War I', *History Compass*, 11.1 (2013): 14–23

Harrison, Mark, *The Medical War: British Military Medicine in the First World War* (Oxford: Oxford University Press, 2010)

Haste, Cate, *Keep the Home Fires Burning: Propaganda in the First World War* (London: Allen Lane, 1977)

Hawkins, Sue, 'From Maid to Matron: Nursing as a Route to Social Advancement in Nineteenth-Century England', *Women's History Review*, 19.1 (2010): 125–43

Hawkins, Sue, *Nursing and Women's Labour in the Nineteenth Century: The Quest for Independence* (London: Routledge, 2010)

Hector, Winifred, *The Work of Mrs Bedford Fenwick and the Rise of Professional Nursing* (London: Royal College of Nursing, 1973)

Helmstadter, Carol, 'Old Nurses and New: Nursing in the London Teaching Hospitals before and after the Mid-Ninteenth-Century Reforms', *Nursing History Review*, 1 (1993): 43–70

Helmstadter, Carol, 'Doctors and Nurses in the London Teaching Hospitals: Class, Gender, Religion and Professional Expertise, 1850–1890', *Nursing History Review*, 5 (1997): 61–97

Helmstadter, Carol, 'From the Private to the Public Sphere: The First Generation of Lady Nurses in England', *Nursing History Review*, 9 (2001): 127–40

Helmstadter, Carol, '"A Real Tone": Professionalizing Nursing in Nineteenth-Century London', *Nursing History Review*, 11 (2003): 3–30

Henty, G. A., *The Collected Works of G. A. Henty*, 7 vols (Alvin, TX: Halcyon Classics, 2011)

Higonnet, Margaret, 'Not So Quiet in No-Woman's Land', in Miriam Cooke and Angela Woollacott (eds), *Gendering War Talk* (Princeton, NJ: Princeton University Press, 1993): 205–26

Higonnet, Margaret, *Lines of Fire: Women Writers of World War I* (Harmondsworth: Penguin, 1999)

Higonnet, Margaret, *Nurses at the Front: Writing the Wounds of the Great War* (Boston, MA: Northeastern University Press, 2001)

Higonnet, Margaret, 'Authenticity and Art in Trauma Narratives of World War I', *Modernism/Modernity*, 9.1 (2002): 91–107

Higonnet, Margaret, 'Cubist Vision in Nursing Accounts', in Alison S. Fell and Christine E. Hallett (eds), *First World War Nursing: New Perspectives* (New York: Routledge, 2013): 156–72

Higonnet, Margaret and Patrice Higonnet, 'The Double Helix', in Margaret Randolph Higonnet, Jane Jenson, Sonya Michel, and Margaret Collins Weitz (eds), *Behind the Lines: Gender and the Two World Wars* (New Haven: Yale University Press, 1987): 31–47

Higonnet, Margaret Randolph, Jane Jenson, Sonya Michel, and Margaret Collins Weitz (eds), *Behind the Lines: Gender and the Two World Wars* (New Haven: Yale University Press, 1987)

Hokanson, Katya, 'Russian Women Travellers in Central Asia and India', *Russian Review*, 70.1 (2011): 1–19

Holtz, William (ed.), *Travels with Zenobia: Paris to Albania by Model T Ford* (Columbia and London: University of Missouri Press, 1983)

Howell, Jessica, Anne Marie Rafferty, and Anna Snaith, '(Author)ity Abroad: The Life Writing of Colonial Nurses', *International Journal of Nursing Studies*, 48.9 (2011): 1155–62

Hurley, Frank, *South with Endurance: Shackleton's Antarctic Expedition 1914–1917* (London: Bloomsbury, 2004)

Hutchison, Hazel, 'The Theater of Pain: Observing Mary Borden in *The Forbidden Zone*,' in Alison S. Fell and Christine E. Hallett (eds), *First World War Nursing: New Perspectives* (New York: Routledge, 2013): 139–55

Hynes, Samuel, *A War Imagined: The First World War and English Culture* (London: Pimlico, 1992)

Hynes, Samuel, *The Soldier's Tale: Bearing Witness to a Modern War* (London: Penguin, 1998)

Jensen, Kimberly, 'A Base Hospital Is Not a Coney Island Dance Hall: American Women Nurses, Hostile Work Environment, and Military Rank in the First World War', *Frontiers*, 26.2 (2005): 206–35

Jensen, Kimberly, *Mobilizing Minerva: American Women in the First World War* (Urbana and Chicago: University of Illinois Press, 2008)

Jones, Angela, 'Romantic Women Travel Writers and the Representation of Everyday Experience, *Women's Studies*, 26.5 (1997): 497–522

Joule, Victoria, '"Heroines of Their Own Romance": Creative Exchanges between Life-Writing and Fiction, the "Scandalous Memoirists" and Charlotte Lennox', *Journal for Eighteenth-Century Studies*, 37.1 (2014): 37–52

Kahn, Richard J., 'Women and Men at Sea: Gender Debate aboard the Hospital Ship "Maine" during the Boer War, 1899–1900', *Journal of the History of Medicine and Allied Sciences*, 56 (2001): 111–139

Kaplan, Laurie, 'Deformities of the Great War: The Narratives of Mary Borden and Helen Zenna Smith', *Women and Language*, 27.2 (2004): 35–43

Kendall, Sherayl and David Corbett, *New Zealand Military Nursing: A History of the RNZNC Boer War to the Present Day* (Auckland: S. Kendall and D. Corbett, 1990)

Khazeni, Arash, 'Across the Black Sands, and the Red: Travel Writing, Nature and the Reclamation of the Eurasian Steppe circa 1850', *International Journal of Middle East Studies*, 42.4 (2010): 591–614

Kilbride, Daniel, 'Travel Writing as Evidence with Special Attention to Nineteenth-Century Anglo-America', *History Compass*, 9.4 (2011): 339–50

Kramer, Alan, *Dynamic of Destruction: Culture and Mass Killing in the First World War* (Oxford: Oxford University Press, 2007)

Laffin, J. *British Butchers and Bunglers of World War One* (Stroud: Sutton, 1988)

Lawson, John and Harold Silver, *A Social History of Education in England* (London: Methuen, 1973)

Layton, Lynne, 'Vera Brittain's Testament(s)', in Margaret Randolph Higonnet, Jane Jenson, Sonya Michel, and Margaret Collins Weitz (eds), *Behind the Lines: Gender and the Two World Wars* (New Haven: Yale University Press, 1987): 70–83

Lee, Janet, *War Girls: The First Aid Nursing Yeomanry in the First World War* (Manchester: Manchester University Press, 2005)

Leed, Eric, *No Man's Land: Combat and Identity in World War One* (New York: Cambridge University Press, 1979)

Leneman, Leah, *In the Service of Life: The Story of Elsie Inglis and the Scottish Women's Hospitals* (Edinburgh: Mercat Press, 1994)

Liddle, Peter, *Captured Memories 1900–1918: Across the Threshold of War* (Barnsley: Pen and Sword, 2010)

Light, Sue, 'British Military Nurses and the Great War: A Guide to the Services', *The Western Front Association Forum* (7 February 2010): 4, available at www.westernfrontassociation.com (accessed 30 October 2012)

Logan, Mawuena Kossi, *Narrating Africa: George Henty and the Fiction of Empire* (London: Taylor and Francis, 2007)

Luard, Kate, *Unknown Warriors: The Letters of Kate Luard, R.R.C. and Bar., Nursing Sister in France 1914–1918*, ed. John Stevens and Caroline Stevens (Stroud: History Press, 2014)

MacDonald, Lyn, *The Roses of No Man's Land* (Harmondsworth: Penguin, 1993 [1980])

Maggs, Christopher, *The Origins of General Nursing* (London: Coom Helm, 1983)

Mann, Susan, *Margaret Macdonald: Imperial Daughter* (Montreal and Kingston: McGill-Queens University Press, 2005)

Marcus, Jane, 'Corpus/Corps/Corpse: Writing the Body in/at War', in Helen M. Cooper, Adrienne Auslander Munich, and Susan Merrill Squier (eds), *Arms and the Woman: War, Gender and Literary Representation* (Chapel Hill: University of North Carolina Press, 1989): 124–67

McDermid, Jane, 'What's in a Name? The Scottish Women's Hospitals in the First World War', *Minerva: Women and War*, 1.1 (2007): 102–14

McEnroe, Natasha and Tig Thomas, *The Hospital in the Oatfield* (London: Florence Nightingale Museum, 2014)

McGann, Susan, *The Battle of the Nurses: A Study of Eight Women who Influenced the Development of Professional Nursing, 1880–1930* (London: Scutari Press, 1992)

McGann, Susan, 'The Wind of Change Is Blowing', *Nursing History Review*, 10 (2002): 21–32

McPherson, Kathryn, *Bedside Matters: The Transformation of Canadian Nursing, 1900–1990* (Toronto: University of Toronto Press, 2003 [1996])

Mellow, James R., *Charmed Circle: Gertrude Stein and Company* (London: Phaidon Press, 1974)

Mill, Hugh Robert, *The Life of Sir Ernest Shackleton* (London: William Heinemann, 2006)

Mitchell, Sally, 'Helen Dore Boylston', in Lina Mainiero (ed.), *American Women Writers* (New York: Frederick Ungar, 1979)

Nicholson, Juliet, *The Great Silence: 1918–1920. Living in the Shadow of the Great War* (London: John Murray, 2009)

Nicolson, Nigel, 'Bagnold, Enid Algerine [*Married Name* Enid Algerine Jones, Lady Jones] (1889–1981), Novelist and Playwright', in *Oxford Dictionary of National Biography* (Oxford: Oxford University Press, 2004)

Noakes, Lucy, 'Eve in Khaki: Women Working with the British military, 1915–1918', in Krista Cowman and Louise A. Jackson (eds), *Women and Work Culture* (Aldershot: Ashgate, 2004)

Noakes, Lucy, *Women in the British Army: War and the Gentle Sex, 1907–1948* (New York: Routledge, 2006)

Ogden, Alan, 'Romanian Culture in the Twentieth Century: The View of English Travel Writers before the Second World War', *Romanian Civilization*, 19.3 (2000): 44–54

Ouditt, Sharon, *Fighting Forces, Writing Women: Identity and Ideology in the First World War* (London: Routledge, 1994)

Ouditt, Sharon, *Women Writers of the First World War: An Annotated Bibliography* (London: Routledge, 2000)

Panichas, George (ed.), *Promise of Greatness: The War of 1914–1918* (London: Cassell, 1968)

Paris, Michael, *Warrior Nation: Images of War in British Popular Culture, 1850–2000* (London: Reaktion Books, 2000)

Parker, Edith R. and Sheila M. Collins, *Learning to Care: A History of Nursing and Midwifery Education at the Royal London Hospital, 1740–1993* (London: Royal London Hospital Archives and Museum, 1998)

Pedersen, Peter, *The Anzacs: Gallipoli to the Western Front* (London: Penguin, 2007)

Pengelly, Edna, *Nursing in Peace and War* (Wellington, NZ: H. Tombs, 1956)

Peterson, M. Jeanne, 'No Angels in the House: The Victorian Myth and the Paget Women', *The American Historical Review*, 89.3 (1984): 677–708

Philips, Deborah, 'Healthy Heroines: Sue Barton, Lillian Wald, Lavinia Lloyd Dock and the Henry Street Settlement', *Journal of American Studies*, 33.1 (1999): 65–82

Pickles, Katie, *Female Imperialism and National Identity: Imperial Order of the Daughters of the Empire* (Manchester: Manchester University Press, 2002)

Piggott, Juliet, *Queen Alexandra's Royal Army Nursing Corps* (London: Leo Cooper, 1975)

Potter, Jane, ' "I begin to feel as a normal being should, in spite of the blood and anguish in which I move": American Women's First World War Nursing Memoirs', in Alison S. Fell and Christine E. Hallett (eds), *First World War Nursing: New Perspectives* (New York: Routledge, 2013): 51–68

Quiney, Linda, 'Assistant Angels: Canadian Voluntary Aid Detachment Nurses in the Great War', *Canadian Bulletin of Medical History*, 15 (1998): 189–206

Quinn, Shawna, *Agnes Warner and the Nursing Sisters of the Great War* (Fredericton, NB: Goose Lane Editions with New Brunswick Military Heritage Project, 2010)

Rae, Ruth, 'Reading between Unwritten Lines: Australian Army Nurses in India, 1916–19', *Journal of the Australian War Memorial*, 36 (2001): 1

Rae, Ruth, *Scarlet Poppies: The Army Experience of Australian Nurses during World War One* (Burwood, NSW: College of Nursing, 2004)

Rae, Ruth, *Veiled Lives: Threading Australian Nursing History into the Fabric of the First World War* (Burwood, NSW: College of Nursing, 2009)

Rafferty, Anne Marie, *The Politics of Nursing Knowledge* (London: Routledge, 1996)

Rafferty, Anne Marie, 'The Seductions of History and the Nursing Diaspora', *Health and History: Journal of the Australian and New Zealand Society for the History of Medicine*, 7.2 (2005): 2–6

Rafferty, Anne Marie and Diana Solano, 'The Rise and Demise of the Colonial Nursing Service: British Nurses in the Colonies, 1896–1966', *Nursing History Review*, 15 (2007): 147–54

Rainey, Lawrence, *Modernism: An Anthology* (Oxford: Blackwell Publishing, 2005)

Reilly, Catherine (ed.), *Scars upon my Heart: Women's Poetry and Verse of the First World War* (London: Virago, 1981)

Reznick, Jeffrey, *Healing the Nation: Soldiers and the Culture of Caregiving in Britain during the Great War* (Manchester: Manchester University Press, 2004)

Robbins, Jessica M., 'Class Struggles in the Tubercular World: Nurses, Patients, and Physicians, 1903–1915', *Bulletin of the History of Medicine*, 71.3 (1997): 412–34

Rodgers, Jan, 'Potential for Professional Profit: The Making of the New Zealand Army Nursing Service 1914–1915', *Nursing Praxis in New Zealand*, 11.2 (1996): 4–12

Rogers, Anna, *While You're Away: New Zealand Nurses at War 1899–1948* (Auckland: Auckland University Press, 2003)

Roper, Michael, *The Secret Battle: Emotional Survival in the Great War* (Manchester: Manchester University Press, 2009)

Rowbotham, Sheila, *Dreamers of a New Day: Women who Invented the Twentieth Century* (London: Verso, 2010)

Sarnecky, Mary T., *A History of the US Army Nurse Corps* (Philadelphia: University of Pennsylvania Press, 1999)

Saunders, Max, *Self Impressions: Life-Writing, Autobiografiction and the Forms of Modern Literature* (Oxford: Oxford University Press, 2013)

Schneider, Dorothy and Carl Schneider, *American Women in the Progressive Era: 1900–1920* (New York: Facts on File, 1993)

Schultheiss, Katrin, *Bodies and Souls: Politics and the Professionalization of Nursing in France, 1880–1922* (Cambridge, MA: Harvard University Press, 2001)

Schultz, Jane E., *Women at the Front: Hospital Workers in Civil War America* (Chapel Hill: University of North Carolina Press, 2004)

Scott, Eric (ed.), *Nobody Ever Wins a War: The World War I Diaries of Ella Mae Bongard, R.N.* (Ottawa: Janeric Enterprises, 1997)

Scott, Joan, 'Rewriting History', in Margaret Randolph Higonnet, Jane Jenson, Sonya Michel, and Margaret Collins Weitz (eds), *Behind the Lines: Gender and the Two World Wars* (New Haven: Yale University Press, 1987): 21–30

Scott, Joan, 'Experience', in Sidonie Smith and Julia Watson (eds), *Women, Autobiography, Theory* (Madison: University of Wisconsin Press, 1998): 57–71

Simnett, Anne, 'The Pursuit of Respectability: Women and the Nursing Profession', in Rosemary White (ed.), *Political Issues in Nursing: Past, Present and Future, 3 vols* (Chichester: John Wiley and Sons, 1986–88)

Smith, Angela, *The Second Battlefield: Women, Modernism and the First World War* (Manchester: Manchester University Press, 2000)

Smith, Angela, *Women's Writings of the First World War: An Anthology* (Manchester: Manchester University Press, 2000)

Smith, Angela, 'The Woman who Dared: Major Mabel St Clair Stobart', in Alison S. Fell and Ingrid Sharp (eds), *The Women's Movement in Wartime: International Perspectives 1914–1918* (Basingstoke: Palgrave, 2007): 158–74

Smith, Angela K., ' "Beacons of Britishness": British Nurses and Female Doctors as Prisoners of War', in Alison S. Fell and Christine E. Hallett (eds), *First World War Nursing: New Perspectives* (London: Routledge, 2013): 35–50

Smith, Michelle, 'Adventurous Girls of the British Empire: The Pre-War Novels of Bessie Marchant', *The Lion and the Unicorn*, 33.1 (2009): 1–25

Smith, Michelle, *Empire in British Girls' Literature and Culture: Imperial Girls 1880–1915* (London: Palgrave Macmillan, 2011)

Smith, Sidonie, *Interfaces: Women, Autobiography, Image, Performance* (Ann Arbor: University of Michigan Press, 2002)

Smith, Sidonie and Julia Watson, 'Introduction: Situating Subjectivity in Women's Autobiographical Practices', in Sidonie Smith and Julia Watson (eds), *Women, Autobiography, Theory* (Madison: University of Wisconsin Press, 1998): 3–52

Smith, Sidonie and Julia Watson, *Reading Autobiography: A Guide for Interpreting Life Narratives* (Minneapolis: University of Minnesota Press, 2010)

Somerfield, Muriel and Ann Bellingham, *Violetta Thurstan: A Celebration* (Penzance: Jamieson Library, 1993)

Souhami, Diana, *Edith Cavell* (London: Quercus, 2010)

Starns, Penny, *The March of the Matrons: Military Influence on the British Civilian Nursing Profession, 1939–1969* (Peterborough: DSM, 2000)

Bibliography

Stoff, Laurie, 'The "Myth of the War Experience" and Russian Wartime Nursing in World War I', *Aspasia: The International Yearbook of Central, Eastern, and Southeastern European Women's and Gender History*, 5 (2012): 96–116

Stuart, Denis, *Dear Duchess: Millicent, Duchess of Sutherland (1867–1955)* (Newton Abbot: David and Charles, 1982)

Sugiyama, Keiko, 'Ellen La Motte, 1873–1961: Gender and Race in Nursing', *The Japanese Journal of American Studies*, 17 (2006): 129–41

Summerfield, Penny, *Reconstructing Women's Wartime Lives* (Manchester: Manchester University Press, 1998)

Summers, Anne, 'Pride and Prejudice: Ladies and Nurses in the Crimean War', *History Workshop*, 16 (1983): 33–56

Summers, Anne, *Angels and Citizens: British Women as Military Nurses, 1854–1914* (London: Routledge and Kegan Paul, 1988)

Summers, Anne, *Angels and Citizens: British Women as Military Nurses, 1854–1914*, rev. edn (Newbury: Threshold Press, 2000)

Tate, Trudi, *Modernism, History and the First World War* (Manchester: Manchester University Press, 1998)

Taylor, A. J. P., *The First World War: An Illustrated History* (Harmondsworth: Penguin, 1963)

Toman, Cynthia, ' "Help Us, Serve England": First World War Military Nursing and National Identities', *Canadian Bulletin of Medical History*, 30.1 (2013): 156–7

T'Serclaes, Baroness de, *Flanders and Other Fields* (London: George G. Harrap, 1964)

Tylee, Claire, *The Great War and Women's Consciousness: Images of Militarism and Womanhood in Women's Writings, 1914–64* (Houndmills and London: Macmillan, 1990)

Van Bergen, Leo, *Before My Helpless Sight: Suffering, Dying and Military Medicine on the Western Front, 1914–1918* (Farnham: Ashgate, 2009)

Vining, Margaret and Barton C. Hacker, 'From Camp Follower to Lady in Uniform: Women, Social Class and Military Institutions before 1920', *Contemporary European History*, 10.3 (2001): 353–73

Vuic, Kara Dixon, 'Wartime Nursing and Power', in Patricia D'Antonio, Julie A. Fairman, and Jean C. Whelan (eds), *Routledge Handbook on the Global History of Nursing* (London: Routledge, 2013): 22–34

Walton, Liz, 'Nurse Violetta Thurstan', *Channel Islands Great War Study Group Journal*, 15 (August 2007): 6–11 (6)

Ward, Chris, *Russia's Cotton Workers and the New Economic Policy: Shop Floor Culture and State Policy, 1921–1929* (Cambridge: Cambridge University Press, 2002)

Watson, Janet S. K., 'Wars in the Wards: The Social Construction of Medical Work in First World War Britain', *Journal of British Studies*, 41 (2002): 484–510

Watson, Janet S. K., *Fighting Different Wars: Experience, Memory and the First World War* (Cambridge: Cambridge University Press, 2004)

West, Rebecca, *The Fountain Overflows* (London: Virago, 1984 [1957])

West Rebecca, *The Birds Fall Down* (London: Macmillan, 1966)

White, Rosemary, *Social Change and the Development of the Nursing Profession: A Study of the Poor Law Nursing Service, 1848–1948* (London: Kimpton, 1978)

Willis, L. Ida G., *A Nurse Remembers* (Lower Hutt, NZ: A. K. Wilson, 1968)

Winter, Jay, *Sites of Memory, Sites of Mourning: The Great War in European Cultural History* (Cambridge: Cambridge University Press, 1995)

Winter, Jay, 'Shell Shock and the Cultural History of the Great War', *Journal of Contemporary History*, 35.1 (2000): 7–11

Woollacott, Angela, 'Sisters and Brothers in Arms: Family, Class and Gendering in World War I Britain', in Miriam Cooke and Angela Woollacott (eds), *Gendering War Talk* (Princeton, NJ: Princeton University Press, 1993)

Woollacott, Angela, 'Khaki Fever and Its Control: Gender, Class, Age and Sexual Morality on the British Home Front in the First World War', *Journal of Contemporary History*, 29 (1994): 325–47

Young, Arlene, 'Entirely a Woman's Question? Class, Gender and the Victorian Nurse', *Journal of Victorian Culture*, 13.1 (2008): 18–41

Young, Margaret (ed.), *We Are Here Too: The Diaries and Letters of Sister Olive L. C. Haynes, November 1914 to February 1918* (Adelaide: Down Syndrome Association, 1991)

Zino, Bart, 'A Kind of Round Trip: Australian Soldiers and the Tourist Analogy, 1914–1918', *War and Society*, 25.2 (2006): 39–52

Theses and dissertations

Adams, Sara Amy Zackheim, 'Creating Amateur Professionals: British Voluntary Aid Detachment Nurses and the First World War' (unpublished Ph.D. thesis, University of Rochester, NY, 1998)

Basford, Hazel Bruce, 'Kent VAD: The Work of Voluntary Aid Detachments in Kent during the First World War' (unpublished M.Phi.l thesis, University of Kent, 2004)

Harris, Kirsty, 'Not Just "Routine Nursing": The Roles and Skills of the Australian Army Nursing Service during World War I' (unpublished Ph.D. thesis, University of Melbourne, 2006)

Yamaguchi, Midori, '"Unselfish" Desires: Daughters of the Anglican Clergy, 1830–1914' (unpublished Ph.D. thesis, University of Essex, 2001)

Index

Index